# THE ULTIMATE AIR FRYER COOKBOOK

## 575 Best Air Fryer Recipes of All Time

~ Rachel Collins

## Copyright © 2019 by Rachel Collins

All rights reserved. No part of this publication may be reproduced, distributed, or transmitted in any form or by any means, including photocopying, recording, or other electronic or mechanical methods, without the prior written permission of the publisher, except in the case of brief quotations embodied in critical reviews and certain other non-commercial uses permitted by copyright law.

Limit of liability/Disclaimer of Warranty: The publisher and the author make no representations or warranties with respect to the accuracy or completeness of the contents of this work and specifically disclaim all warranties, including without limitation warranties of fitness for a particular purpose. No warranty may be created or extended by sales or promotional materials. The advice and strategies contained herein may not be suitable for every situation. This work is sold with the understanding that the author is not engaged in rendering medical, legal or other professional advice or services. If professional assistance is required, the services of a competent professional person should be sought. Neither the publisher nor the author shall be liable for damages arising herefrom. The fact that an individual, organization, or website is referred to in this work as a citation and/or potential source of further information does not mean that the author or the publisher endorses the information the individual, organization, or website may provide or recommendations they/it may make.

Illustrations © James Foster

Cover design by Neil Bercow

# *Dedication*

*To all my Air Fryer Cookbook fans, this book is dedicated to you. Without your loyalty and support, this book would never have been possible.*

*To my favorite taste-testers – my husband, John, and my lovely girls Amelia and Ava – thanks for trying all my cooking experiments (the good and the bad!) and for your love and throughout this amazing journey!*

# TABLE OF CONTENTS

**INTRODUCTION** 1

**AIR FRYER BASICS** 2

**CHAPTER 1**
BREAD AND BREAKFAST 17

**CHAPTER 2**
SNACKS AND APPETIZERS 56

**CHAPTER 3**
CHICKEN AND POULTRY 92

**CHAPTER 4**
BEEF, PORK AND LAMB 136

**CHAPTER 5**
FISH AND SEAFOOD 177

**CHAPTER 6**
VEGETARIAN AND VEGAN 215

**CHAPTER 7**
DESSERTS 273

**AIR FRYER COOKING CHARTS** 316

**MEASUREMENT CONVERSION CHARTS** 318

**ABOUT THE AUTHOR** 321

**RECIPE INDEX** 322

# Introduction

Eating fresh salads, sandwiches, and choosing healthy foods can be easy for some but difficult for the rest of us. The thought of not being able to eat fried chicken wings or beloved French fries is a nightmare for those who have spent their whole lives eating deep-fried foods. For people who still want their deep-fried foods but want to have a healthier lifestyle, they now have the option to do so, thanks to recent innovations such as the Air Fryer.

The hot air fryer is a modern kitchen appliance that allows you to fry food without oil. Now, how is that possible? Well, the hot air fryer cooks fried foods without using oil. If you were to tell that to your grandmother, she would most likely tell you that the food will come out horribly dry and tasteless. After all, deep frying in a large amount of oil has always been the way to eat fried foods. It delivers that nice crunch on the outside, while being moist and tender on the inside.

I don't know about you, but I love eating fried foods. What I don't like is the unhealthy aftereffects that I get such as weight gain, digestive problems, and the oil that comes oozing out of my pores. I think everyone should be able to eat fries, chicken, and other fried foods without having to worry about dealing with all of the health issues. Apparently so does the maker of the air fryer, which is why they have come out with this modern innovation in cooking technology.

In this cookbook, you will find 575 recipes that don't just claim to be healthy, but are truly heart healthy along with having the nutritional information to back up their claim. You'll also find tips for using your air fryer, information on buying the best air fryer for yourself and your family, a step-by-step guide on how to use your air fryer, and even more ways to reduce fat and salt while increasing flavor in your favorite foods.

Happy Cooking!

# Air Fryer Basics

## What is an Air Fryer?

Today's air fryer technology is still relatively new when compared to other well-known kitchen appliances. While this device has indeed penetrated into the hearts of many, there are still countless people out there who are unaware of this modern marvel.

If you are one of them, then you are going to appreciate the information provided in this chapter. I will be walking you through the very basics of how to use an air fryer.

Let's start with what truly makes the air fryer so "unique" … its cooking mechanism.

While other kitchen appliances out there mostly rely on conduction for preparing meals, air fryers differentiate themselves by incorporating airflow into their cooking process in a technique called "convection."

Using "rapid air technology," the air fryer can prepare meals quickly with a very minimal amount of oil.

## The Rapid Air Technology

For those of you who are wondering what "rapid air technology" is, let me give you a brief overview.

Once the air fryer has pulled in the air from outside, the appliance immediately superheats the air to a temperature of 392 degrees Fahrenheit, after which it is passed into a very specialized heating chamber where the actual cooking happens.

This whole process is referred to as "rapid air technology" as it eliminates the need to use a heavy amount of oil during frying, baking, grilling or even roasting and completes the cooking over a very short period of time.

# The Structure of an Air Fryer

Different brands of air fryers out there will definitely have some "flair" of their own! However, the following features are common staples of every air fryer.

In general, an air fryer consists of:

- **The Cooking Chamber:** This is the actual chamber where the cooking takes place. The difference between various models usually comes in the form of holding capacity. Some air fryers have the capacity to hold two cooking baskets, while some can hold only one.

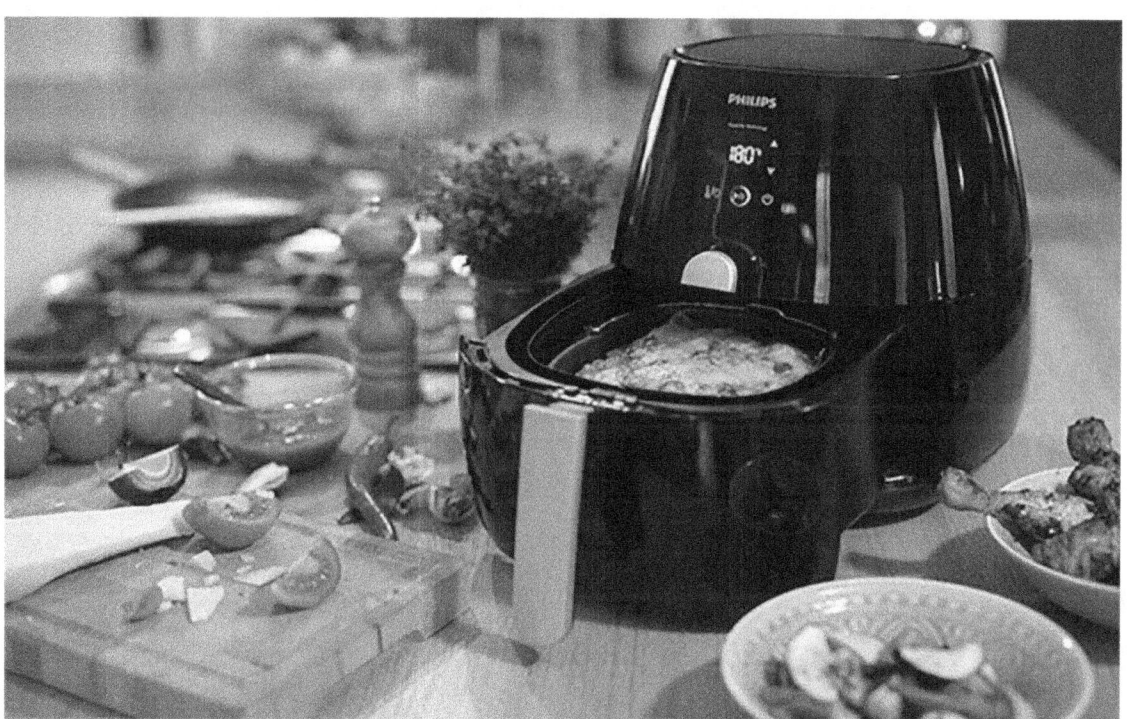

- **Heating Element:** The heating element of an air fryer is the coil inside the fryer that produces the heat once electricity passes through it. Once the heating element reaches the desired temperature, air is passed through this coil, where it gets heated up and is passed towards the fan and grill.

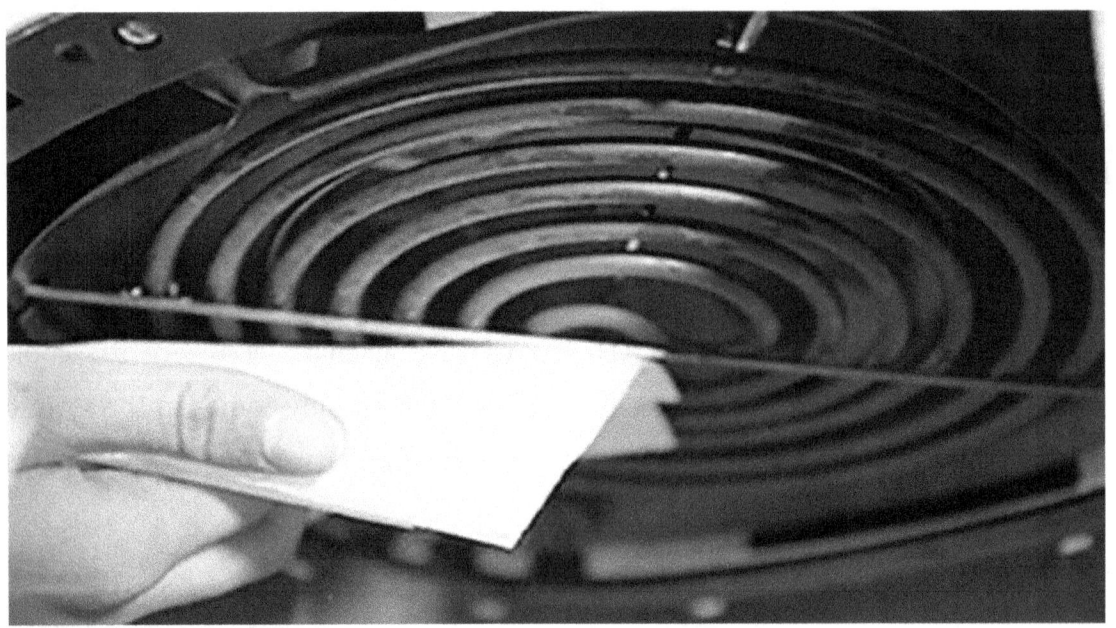

- **Fan and Grill:** The fan and grill of the air fryer work together in order to ensure that the heated air is distributed evenly throughout the cooking basket. The air fryer is able to adjust the direction of the air, which plays a significant role in cooking the meal consistently.

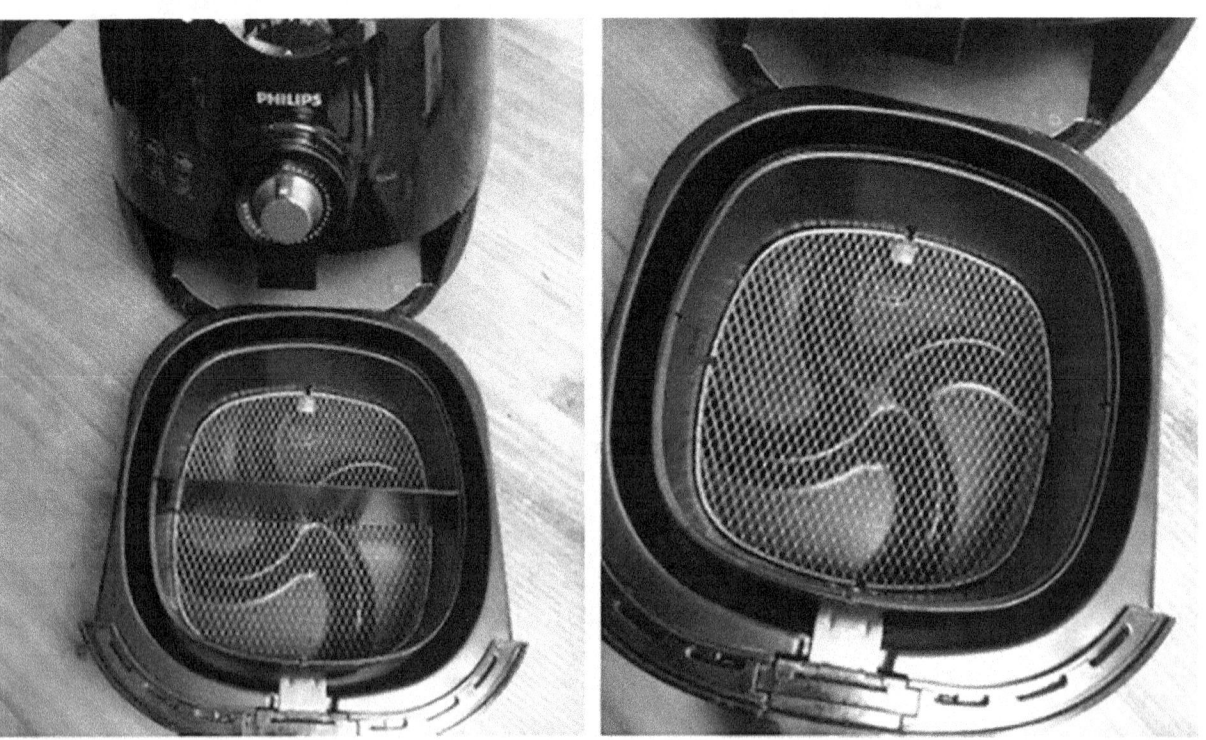

- **Exhaust System:** The exhaust system of an air fryer is responsible for maintaining a stable internal pressure and preventing the buildup of any harmful air. Some air fryer models tend to have a filter installed with the exhaust that cleans the exhausted air, making it free from any harmful particles or unpleasant odors.

- **Transferable Food Tray:** The food tray is also known as the cooking basket. This is where you place the food in the air fryer to be cooked. Some newer models of air fryers tend to include a cooking basket with multiple walls built inside. This makes the cooking baskets much more versatile and allows the users to cook multiple items in one go. Some models even include a universal handle that allows the cooking basket to be handled with ease.

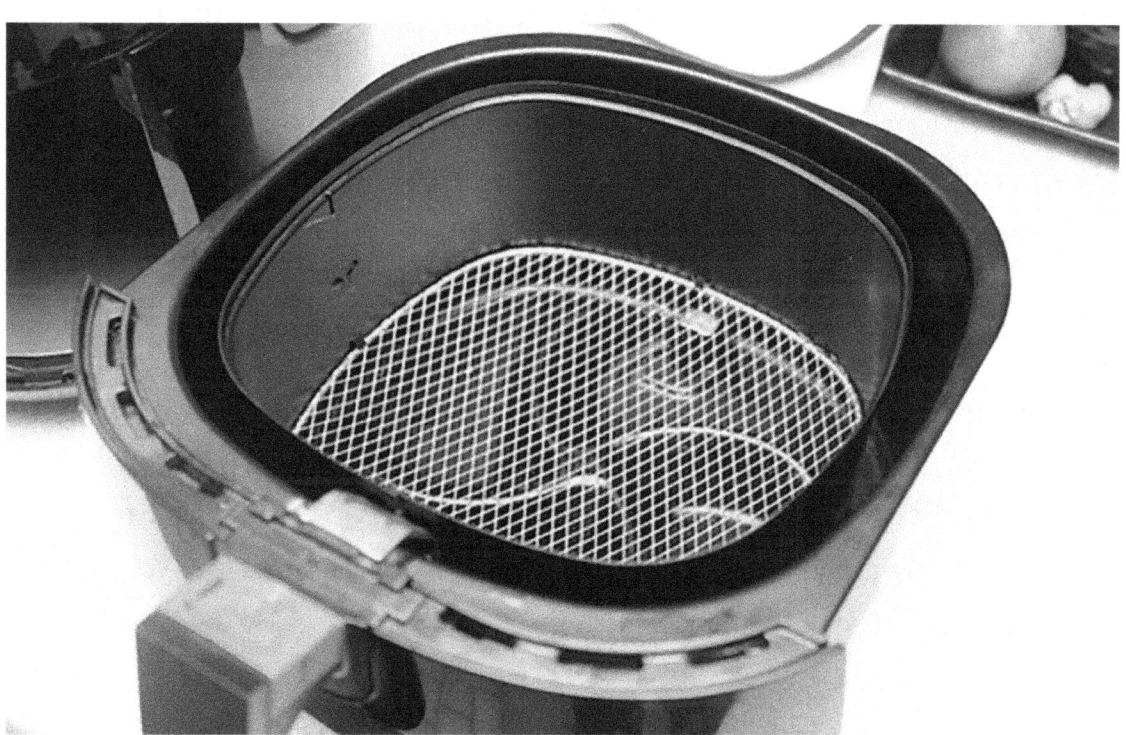

# The Basic Features of an Air Fryer

Again, different brands of air fryers tend to add something special regarding their functionality in order to make their device stand out. However, the following features are common to almost all air fryers.

- **Automated Temperature Control System:** This is one of the more crucial and essential elements of an air fryer. The automated temperature control system plays a great role in determining how the final product turns out. The automatic temperature control system allows the appliance to keep track of the temperature and turn off the system when the airflow reaches a specific temperature. This allows each and every meal to be created according to the user's personal preferences.

- **Digital Screen and Touch Panel:** In our modern "digitized" generation, touch screen and digital controls are generating all the buzz! If you don't have a device with a touch screen panel, then you might as well be living in the past! Air fryer manufacturers are fully aware of this trend and have recently added a fully functional touchscreen interface into many fryers! This allows the users to seamlessly control the device without any hassle.

- **A Convenient Buzzer:** Most air fryers come with a buzzer that makes it extremely simple for users to know whenever their meals are ready. When cooking with an air fryer, you won't have to stand in front of the device all day just to make sure that your meals aren't burnt! All you have to do is set the timer and your air fryer will let you know once the cooking is done!

- **An Assorted Selection of Cooking Presets:** Air fryer companies fully understand that the majority of their users are not amazing chefs or prodigies when it comes to cooking. Some people out there are still amateur, but they want to cook and prepare amazing meals. For these people, the air fryer comes with a plethora of different preset parameters that ensure it is easy for inexperienced individuals to cook meals they can be proud of.

| PRESET BUTTON COOKING CHART | | |
|---|---|---|
| PRESET BUTTON | TEMPERATURE | TIME |
| French Fries | 400°F | 20 min |
| Roasts | 370°F | 15 min |
| Shrimp | 330°F | 15 min |
| Baked Goods | 350°F | 25 min |
| Chicken | 380°F | 25 min |
| Steak | 380°F | 25 min |
| Fish | 390°F | 25 min |

## **Amazing Benefits of Using an Air Fryer**

Preparing meals using an air fryer will reduce the amount of oil used by 80%, but that's not the only advantage here.

- An air fryer is very convenient and easy to use
- Cleaning an air fryer does not make any mess
- Oil- free meals produced by the air fryer will help with weight loss and improve overall health
- Cooking with an air fryer will allow you to cook meals rapidly

## **Cleaning Instructions and Some Helpful Tips**

Some people think that cleaning an air fryer might be an exceptionally herculean task! However, cleaning an air fryer is actually very easy.

Just make sure to keep the following steps in mind after use:

- Remove the plug from the wall and give your air fryer time to cool down.
- Gently wipe the external parts of the air fryer using a moist cloth. (dipped in a mixture of water and mild detergent)
- Clean the outer basket of the air fryer using hot water mixed with mild detergent and a soft sponge.
- If you see that any residual food particles are stuck to the heating element, use a dish cleaning brush to remove them.

Some additional tips when cleaning:

- ✓ For maximum efficiency, soak the basket with water and dish detergent for a few minutes and rinse it thoroughly under hot water.
- ✓ Keep in mind that metal utensils and cleaning brushes may leave scratches on the body of the fryer, so refrain from using brushes, sponges or harsh products on the air fryer and its parts.

## **Some Amateur Mistakes to Avoid**

If you are just getting comfortable with your new air fryer, then you should really follow the following tips to increase the longevity of your device:

- ❖ Make sure to keep your device in a well-ventilated place for maximum airflow. Keeping your air fryer in a corner will restrict airflow, which will damage your device in the long run.
- ❖ When you are not using your air fryer, make sure to remove the power cables to prevent any internal damage.
- ❖ Keep in mind that the air fryer does not take long to heat up, so preheat it just before cooking.
- ❖ When using frozen foods, make sure to thaw them thoroughly before placing them in your cooking basket (unless specifically asked by a recipe).

## **The basic Steps for Using an Air Fryer**

Some people imagine that using an air fryer might be extremely difficult! However, it is the exact opposite.

The creators of modern air fryers have spent years upon years perfecting these devices to ensure that they are as accessible and easy to use as possible.

As a result, the air fryer can get working with some very basic steps:

- Take your cooking basket and drizzle a bit of oil in it
- Prepare the ingredients of the meal accordingly
- Transfer the prepared tray to your cooking basket and follow any additional instructions

- Alternatively, if you are baking a cake then you might want to put the batter in a separate dish and place this inside your cooking tray
- Set your temperature to the specified temperature and set your timer
- Make sure to check if the recipe requires you to shake your basket. If so, do it accordingly.
- Wait until the timer runs out. Bon Appétit!

Most recipes will require little to no oil! Overall, the oil intake will be lowered by almost 80%.

## **Choosing The Best Air Fryer for You**

If you are a fast food aficionado who often likes to stroll down to the local burger joint to grab a plate of delicious crispy French fries (just like me), then a modern oil-free hot air fryer is just what you are looking for!

Not only will it help to satisfy your desire for French fries, but it will do so in a very friendly and healthy way, thanks to the fact that cooking in these fryers is done through the circulation of hot air as opposed to cooking with oil.

However, with the plethora of options out there, it might be a little difficult to actually go out there and decided on that first air fryer.

Keeping that in mind, this section of the book has been designed to help those individuals in need and educate them, so that they can seamlessly purchase their first air fryer with ease.

So, the basic rule of thumb when going out to buy your first air fryer is to keep certain parameters in mind. Namely:

- Capacity
- Accessibility
- Accessories
- Price
- Pros and cons of the device that you are considering

I will be going through each of these step by step and will break them down to you for your convenience.

But keep in mind that despite these factors, the decision will ultimately come down to your personal requirements and budget.

With that being said, let's start with the most basic one first.

**Capacity**

When it comes to choosing the capacity of your air fryer, you will have to choose between a small one or a large device. This decision should be made based on the size of your family.

To give you an idea,

- Philips air fryers tend to have a capacity between 1.8 pounds to 2.6 pounds
- Tefal Actifry holds up to 2.2 pounds
- Larger air fryers such as the Lidore air fryer come with a whopping 22-pound capacity
- Avalon Bay's air fryer has a capacity of 3.2 pounds

**Accessibility**

The different models of air fryers generally have two different modes of operation.

- Analog button
- Digital interface with interactive touchscreen

The air fryer devices with analog buttons are mostly the old ones. They get the job done but don't pack that many functionalities under their hood.

On the other hand, modern air fryers such as the Philips air fryers are now produced with digital touchpad controls and a plethora of different programmable cooking options. These cooking options give you multiple preset temperature settings for various types of meals and cooking methods such as warming up, making steak, cooking chicken and so on.

Simple analog air fryers mostly tend to have only one fixed temperature setting and a timer.

You should keep both of these options under consideration when making a purchase and choose the one that best suits you. Analog air fryers are extremely simple to use but lack the extra functions that you might enjoy with a digital air fryer.

**The Accessories**

Every air fryer model comes with some additional accessories aside from the core cooking basket. These accessories will help to expand your cooking options and increase the versatility of the device.

Aside from your standard fries, using certain air fryers and provided accessories will allow you to grill pork chops, roast chicken wings, and even bake muffins!

Generally, the accessories that you should be looking for include:

- Double Layer Rack
- Grill Pan
- Skewers
- Cake Pan
- Rotisserie Fork
- Fry Cage
- Steak Cage

Rarely will you get all of the accessories in a single package. Therefore, while buying your air fryer, you should keep an eye out for one that provides you with the best value.

Certain models such as a Gourmia GTA1500 come with 4 accessories while the Philips air fryer doesn't necessarily come with a plethora of accessories. However, many accessories can be bought separately.

When it comes to buying accessories though, the brand doesn't really mean that much. Just go for ones that fit easily in the air fryer that you are using, and you will be good to go!

**The Price**

When considering the price of an air fryer, it is better that you check out the different models available on the web (or have a look at the top air fryer list I have included) in order to compare and make the best decision.

## General Pros and Cons of the Air Fryer

Since the core technology used in an air fryer is pretty much the same, there are some general pros and cons that you should keep in mind.

### The Good Aspects

- Very minimal or no oil is used while cooking
- The devices are very accessible and easy to use
- Meals can be cooked at a faster rate using Air Fryer
- The device is very convenient to use
- It is easy to clean
- Modern Air Fryers come with multiple cook modes

### The Not-So-Good Aspects

- The air fryer made for general usages are not huge. So, when it comes to providing for a large family, meals are generally required to be cooked in batches.
- The size of the actual device is somewhat bulky, so this might be problematic for some people.

## The Top 3 Air Fryers Right Now

### The Philips Viva Collection HD9641/96

Philips air fryers are well known for their versatility—and this device is no exception! With the ability to bake, fry, grill, and even roast, Philips's latest attempt at the air fryer market has achieved greatness. Boasting a high capacity (28 ounces) cooking chamber and a form factor that is 20% smaller than the previous iteration, you just can't go wrong with this one! In short, this is the perfect air fryer for a family of 4 or less.

**Price:** $249 (at the time of writing)

### Tefal Actifry Express XL

The Tefal Actifry Express XL is great for feeding a large family. With this air fryer, you will be able to cook almost 4 pounds of food per batch. With user-friendly and easy-to-use controls, this device makes cooking with an air fryer a breeze.

**Price:** $151 (at the time of writing)

**NuWave Brio Digital**

This is a device that has made quite a name for itself in the US market and for good reason! The Air Flow Technology implemented in this product is really top notch, which allows for the food to be cooked evenly from all directions (unlike most other models that cook from only one direction, resulting in uneven cooking). The device comes with a large (approximately 6 pound) capacity basket, so that it can feed a moderately big family as well.

**Price:** $172 (at the time of writing)

# Air Fryer Troubleshooting Guide

| Trouble | What to do |
| --- | --- |
| **Air Fryer is not working properly** | Make sure to check that the device is plugged in properly and the preparation time and temperature are set correctly. |
| **Food is not cooked properly** | Make sure to cook in small batches when needed to ensure that everything is fried evenly. |
| **Food is not evenly fried** | Some meals might require you to shake the basket from time to time to ensure proper cooking. This will be given in the recipe instructions. |
| **Basket won't slide in properly** | One reason for this might be the basket is overfilled or the basket is not appropriately placed inside. Make sure that you don't exceed the maximum specified limit of your basket. Also, while putting the basket back into the Fryer, make sure to keep pushing it until you hear a "Click" sound. |
| **White smoke emitted from the fryer** | This happens when you have accidentally used too much oil. |

# Healthy Oils

While the main selling point of an air fryer is the fact that it uses a very small amount of oil, it still uses a bit of it.

So, if you want to maximize the "health" factor of your meals, it is of paramount importance that you use the healthiest oil possible!

To save you some time and effort, I have listed the five healthiest oil that you can use while cooking using your air fryer.

**Coconut Oil:** When it comes to high heat cooking, coconut oil is the best with over 90% of the fatty acids being saturated, which makes it very resistant to heat. This particular oil is semi-solid at room temperature and can be used for months without it turning rancid.

This particular oil also has a lot of health benefits! Since this oil is rich in a fatty acid known as lauric acid, it can help to improve cholesterol levels and kill various pathogens.

**Extra-Virgin Olive Oil:** Olive oil is very well known for its heart health benefits. In fact, this is one of the main reasons why the Mediterranean diet uses olive oil as a key ingredient.

Some recent studies have shown that olive oil can even help to improve health biomarkers such as increasing HDL cholesterol and lowering the amount of bad LDL cholesterol.

**Avocado Oil:** The composition of Avocado oil is very similar to olive oil and as such it holds similar health benefits. It can be used for many purposes including as an alternative to olive oil.

**Fish Oil:** Fish oil is extremely rich in omega-3 fatty acids such as EPA and DHA. Just a tablespoon of fish oil is enough to satisfy the body's daily needs.

If you are looking for the best fish oil, then cod fish liver oil is your best option—plus, it I also rich in Vitamin D3.

But here is the thing, since fish oil has a high concentration of polyunsaturated fats, it should not be used for cooking. The best way to use this oil is as a supplement.

**Grapeseed Oil:** Grapeseed oil is a very versatile cooking oil that is extracted from grape seeds that are left behind after winemaking. This is a favorite oil among chefs and foodies! This oil has a very mild flavor that can be added with other ingredients that give a very strong flavor to meals.

Grapeseed has a very high percentage of polyunsaturated fat and has a similar fatty acid profile to soybean oil.

According to multiple sources, grapeseed oil has a good number of positive effects on the heart.

# Frequently Asked Questions Regarding Air Fryers

**Do we need to add oil before we start cooking?**

Not really. If you like you can add one spoon of olive oil to your fries or chicken breast and massage it. But you really don't need to. For meat that is not lean such as chicken leg or dark meat, you will get pretty juicy results without any oil.

**How many people does this cook for? We are a family of 3.**

It depends on what you're cooking in terms of the size of each portion. Most air fryers can cook enough food for 5 people. If you would like larger portions or to double the recipe, you might need to cook another round. Since timing for fish, veggies, fries, onion rings, etc., is generally less than 10 minutes, it is not a big deal to run two rounds. I would recommend getting an air fryer that is at least 5.8 quarts.

**Can you fry fresh chicken?**

Yes, I like to lightly spray the chicken with oil, use the chicken preset, and cook for 60 minutes. Always check halfway through. It should come out nicely browned and crispy chicken.

**Is it dishwasher safe?**

The pans and racks are dishwasher safe, but they are also easily cleaned up by hand as they are nonstick. The unit itself cannot be put in the dishwasher.

**I bought a new air fryer! What's the first thing I should cook in it?**

Let's see, this is a tough one to answer because most foods taste great when cooked in an air fryer. The most common ones to start with are French fries, and also chicken drumsticks. The best advice I can give you is to experiment, and to check the food often.

**What shouldn't we put in an air fryer?**

Because the air fryer will be blowing hot air around the cooking cavity, you want to make sure any food that is light in weight or that is at risk of being blown around should be avoided. Also avoid any wet batters because the air flow will blow the batter off the food and all around the cavity.

# CHAPTER 1 | BREAD AND BREAKFAST

## Sourdough Bread

**(Yields:** 8 servings / **Prep Time:** 20 minutes / **Cooking Time:** 20 minutes)

### Ingredients

- 1 cup sourdough starter
- 1 cup unbleached all-purpose flour
- ¼ cup whole-wheat flour
- 1 tablespoon white sugar
- ½ teaspoon salt
- 1 tablespoon canola oil

### Instructions

1. In the baking pan of a bread machine, place all the ingredients in the order recommended by the manufacturer.
2. Place the baking pan in bread machine and close with the lid.
3. Select the Dough cycle and press Start button.
4. Once the cycle is completed, remove the paddles from bread machine but keep the dough inside for about 4 hours to proof.
5. Now, transfer the dough into a floured proofing basket and set aside to rise for about 3 hours.
6. Set the temperature of air fryer to 390 degrees F.
7. Carefully, arrange the dough onto the grill insert of an air fryer.
8. Air fry for about 20 minutes, turning the pan once halfway through.
9. Remove the bread from air fryer and place onto a wire rack for about 2-3 hours before slicing.
10. Cut the bread into desired size slices and serve.

### Nutrition Values (Per Serving)

- Calories: 162
- Carbohydrate: 25.3g
- Protein: 11.3g
- Fat: 3.1g
- Sugar: 1.6g
- Sodium: 160mg

# Cream Bread

**(Yields:** 12 servings / **Prep Time:** 20 minutes / **Cooking Time:** 55 minutes)

## Ingredients

- 1 cup milk
- ¾ cup whipping cream
- 1 large egg
- 4½ cups bread flour
- ½ cup all-purpose flour
- 2 tablespoons milk powder
- 1 teaspoon salt
- ¼ cup fine sugar
- 3 teaspoons dry yeast

## Instructions

1. In the baking pan of a bread machine, place all the ingredients in the order recommended by the manufacturer.
2. Place the baking pan in bread machine and close with the lid.
3. Select the Dough cycle and press Start button.
4. Once the cycle is completed, remove the paddles from bread machine but keep the dough inside for about 45-50 minutes to proof.
5. Set the temperature of air fryer to 375 degrees F. Grease 2 loaf pans.
6. Remove the dough from pan and place onto a lightly floured surface.
7. Divide the dough into four equal-sized balls and then, roll each into a rectangle.
8. Tightly, roll each rectangle like a Swiss roll.
9. Place two rolls into each prepared loaf pan.
10. Set aside for about 1 hour.
11. Arrange the loaf pans into an air fryer basket.
12. Air fry for about 50-55 minutes or until a toothpick inserted in the center comes out clean.
13. Remove the pans from air fryer and place onto a wire rack for about 10-15 minutes.
14. Then, remove the bread rolls from pans and place onto a wire rack until they are completely cool before slicing.
15. Cut each roll into desired size slices and serve.

## Nutrition Values (Per Serving)

- Calories: 215
- Carbohydrate: 36.9g
- Protein: 6.5g
- Fat: 3.1g
- Sugar: 5.2g
- Sodium: 189mg

# Sunflower Seeds Bread

**(Yields:** 4 servings / **Prep Time:** 15 minutes / **Cooking Time:** 18 minutes)

## Ingredients

- 2/3 cup whole-wheat flour
- 2/3 cup plain flour
- 1/3 cup sunflower seeds
- ½ sachet instant yeast
- 1 teaspoon salt
- 2/3-1 cup lukewarm water

## Instructions

1. In a bowl, mix together the flours, sunflower seeds, yeast, and salt.
2. Slowly, add in the water, stirring continuously until a soft dough ball forms.
3. Now, move the dough onto a lightly floured surface and knead for about 5 minutes using your hands.
4. Make a ball from the dough and place into a bowl.
5. With a plastic wrap, cover the bowl and place at a warm place for about 30 minutes.
6. Set the temperature of air fryer to 390 degrees F. Grease a cake pan. (6"x 3")
7. Coat the top of dough with water and place into the prepared cake pan.
8. Arrange the cake pan into an air fryer basket.
9. Air fry for about 18 minutes or until a toothpick inserted in the center comes out clean.
10. Remove from air fryer and place the pan onto a wire rack for about 10-15 minutes.
11. Carefully, take out the bread from pan and put onto a wire rack until it is completely cool before slicing.
12. Cut the bread into desired size slices and serve.

## Nutrition Values (Per Serving)

- Calories: 177
- Carbohydrate: 33g
- Protein: 5.5g
- Fat: 2.4g
- Sugar: 0.2g
- Sodium: 580mg

# Date Bread

**(Yields:** 10 servings / **Prep Time:** 15 minutes / **Cooking Time:** 22 minutes)

## Ingredients

- 2½ cup dates, pitted and chopped
- ¼ cup butter
- 1 cup hot water
- 1½ cups flour
- ½ cup brown sugar
- 1 teaspoon baking powder
- 1 teaspoon baking soda
- ½ teaspoon salt
- 1 egg

## Instructions

1. In a large bowl, add the dates, butter and top with the hot water.
2. Set aside for about 5 minutes.
3. In a separate bowl, mix together the flour, brown sugar, baking powder, baking soda, and salt.
4. In the same bowl of dates, mix well the flour mixture, and egg.
5. Set the temperature of air fryer to 340 degrees F. Grease an air fryer non-stick pan.
6. Place the mixture into the prepared pan.
7. Arrange the pan into an air fryer basket.
8. Air fry for about 22 minutes or until a toothpick inserted in the center comes out clean.
9. Remove from air fryer and place the pan onto a wire rack for about 10-15 minutes.
10. Carefully, take out the bread from pan and put onto a wire rack until it is completely cool before slicing.
11. Cut the bread into desired size slices and serve.

## Nutrition Values (Per Serving)

- Calories: 269
- Carbohydrate: 55.1g
- Protein: 3.6g
- Fat: 5.4g
- Sugar: 35.3
- Sodium: 585mg

# Banana Bread

(**Yields:** 8 servings / **Prep Time:** 10 minutes / **Cooking Time:** 20 minutes)

## Ingredients

- 1 1/3 cups flour
- 2/3 cup sugar
- 1 teaspoon baking soda
- 1 teaspoon baking powder
- 1 teaspoon ground cinnamon
- 1 teaspoon salt
- ½ cup milk
- ½ cup olive oil
- 3 bananas, peeled and sliced

## Instructions

1. Take the bowl of a stand mixer and mix well all the listed ingredients.
2. Set the temperature of air fryer to 330 degrees F. Grease a loaf pan.
3. Place the mixture into the prepared pan.
4. Arrange the loaf pan into an air fryer basket.
5. Air fry for about 20 minutes or until a toothpick inserted in the center comes out clean.
6. Remove from air fryer and place the pan onto a wire rack for about 10-15 minutes.
7. Carefully, take out the bread from pan and put onto a wire rack until it is completely cool before slicing.
8. Cut the bread into desired size slices and serve.

## Nutrition Values (Per Serving)

- Calories: 295
- Carbohydrate: 44g
- Protein: 3.1g
- Fat: 13.3g
- Sugar: 22.8g
- Sodium: 458mg

---

# Nutty Banana Bread

(**Yields:** 10 servings / **Prep Time:** 15 minutes / **Cooking Time:** 25 minutes)

## Ingredients

- 1½ cups self-rising flour
- ¼ teaspoon bicarbonate of soda
- 5 tablespoons plus 1 teaspoon butter
- 2/3 cup plus ½ tablespoon caster sugar
- 2 medium eggs

- 3½ ounces walnuts, chopped
- 2 cups bananas, peeled and mashed

## Instructions

1. In a bowl, mix together the flour and bicarbonate of soda.
2. In another bowl, add the butter, and sugar. Beat until pale and fluffy.
3. Put the eggs, one at a time along with a little flour and mix them well.
4. Stir in the remaining flour and walnuts.
5. Now, add the bananas and mix until well combined.
6. Set the temperature of air fryer to 355 degrees F. Grease a loaf pan.
7. Place the mixture evenly into the prepared pan.
8. Arrange the loaf pan into an air fryer basket.
9. Air fry for 10 minutes on 355 degrees F, then 15 minutes for 338 degrees F.
10. Once done, remove from air fryer and place the pan onto a wire rack for about 10-15 minutes.
11. Carefully, take out the bread from pan and put onto a wire rack until it is completely cool before slicing.
12. Cut the bread into desired size slices and serve.

## Nutrition Values (Per Serving)

- Calories: 337
- Carbohydrate: 44.5g
- Protein: 7.3g
- Fat: 16g
- Sugar: 21.6g
- Sodium: 106mg

---

# Yogurt Banana Bread

(**Yields:** 5 servings / **Prep Time:** 15 minutes / **Cooking Time:** 35 minutes)

## Ingredients

- ½ cup all-purpose flour
- ¼ cup whole-wheat flour
- ¼ teaspoon baking soda
- ½ teaspoon salt
- 1 large egg
- ½ cup granulated sugar
- ¼ cup plain yogurt
- ¼ cup vegetable oil
- ½ teaspoon pure vanilla extract
- 2 ripe bananas, peeled and mashed
- 2 tablespoons turbinado sugar

## Instructions

1. In a bowl, sift together the flours, baking soda, and salt.

2. In another large bowl, mix well the egg, granulated sugar, yogurt, oil, and vanilla extract.
3. Add in the bananas and beat until well combined.
4. Now, add the flour mixture and mix until just combined.
5. Set the temperature of Air Fryer to 310 degrees F.
6. Place the mixture evenly into a cake pan and sprinkle with the turbinado sugar.
7. Arrange the cake pan into an Air Fryer basket.
8. Air Fry for about 30-35 minutes or until a toothpick inserted in the center comes out clean, turning the pan once halfway through.
9. Carefully, take out the bread from pan and put onto a wire rack until it is completely cool before slicing.
10. Cut the bread into desired size slices and serve.

## **Nutrition Values (Per Serving)**

- Calories: 317
- Carbohydrate: 49.2g
- Protein: 7.3g
- Fat: 16g
- Sugar: 21.6g
- Sodium: 106mg

## **Peanut Butter Banana Bread**

(**Yields:** 6 servings / **Prep Time:** 15 minutes / **Cooking Time:** 40 minutes)

## **Ingredients**

- 1 cup plus 1 tablespoon all-purpose flour
- 1 teaspoon baking powder
- ¼ teaspoon baking soda
- ¼ teaspoon salt
- 1 large egg
- 1/3 cup granulated sugar
- ¼ cup canola oil
- 2 tablespoons creamy peanut butter
- 2 tablespoons sour cream
- 1 teaspoon vanilla extract
- 2 medium ripe bananas, peeled and mashed
- ¾ cup walnuts, roughly chopped

## **Instructions**

1. Take a bowl and mix together the flour, baking powder, baking soda, and salt.
2. In another large bowl, add the egg, sugar, oil, peanut butter, sour cream, and vanilla extract. Beat until well combined.
3. Add in the bananas and beat until well combined.
4. Now, add the flour mixture and mix until just combined.
5. Gently, fold in the walnuts.

6. Set the temperature of Air Fryer to 330 degrees F. Grease a non-stick baking dish.
7. Transfer the mixture evenly into the prepared baking dish.
8. Arrange the baking dish in an Air Fryer basket.
9. Air Fry for about 30-40 minutes or until a toothpick inserted in the center comes out clean.
10. Remove the dish from Air Fryer and place onto a wire rack for about 10-15 minutes.
11. Carefully, take out the bread from dish and place onto a wire rack until it is completely cool before slicing.
12. Cut the bread into desired size slices and serve.

## **Nutrition Values (Per Serving)**

- Calories: 384
- Carbohydrate: 39.3g
- Protein: 8.9g
- Fat: 2.6g
- Sugar: 16.6g
- Sodium: 189mg

# **Chocolate Banana Bread**

(**Yields:** 10 servings / **Prep Time:** 6 minutes / **Cooking Time:** 20 minutes)

## **Ingredients**

- 2 cups flour
- ½ teaspoon baking soda
- ½ teaspoon baking powder
- ½ teaspoon salt
- ¾ cup sugar
- 1/3 cup butter, softened
- 3 eggs
- 1 tablespoon vanilla extract
- 1 cup milk
- ½ cup bananas, peeled and mashed
- 1 cup chocolate chips

## **Instructions**

1. Take a bowl and mix together the flour, baking soda, baking powder, and salt.
2. In another large bowl, add the butter, and sugar. Beat until light and fluffy.
3. Now, add in the eggs, and vanilla extract. Beat until well combined.
4. Add the flour mixture and mix until well combined.
5. Add in the milk, and mashed bananas and mix them well.
6. Gently, fold in the chocolate chips.
7. Set the temperature of Air Fryer to 360 degrees F. Grease a loaf pan.
8. Place the mixture evenly into the prepared pan.
9. Arrange the loaf pan into an Air Fryer basket.
10. Air Fry for about 20 minutes or until a toothpick inserted in the center comes out clean.

11. Remove from Air Fryer and place the pan onto a wire rack for about 10-15 minutes.
12. Carefully, take out the bread from pan and put onto a wire rack until it is completely cool before slicing.
13. Cut the bread into desired size slices and serve.

## **Nutrition Values (Per Serving)**

- Calories: 333
- Carbohydrate: 47.4g
- Protein: 6.5g
- Fat: 13.2g
- Sugar: 26g
- Sodium: 267mg

---

# **Nutty Zucchini Bread**

(**Yields:** 16 servings / **Prep Time:** 15 minutes / **Cooking Time:** 20 minutes)

## **Ingredients**

- 3 cups all-purpose flour
- 1 teaspoon baking powder
- 1 teaspoon baking soda
- 1 tablespoon ground cinnamon
- 1 teaspoon salt
- 2¼ cups white sugar
- 1 cup vegetable oil
- 3 eggs
- 3 teaspoons vanilla extract
- 2 cups zucchini, grated
- 1 cup walnuts, chopped

## **Instructions**

1. Take a bowl and mix together the flour, baking powder, baking soda, cinnamon, and salt.
2. In another large bowl, add the sugar, oil, eggs, and vanilla extract. Beat until well combined.
3. Then, add in the flour mixture and stir until just combined.
4. Gently, fold in the zucchini and walnuts.
5. Set the temperature of Air Fryer to 320 degrees F. Grease and flour two (8x4-inch) loaf pans.
6. Place the mixture evenly into the prepared pans.
7. Arrange the loaf pans into an Air Fryer basket.
8. Air Fry for about 20 minutes or until a toothpick inserted in the center comes out clean.
9. Remove the pans from Air Fryer and place onto a wire rack for about 10-15 minutes.

10. Carefully, take out the bread from pans and put onto a wire rack until it is completely cool before slicing.
11. Cut the breads into desired size slices and serve.

## **Nutrition Values (Per Serving)**

- Calories: 377
- Carbohydrate: 47.9g
- Protein: 5.5g
- Fat: 19.3g
- Sugar: 28.7g
- Sodium: 241mg

---

# **Zucchini & Apple Bread**

(**Yields:** 8 servings / **Prep Time:** 15 minutes / **Cooking Time:** 30 minutes)

## **Ingredients**

### For Bread:

- 1 cup all-purpose flour
- ¾ teaspoon baking powder
- ¼ teaspoon baking soda
- 1¼ teaspoons ground cinnamon
- ¼ teaspoon salt
- 1/3 cup vegetable oil
- 1/3 cup sugar
- 1 egg
- 1 teaspoon vanilla extract
- ½ cup zucchini, shredded
- ½ cup apple, cored and shredded
- 5 tablespoons walnuts, chopped

### For Topping:

- 1 tablespoon walnuts, chopped
- 2 teaspoons brown sugar
- ¼ teaspoon ground cinnamon

## **Instructions**

1. For bread: in a bowl, mix together the flour, baking powder, baking soda, cinnamon, and salt.
2. In another large bowl, mix well the oil, sugar, egg, and vanilla extract.
3. Then, add in the flour mixture and mix until just combined
4. Gently, fold in the zucchini, apple and walnuts.
5. For the topping: in a small bowl, add all the ingredients and whisk them well.
6. Preheat the Air Fryer to 325 degrees F. Grease and flour an 8 x 4-inch loaf pan.
7. Place the bread mixture evenly into the prepared pan and sprinkle with the topping mixture.
8. Arrange the loaf pan into an Air Fryer basket.
9. Air Fry for about 30 minutes or until a toothpick inserted in the center comes out clean.

10. Remove from Air Fryer and place the pan onto a wire rack for about 10-15 minutes.
11. Carefully, take out the bread from pan and put onto a wire rack until it is completely cool before slicing.
12. Cut the bread into desired size slices and serve.

## **Nutrition Values (Per Serving)**

- Calories: 207
- Carbohydrate: 24.4g
- Protein: 3.9g
- Fat: 13.3g
- Sugar: 10.9g
- Sodium: 140mg

---

# **Pumpkin & Yogurt Bread**

**(Yields:** 4 servings / **Prep Time:** 10 minutes / **Cooking Time:** 15 minutes)

## **Ingredients**

- 2 large eggs
- 8 tablespoons pumpkin puree
- 6 tablespoons banana flour
- 4 tablespoons honey
- 4 tablespoons plain Greek yogurt
- 2 tablespoons vanilla essence
- Pinch of ground nutmeg
- 6 tablespoons oats

## **Instructions**

1. Take a bowl, add in all the ingredients except oats and with a hand mixer, mix until smooth.
2. Add the oats and mix them well using a fork.
3. Set the temperature of Air Fryer to 360 degrees F. Grease and flour a loaf pan.
4. Place the mixture evenly into the prepared pan.
5. Arrange the loaf pan into an Air Fryer basket.
6. Air Fry for about 15 minutes or until a toothpick inserted in the center comes out clean.
7. Remove the pans from Air Fryer and place onto a wire rack for about 5 minutes.
8. Carefully, take out the bread from pan and put onto a wire rack to cool for about 5-10 minutes before slicing.
9. Cut the bread into desired size slices and serve.

## Nutrition Values (Per Serving)

- Calories: 212
- Carbohydrate: 36g
- Protein: 6.6g
- Fat: 3.4g
- Sugar: 20.5g
- Sodium: 49mg

---

# Spiced Pumpkin Bread

**(Yields:** 4 servings / **Prep Time:** 15 minutes / **Cooking Time:** 25 minutes)

## Ingredients

- ¼ cup coconut flour
- 2 tablespoons stevia blend
- 1 teaspoon baking powder
- ¾ teaspoon pumpkin pie spice
- ¼ teaspoon ground cinnamon
- 1/8 teaspoon salt
- ¼ cup canned pumpkin
- 2 large eggs
- 2 tablespoons unsweetened almond milk
- 1 teaspoon vanilla extract

## Instructions

1. In a bowl, mix together the flour, stevia, baking powder, spices, and salt.
2. In another large bowl, add the pumpkin, eggs, almond milk, and vanilla extract. Beat until well combined.
3. Then, add in the flour mixture and mix until just combined
4. Set the temperature of air fryer to 350 degrees F. Line a cake pan with a greased parchment paper.
5. Place the mixture evenly into the prepared pan.
6. Arrange the pan into an air fryer basket.
7. Air fry for about 25 minutes or until a toothpick inserted in the center comes out clean.
8. Remove the pans from air fryer and place onto a wire rack for about 5 minutes.
9. Carefully, take out the bread from pan and put onto a wire rack to cool for about 5-10 minutes before slicing.
10. Cut the bread into desired size slices and serve.

## Nutrition Values (Per Serving)

- Calories: 67
- Carbohydrate: 9g
- Protein: 3.5g
- Fat: 2.8g
- Sugar: 6.9g
- Sodium: 118mg

# Chocolate Peanut Butter Bread

**(Yields:** 8 servings / **Prep Time:** 15 minutes / **Cooking Time:** 30 minutes)

## Ingredients

- ¾ cup all-purpose flour
- ¼ cup cocoa powder
- ¼ cup sugar
- ½ teaspoon baking soda
- ½ teaspoon baking powder
- 1/8 teaspoon salt
- 1 egg
- 1/3 cup unsweetened applesauce
- ¼ cup plain Greek yogurt
- ½ teaspoon vanilla extract
- 1/3 cup creamy peanut butter
- 1/3 cup mini chocolate chips

## Instructions

1. In a bowl, mix together the flour, cocoa powder, sugar, baking soda, baking powder, and salt.
2. In another bowl, add the egg, applesauce, yogurt, and vanilla extract. Beat until well combined.
3. Then, add in the flour mixture and mix until just combined.
4. Add the peanut butter and mix until smooth.
5. Gently, fold in the chocolate chips.
6. Set the temperature of Air Fryer to 350 degrees F. Grease a loaf pan.
7. Place the mixture evenly into the prepared pan.
8. Arrange the loaf pan into an Air Fryer basket.
9. Air Fry for about 30 minutes or until a toothpick inserted in the center comes out clean.
10. Remove from Air Fryer and place the pan onto a wire rack for about 10-15 minutes.
11. Carefully, take out the bread from pan and put onto a wire rack until it is completely cool before slicing.
12. Cut the bread into desired size slices and serve.

## Nutrition Values (Per Serving)

- Calories: 191
- Carbohydrate: 24.9g
- Protein: 6.1g
- Fat: 8.6g
- Sugar: 12.6g
- Sodium: 183mg

# Simple Cornbread

**(Yields:** 8 servings / **Prep Time:** 15 minutes / **Cooking Time:** 25 minutes)

## Ingredients

- 1 cup cornmeal
- ¾ cup all-purpose flour
- 1 tablespoon sugar
- 1½ teaspoons baking powder
- ½ teaspoon baking soda
- ¼ teaspoon salt
- 1½ cups buttermilk
- 6 tablespoons unsalted butter, melted
- 2 large eggs, lightly beaten

## Instructions

1. In a bowl, mix together the cornmeal, flour, sugar, baking soda, baking powder, and salt.
2. Take a separate bowl, mix well the buttermilk, butter, and eggs.
3. Then, add in the flour mixture and mix until just combined.
4. Set the temperature of Air Fryer to 360 degrees F. Lightly, grease an 8-inch baking dish.
5. Transfer the flour mixture evenly into the prepared baking dish.
6. Place the dish into an Air Fryer basket.
7. Air Fry for about 25 minutes or until a toothpick inserted in the center comes out clean, turning the dish once halfway through.
8. Remove from Air Fryer and place the dish onto a wire rack for about 10-15 minutes.
9. Carefully, take out the bread from dish and put onto a wire rack until it is completely cool before slicing.
10. Cut the bread into desired size slices and serve.

## Nutrition Values (Per Serving)

- Calories: 217
- Carbohydrate: 24.9g
- Protein: 5.6g
- Fat: 10.9g
- Sugar: 3.9g
- Sodium: 286mg

# Pineapple Cornbread

**(Yields:** 5 servings / **Prep Time:** 10 minutes / **Cooking Time:** 15 minutes)

## Ingredients

- 1 (8½-ounces) package Jiffy corn muffin
- 7 ounces canned crushed pineapple
- 1/3 cup canned pineapple juice
- 1 egg

## Instructions

1. In a bowl, mix together all the ingredients.
2. Set the temperature of Air Fryer to 330 degrees F. Grease a round cake pan. (6"x 3")
3. Place the mixture evenly into the prepared pan.
4. Arrange the cake pan into an Air Fryer basket.
5. Air Fry for about 15 minutes or until a toothpick inserted in the center comes out clean.
6. Remove from Air Fryer and place the pan onto a wire rack for about 10-15 minutes.
7. Carefully, take out the bread from pan and put onto a wire rack until it is completely cool before slicing.
8. Cut the bread into desired size slices and serve.

## Nutrition Values (Per Serving)

- Calories: 220
- Carbohydrate: 40g
- Protein: 3.8g
- Fat: 6.4g
- Sugar: 14.1g
- Sodium: 423mg

# Sweet Rosemary Cornbread

**(Yields:** 4 servings / **Prep Time:** 15 minutes / **Cooking Time:** 25 minutes)

## Ingredients

- ¾ cup fine yellow cornmeal
- ½ cup sorghum flour
- ¼ cup tapioca starch
- ½ teaspoon xanthan gum*
- ¼ cup granulated sugar
- 2 teaspoons baking powder
- ¼ teaspoon salt
- 1 cup plain almond milk
- 3 tablespoons olive oil
- 2 teaspoons fresh rosemary, minced

## Instructions

1. In a large bowl, mix together the cornmeal, sorghum flour, tapioca starch, xanthan gum, sugar, baking powder, and salt.
2. Add the almond milk, oil, and rosemary. Mix until well combined.
3. Set the temperature of Air Fryer to 400 degrees F. Grease 4 ramekins.
4. Put the mixture evenly into the prepared ramekins.
5. Place the ramekins into an Air Fryer basket.
6. Air Fry for about 20-25 minutes or until a toothpick inserted in the center comes out clean.
7. Remove from Air Fryer and place the ramekins onto a wire rack for about 10-15 minutes.
8. Carefully, invert the breads into serving plates.
9. Enjoy!

## Nutrition Values (Per Serving)

- Calories: 458
- Carbohydrate: 56.3g
- Protein: 5.3g
- Fat: 26.2g
- Sugar: 15g
- Sodium: 176mg

(**Note: Xanthan gum*** - Xanthan gum is a polysaccharide with many industrial uses, including as a common food additive. It is an effective thickening agent and stabilizer to prevent ingredients from separating. Cornstarch can make an ideal substitute for xanthan gum when used in baked goods, gravies and sauces.)

---

## Sweet Jalapeño Cornbread

(**Yields:** 10 servings / **Prep Time:** 15 minutes / **Cooking Time:** 18 minutes)

## Ingredients

- 1 cup flour
- 1 cup yellow cornmeal
- ½ cup white sugar
- 2 teaspoons baking powder
- ½ teaspoon baking soda
- 1 teaspoon salt
- 2 large eggs
- ¾ cup sour cream
- ½ cup buttermilk
- 3 tablespoons butter, melted
- 2 tablespoons vegetable oil
- ¼ cup pepper jack cheese, grated
- ½ of jalapeño pepper, finely chopped

### Instructions

1. In a bowl, mix together the flour, cornmeal, sugar, baking powder, baking soda, and salt.
2. In another large bowl, mix well the eggs, sour cream, buttermilk, butter, and oil.
3. Then, add in the flour mixture and mix until well combined.
4. Add the cheese, and jalapeño and stir to combine.
5. Set the temperature of Air Fryer to 300 degrees F. Grease a round cake pan.
6. Put the mixture evenly into the prepared pan.
7. Arrange the cake pan into an Air Fryer basket.
8. Air Fry for about 18 minutes or until a toothpick inserted in the center comes out clean, turning the pan once halfway through.
9. Remove from Air Fryer and place the pan onto a wire rack for about 10-15 minutes.
10. Carefully, take out the bread from pan and put onto a wire rack until it is completely cool before slicing.
11. Cut the bread into desired size slices and serve.

### Nutrition Values (Per Serving)

- Calories: 238
- Carbohydrate: 30.8g
- Protein: 4.6g
- Fat: 11.6g
- Sugar: 10.6g
- Sodium: 363mg

## Fried Flatbreads

(**Yields:** 8 servings / **Prep Time:** 15 minutes / **Cooking Time:** 9 minutes)

### Ingredients

- 1½ tablespoons granulated sugar
- 1 tablespoon active dry yeast
- ½ teaspoon salt
- 1 2/3 cups whole milk
- 1½ tablespoons shortening*
- 1 egg, beaten
- 4-4½ cups bread flour
- 1 cup vegetable oil

### Instructions

1. In a small bowl, mix well sugar, yeast, and salt.
2. In a small pan, add the milk and shortening over medium heat and cook for about 2-3 minutes or until shortening just melts, stirring continuously.
3. Once done, move away the pan from the heat and set aside until just warm.
4. Take the bowl of a stand mixer, attached with the dough hook, add in the yeast mixture, and milk mixture. Mix them well and set aside for about 10 minutes.

5. Add the egg and 1½ cups of flour and mix on low speed until combined.
6. Gradually, add the remaining flour and blend until non-sticky dough ball forms.
7. Place the dough into a lightly greased bowl and turn to coat.
8. With a clean kitchen towel, cover the bowl and set aside for about 1-2 hours or until doubled in size.
9. Set the temperature of Air Fryer to 300 degrees F.
10. Make 2 golf ball sized balls from the dough and place on a lightly floured surface.
11. Now, roll each ball into a circle using a rolling pin and coat both sides with a little oil.
12. Arrange both rolled knead in an Air fryer basket.
13. Air Fry for about 9 minutes or until puffy and browned.
14. Repeat with the remaining dough.
15. Serve warm.

## Nutrition Values (Per Serving)

- Calories: 569
- Carbohydrate: 58.8g
- Protein: 10.2g
- Fat: 32.6g
- Sugar: 5.2g
- Sodium: 177mg

(**Note: Shortening\*** -Shortening is any fat that is a solid at room temperature and used to make crumbly pastry and other food products. Although butter is solid at room temperature and is frequently used in making pastry, the term "shortening" seldom refers to butter, but is more closely related to margarine)

---

# Banana Muffins

(**Yields:** 12 servings / **Prep Time:** 15 minutes / **Cooking Time:** 25 minutes)

## Ingredients

- 1 2/3 cups plain flour
- 1 teaspoon baking soda
- 1 teaspoon baking powder
- 1 teaspoon ground cinnamon
- 1 teaspoon salt
- 4 ripe bananas, peeled and mashed
- 2 eggs
- ½ cup brown sugar
- 1 teaspoon vanilla essence
- 3 tablespoon milk
- 1 tablespoon Nutella
- ¼ cup walnuts

## Instructions

1. In a large bowl, sift the flour, baking soda, baking powder, cinnamon, and salt.
2. In another bowl, mix together the remaining ingredients except walnuts.

3. Add the banana mixture into flour mixture and mix until just combined.
4. Fold in the walnuts.
5. Set the temperature of Air Fryer to 248 degrees F. Grease 12 muffin molds.
6. Put the mixture evenly into the prepared muffin molds.
7. Arrange the molds into an Air Fryer basket.
8. Air Fry for about 20-25 minutes or until a toothpick inserted in the center comes out clean.
9. Remove the muffin molds from Air Fryer and place onto a wire rack to cool for about 10 minutes.
10. Carefully, invert the muffins onto the wire rack to completely cool before serving.
11. Serve.

## **Nutrition Values (Per Serving)**

- Calories: 227
- Carbohydrate: 38.1g
- Protein: 5.2g
- Fat: 6.6g
- Sugar: 15.8g
- Sodium: 364mg

## Apple Muffins

(**Yields:** 12 servings / **Prep Time:** 15 minutes / **Cooking Time:** 25 minutes)

## **Ingredients**

- 1¾ cups plain flour
- 1/3 cup white sugar
- 1½ teaspoons baking powder
- ½ teaspoon ground cinnamon
- ¼ teaspoon ground ginger
- ¼ teaspoon salt
- ¾ cup milk
- 1/3 cup applesauce
- 1 cup apple, cored and chopped

## **Instructions**

1. In a large bowl, mix together the flour, sugar, baking powder, spices, and salt.
2. Add in the milk and applesauce. Beat until just combined.
3. Fold in the chopped apple.
4. Set the temperature of Air Fryer to 390 degrees F. Grease 12 muffin molds.
5. Put the mixture evenly into the prepared muffin molds.

6. Arrange the molds into an Air Fryer basket.
7. Air Fry for about 20-25 minutes or until a toothpick inserted in the center comes out clean.
8. Remove the muffin molds from Air Fryer and place onto a wire rack to cool for about 10 minutes.
9. Carefully, invert the muffins onto the wire rack to completely cool before serving.
10. Serve.

## **Nutrition Values (Per Serving)**

- Calories: 108
- Carbohydrate: 24g
- Protein: 2.4g
- Fat: 0.5g
- Sugar: 8.9g
- Sodium: 59mg

---

# **Blueberry Muffins**

**(Yields:** 12 servings / **Prep Time:** 15 minutes / **Cooking Time:** 12 minutes**)**

## **Ingredients**

- 2 cups plus 2 tablespoons self-rising flour
- 5 tablespoons white sugar
- ½ cup milk
- 2 ounces butter, melted
- 2 eggs
- 2 teaspoons fresh orange zest, finely grated
- 2 tablespoons fresh orange juice
- ½ teaspoon vanilla extract
- ½ cup fresh blueberries

## **Instructions**

1. In a bowl, mix together the flour, and white sugar.
2. In another large bowl, mix well the remaining ingredients except blueberries.
3. Now, add in the flour mixture and mix until just combined.
4. Fold in the blueberries.
5. Set the temperature of Air Fryer to 355 degrees F. Grease 12 muffin molds.
6. Put the mixture evenly into the prepared muffin molds. Arrange the molds into an Air Fryer basket.
7. Air Fry for about 12 minutes or until a toothpick inserted in the center comes out clean.
8. Remove the muffin molds from Air Fryer and place onto a wire rack to cool for about 10 minutes.

9. Carefully, invert the muffins onto the wire rack to completely cool before serving.
10. Serve.

## Nutrition Values (Per Serving)

- Calories: 154
- Carbohydrate: 23.7g
- Protein: 3.7g
- Fat: 5g
- Sugar: 6.4g
- Sodium: 43mg

---

# Raisin & Oat Muffins

**(Yields:** 4 servings / **Prep Time:** 15 minutes / **Cooking Time:** 10 minutes)

## Ingredients

- ½ cup flour
- ¼ cup rolled oats
- 1/8 teaspoon baking powder
- ½ cup powdered sugar
- ½ cup butter, softened
- 2 eggs
- ¼ teaspoon vanilla extract
- ¼ cup raisins

## Instructions

1. In a bowl, mix together the flour, oats, and baking powder.
2. In another bowl, add the sugar, and butter. Beat until you get the creamy texture.
3. Then, add in the egg and vanilla extract and beat until well combined.
4. Add the egg mixture into oat mixture and mix until just combined.
5. Fold in the raisins.
6. Set the temperature of Air Fryer to 355 degrees F. Grease 4 muffin molds.
7. Place the mixture evenly into the prepared muffin molds. Arrange the molds into an Air Fryer basket.
8. Air Fry for 10 minutes or until a toothpick inserted in the center comes out clean.
9. Remove the muffin molds from Air Fryer and place onto a wire rack to cool for about 10 minutes.
10. Carefully, invert the muffins onto the wire rack to completely cool before serving.
11. Serve.

## Nutrition Values (Per Serving)

- Calories: 398
- Carbohydrate: 37.8g
- Protein: 5.6g
- Fat: 25.8g
- Sugar: 20.4g
- Sodium: 196mg

# Savory Carrot Muffins

**(Yields:** 6 servings / **Prep Time:** 15 minutes / **Cooking Time:** 7+7 = 14 minutes)

## Ingredients

**For Muffins:**
- ¼ cup whole-wheat flour
- ¼ cup all-purpose flour
- ½ teaspoon baking powder
- 1/8 teaspoon baking soda
- ½ teaspoon dried parsley, crushed
- ½ teaspoon salt
- ½ cup yogurt
- 1 teaspoon vinegar
- 1 tablespoon vegetable oil
- 3 tablespoons cottage cheese, grated
- 1 carrot, peeled and grated
- 2-4 tablespoons water (if needed)

**For Topping:**
- 7 ounces Parmesan cheese, grated
- ¼ cup walnuts, chopped

## Instructions

1. Set the temperature of Air Fryer to 355 degrees F. Grease 6 medium muffin molds.
2. For muffin: in a large bowl, mix together the flours, baking powder, baking soda, parsley, and salt.
3. In another large bowl, mix well the yogurt, and vinegar.
4. Add the remaining ingredients except water and beat them well. (add some water if needed)
5. Make a well in the center of the yogurt mixture.
6. Slowly, add the flour mixture in the well and mix until well combined.
7. Place the mixture evenly into the prepared muffin molds and top with the Parmesan cheese and walnuts.
8. Place the muffin molds into an Air Fryer basket in 2 batches.
9. Air Fry for about 7 minutes or until a toothpick inserted in the center comes out clean.
10. Remove the muffin molds from Air Fryer and place onto a wire rack to cool for about 10 minutes.
11. Carefully, invert the muffins onto the wire rack to completely cool before serving.
12. Enjoy!

## Nutrition Values (Per Serving)

- Calories: 222
- Carbohydrate: 12.6g
- Protein: 15.2g
- Fat: 12.9g
- Sugar: 2g
- Sodium: 579mg

# Zucchini Fritters

**(Yields:** 4 servings / **Prep Time:** 15 minutes / **Cooking Time:** 7 minutes)

## Ingredients

- 10½ ounces zucchini, grated and squeezed
- 7 ounces Halloumi cheese
- ¼ cup all-purpose flour
- 2 eggs
- 1 teaspoon fresh dill, minced
- Salt and freshly ground black pepper, as needed

## Instructions

1. In a large bowl and mix together all the listed ingredients.
2. Make a small-sized fritters from the mixture.
3. Set the temperature of Air Fryer to 355 degrees F. Grease a baking dish.
4. Place the fritters into the prepared baking dish.
5. Arrange the dish in an Air Fryer basket.
6. Air Fry for about 6-7 minutes.
7. Serve warm.

## Nutrition Values (Per Serving)

- Calories: 250
- Carbohydrate: 10g
- Protein: 15.2g
- Fat: 17.2g
- Sugar: 2.7g
- Sodium: 330mg

---

# Potato Rosti

**(Yields:** 2 servings / **Prep Time:** 15 minutes / **Cooking Time:** 15 minutes)

## Ingredients

- 1 teaspoon olive oil
- ½ pound russet potatoes, peeled and roughly grated
- 1 tablespoon fresh chives, finely chopped
- Salt and ground black pepper, as required
- 2 tablespoons sour cream
- 3½ ounces smoked salmon, cut into slices

### Instructions

1. Set the temperature of Air Fryer to 355 degrees F. Grease a pizza pan with the olive oil.
2. In a large bowl, mix together the potatoes, chives, salt, and black pepper.
3. Place the potato mixture into the prepared pizza pan.
4. Arrange the pan in an Air Fryer basket.
5. Air Fry for about 15 minutes or until the top becomes golden brown.
6. Cut the potato rosti into wedges.
7. Top with the sour cream and smoked salmon slices and serve immediately.

### Nutrition Values (Per Serving)

- Calories: 182
- Carbohydrate: 18.4g
- Protein: 11.4g
- Fat: 7.1g
- Sugar: 1.4g
- Sodium: 885mg

---

## French Toasts

**(Yields:** 2 servings / **Prep Time:** 10 minutes / **Cooking Time:** 3 minutes)

### Ingredients

- 2 eggs
- ¼ cup evaporated milk
- 3 tablespoons sugar
- 2 teaspoons olive oil
- 1/8 teaspoon vanilla extract
- 4 bread slices

### Instructions

1. Set the temperature of Air Fryer to 390 degrees F. Grease an Air Fryer pan and insert in the Air Fryer while heating.
2. In a large bowl, mix together all the above ingredients except bread slices.
3. Coat the bread slices evenly with egg mixture.
4. Arrange the bread slices in the prepared pan.
5. Air Fry for about 2-3 minutes per side.
6. Serve warm.

### Nutrition Values (Per Serving)

- Calories: 261
- Carbohydrate: 30.6g
- Protein: 9.1g
- Fat: 12g
- Sugar: 22.3g
- Sodium: 218mg

# Savory French Toasts

**(Yields:** 2 servings / **Prep Time:** 10 minutes / **Cooking Time:** 4 minutes)

## Ingredients

- ¼ cup chickpea flour
- 3 tablespoons onion, finely chopped
- 2 teaspoons green chili, seeded and finely chopped
- ½ teaspoon red chili powder
- ¼ teaspoon ground turmeric
- ¼ teaspoon ground cumin
- Salt, to taste
- Water, as needed
- 4 bread slices

## Instructions

1. Add all the ingredients except bread slices in a large bowl and mix until a thick mixture forms.
2. Apply the mixture over both sides of the bread slices using a spoon.
3. Set the temperature of Air Fryer to 390 degrees F. Line the Air Fryer pan with a piece of foil.
4. Place the bread slices in the prepared pan.
5. Now, set the Air Fryer to 355 degrees F.
6. Air Fry for about 3-4 minutes.
7. Serve warm.

## Nutrition Values (Per Serving)

- Calories: 151
- Carbohydrate: 26.7g
- Protein: 9.1g
- Fat: 6.5g
- Sugar: 4.1g
- Sodium: 234mg

---

# Cinnamon Toasts

**(Yields:** 6 servings / **Prep Time:** 15 minutes / **Cooking Time:** 5 minutes)

## Ingredients

- ½ cup sugar
- 1½ teaspoons ground cinnamon
- 1½ teaspoons vanilla extract
- ¼ teaspoons freshly ground black pepper
- ½ cup salted butter, softened
- 12 whole wheat bread slices

### Instructions

1. Set the temperature of Air Fryer to 400 degrees F. Grease an Air Fryer pan and insert in the Air Fryer while heating.
2. In a bowl, add the sugar, vanilla, cinnamon, pepper, and butter. Mix until smooth.
3. Spread the butter mixture evenly over each bread slice.
4. Arrange the bread slices in the prepared pan.
5. Air Fry for about 5 minutes or until crispy.
6. Cut the bread slices diagonally and serve.

### Nutrition Values (Per Serving)

- Calories: 341
- Carbohydrate: 9g
- Protein: 7.4g
- Fat: 17.2g
- Sugar: 19.9g
- Sodium: 373mg

---

## Cheesy Mustard Toasts

**(Yields:** 4 servings / **Prep Time:** 15 minutes / **Cooking Time:** 15 minutes)

### Ingredients

- 4 bread slices
- 2 tablespoons cheddar cheese, shredded
- 2 eggs, whites and yolks, separated
- 1 tablespoon mustard
- 1 tablespoon paprika

### Instructions

1. Set the temperature of Air Fryer to 355 degrees F.
2. Place the bread slices in an Air fryer basket.
3. Air Fry for about 5 minutes or until toasted.
4. Add the egg whites in a clean glass bowl and beat until they form soft peaks.
5. In another bowl, mix together the cheese, egg yolks, mustard, and paprika.
6. Gently, fold in the egg whites.
7. Spread the mustard mixture over the toasted bread slices.
8. Air Fry for about 10 minutes.
9. Serve warm!

### Nutrition Values (Per Serving)

- Calories: 164
- Carbohydrate: 11.1g
- Protein: 10.2g
- Fat: 9.2g
- Sugar: 1.7g
- Sodium: 199mg

# Zucchini Omelet

**(Yields:** 2 servings / **Prep Time:** 15 minutes / **Cooking Time:** 14 minutes)

## Ingredients

- 1 teaspoon butter
- 1 zucchini, julienned
- 4 eggs
- ¼ teaspoon fresh basil, chopped
- ¼ teaspoon red pepper flakes, crushed
- Salt and ground black pepper, as required

## Instructions

1. Set the temperature of Air Fryer to 355 degrees F. Grease an Air Fryer pan.
2. Take a skillet, melt the butter over medium heat and cook the zucchini for about 3-4 minutes.
3. Meanwhile, in a bowl, mix together the eggs, basil, red pepper flakes, salt, and black pepper.
4. Add the cooked zucchini and gently, stir to combine.
5. Transfer the mixture into the prepared pan.
6. Air Fry for 10 minutes or until done completely.
7. Serve hot.

## Nutrition Values (Per Serving)

- Calories: 159
- Carbohydrate: 4.1g
- Protein: 12.3g
- Fat: 10.9g
- Sugar: 2.4g
- Sodium: 224mg

---

# Cheese Omelet

**(Yields:** 2 servings / **Prep Time:** 5 minutes / **Cooking Time:** 8 minutes)

## Ingredients

- 4 eggs
- ¼ cup cream
- Salt and freshly ground black pepper, to taste
- ¼ cup cheddar cheese, grated

## Instructions

1. Set the temperature of Air Fryer to 350 degrees F. Lightly, grease a 6"x3" pan.
2. In a bowl, mix together the eggs, cream, salt, and black pepper.

3. Then, pour the egg mixture into the prepared pan and Air Fry for about 4 minutes.
4. Once done, sprinkle the cheese over the top and cook for another 4 minutes at 350° F.
5. When the time is up, take out the pan from air fryer and use a spatula to flip the omelet onto the pan.
6. Serve hot.

## Nutrition Values (Per Serving)

- Calories: 216
- Carbohydrate: 7.9g
- Protein: 15.5g
- Fat: 13.8g
- Sugar: 3.9g
- Sodium: 251mg

---

# Chicken Omelet

**(Yields:** 8 servings / **Prep Time:** 15 minutes / **Cooking Time:** 16 minutes)

## Ingredients

- 1 teaspoon butter
- 1 onion, chopped
- ½ jalapeño pepper, seeded and chopped
- 3 eggs
- Salt and freshly ground black pepper, as needed
- ¼ cup cooked chicken, shredded

## Instructions

1. Take a frying pan, melt the butter over medium heat and sauté the onion for about 4-5 minutes.
2. Add in the jalapeño pepper and sauté for about 1 minute.
3. Add the chicken and stir to combine.
4. Remove from the heat and set aside.
5. Set the temperature of Air Fryer to 355 degrees F. Grease an Air Fryer pan.
6. Meanwhile, in a bowl, mix together the eggs, salt, and black pepper.
7. Place the chicken mixture into the prepared pan.
8. Pour the egg mixture over chicken mixture.
9. Air Fry for 10 minutes or until done completely.
10. Serve hot.

## Nutrition Values (Per Serving)

- Calories: 161
- Carbohydrate: 5.9g
- Protein: 14.1g
- Fat: 3.4g
- Sugar: 3g
- Sodium: 197mg

# Bacon & Hot Dogs Omelet

**(Yields:** 2 servings / **Prep Time:** 10 minutes / **Cooking Time:** 10 minutes)

## Ingredients

- 4 eggs
- 1 bacon slice, chopped
- 2 hot dogs, chopped
- 2 small onions, chopped

## Instructions

1. Set the temperature of Air Fryer to 320 degrees F.
2. In an Air Fryer baking pan, crack the eggs and beat them well.
3. Now, add in the remaining ingredients and gently, stir to combine.
4. Air Fry for about 10 minutes.
5. Serve hot.

## Nutrition Values (Per Serving)

- Calories: 418
- Carbohydrate: 9.7g
- Protein: 23.4g
- Fat: 31.5g
- Sugar: 5.6g
- Sodium: 1000mg

# Tofu & Mushroom Omelet

**(Yields:** 2 servings / **Prep Time:** 15 minutes / **Cooking Time:** 29 minutes)

## Ingredients

- 2 teaspoons canola oil
- ¼ of onion, chopped
- 1 garlic clove, minced
- 8 ounces silken tofu, pressed and sliced
- 3½ ounces fresh mushrooms, sliced
- Salt and freshly ground black pepper, as needed
- 3 eggs, beaten

## Instructions

1. Set the temperature of Air Fryer to 355 degrees F.
2. In an Air Fryer pan, add the oil, onion, and garlic. Air Fry for about 4 minutes.
3. Add the tofu and mushrooms and sprinkle with salt and black pepper.

4. Place the beaten eggs evenly on top.
5. Air Fry for about 25 minutes, opening after every 8 minutes to poke the eggs.
6. Serve hot.

## Nutrition Values (Per Serving)

- Calories: 224
- Carbohydrate: 6.6g
- Protein: 17.9g
- Fat: 14.5g
- Sugar: 3.4g
- Sodium: 214mg

---

# Eggs & Tomatoes Scramble

**(Yields:** 4 servings / **Prep Time:** 15 minutes / **Cooking Time:** 9 minutes)

## Ingredients

- ¾ cup milk
- 4 eggs
- Salt and freshly ground black pepper
- 8 grape tomatoes, halved
- ½ cup Parmesan cheese, grated

## Instructions

1. Set the temperature of Air Fryer to 355 degrees F. Grease an Air Fryer pan with cooking spray.
2. In a bowl, mix together the milk, eggs, salt, and black pepper.
3. Transfer the egg mixture into the prepared pan.
4. Air Fry for about 6 minutes until the edges begin to set.
5. With a wooden spatula, stir the egg mixture.
6. Top with the tomatoes and Air Fry for about 3 minutes or until the eggs are done.
7. Serve warm with the topping of cheese.

## Nutrition Values (Per Serving)

- Calories: 341
- Carbohydrate: 25.2g
- Protein: 26.4g
- Fat: 17g
- Sugar: 17.7g
- Sodium: 422mg

# Egg & Mushroom Scramble

**(Yields:** 2 servings / **Prep Time:** 15 minutes / **Cooking Time:** 10 minutes)

## Ingredients

- 4 eggs
- Salt and freshly ground black pepper, as needed
- 2 tablespoons unsalted butter
- ½ cup fresh mushrooms, finely chopped
- 2 tablespoons Parmesan cheese, shredded

## Instructions

1. Set the temperature of Air Fryer to 285 degrees F.
2. In a bowl, mix together the eggs, salt, and black pepper.
3. In a baking pan, melt the butter and tilt the pan to spread the butter in the bottom.
4. Add the beaten eggs and Air Fry for about 4-5 minutes
5. Add in the mushrooms and cheese and cook for 5 minutes, stirring occasionally.
6. Serve hot.

## Nutrition Values (Per Serving)

- Calories: 254
- Carbohydrate: 2.1g
- Protein: 13.7g
- Fat: 11g
- Sugar: 1.4g
- Sodium: 267mg

---

# Bacon & Egg Cups

**(Yields:** 2 servings / **Prep Time:** 15 minutes / **Cooking Time:** 23 minutes)

## Ingredients

- 1 bacon slice
- 2 eggs
- 2 tablespoons milk
- Freshly ground black pepper, to taste
- 1 teaspoon marinara sauce
- 1 tablespoon Parmesan cheese, grated
- 1 tablespoon fresh parsley, chopped
- 2 bread slices, toasted and buttered

### Instructions

1. Set the temperature of Air Fryer to 355 degrees F.
2. Place the bacon in an Air Fryer basket and Air Fry for about 10-15 minutes or until tender.
3. Remove from the Air Fryer and cut into small pieces.
4. Divide the bacon into 2 ramekins.
5. Crack 1 egg in each ramekin over the bacon.
6. Pour the milk evenly over eggs and sprinkle with black pepper.
7. Top with marinara sauce, followed by the Parmesan cheese.
8. Place the ramekins in an Air Fryer basket and air fryer for 8 minutes or until desired doneness.
9. Sprinkle with parsley and serve alongside the toasts.

### Nutrition Values (Per Serving)

- Calories: 186
- Carbohydrate: 6.8g
- Protein: 13.2g
- Fat: 11.7g
- Sugar: 1.7g
- Sodium: 498mg

---

## Spinach & Egg Cups

**(Yields:** 4 servings / **Prep Time:** 15 minutes / **Cooking Time:** 23 minutes)

### Ingredients

- 1 tablespoon unsalted butter, melted
- 1 tablespoon olive oil
- 1 pound fresh baby spinach
- 4 eggs
- 7 ounces ham, sliced
- 4 teaspoons milk
- Salt and freshly ground black pepper

### Instructions

1. Set the temperature of Air Fryer to 355 degrees F. Grease 4 ramekins with butter.
2. Take a skillet, heat the oil over medium heat and sauté the spinach for about 2-3 minutes or until just wilted.
3. Drain the liquid completely from the spinach.
4. Divide the spinach into the prepared ramekins, followed by the ham slices.
5. Crack 1 egg into each ramekin over ham slices.
6. Drizzle evenly with milk and sprinkle with salt and black pepper.
7. Air Fry for about 16-20 minutes or until the desired doneness of eggs.
8. Serve hot.

### Nutrition Values (Per Serving)

- Calories: 228
- Carbohydrate: 6.6g
- Protein: 17.2g
- Fat: 15.8g
- Sugar: 1.1g
- Sodium: 821mg

---

## Bread & Bacon Cups

**(Yields:** 2 servings / **Prep Time:** 10 minutes / **Cooking Time:** 10 minutes)

### Ingredients

- ½ teaspoon butter
- 2 bread slices
- 1 bacon slice, chopped
- 4 tomato slices
- 1 tablespoon Mozzarella cheese, shredded
- 2 eggs
- 1/8 teaspoon maple syrup
- 1/8 teaspoon balsamic vinegar
- ¼ teaspoon fresh parsley, chopped
- Salt and freshly ground pepper, to taste
- 2 tablespoons mayonnaise

### Instructions

1. Set the temperature of Air Fryer to 320 degrees F. Lightly, grease 2 ramekins.
2. Line each prepared ramekin with 1 bread slice.
3. Divide evenly the bacon and tomato slices over bread slice in each ramekin.
4. Top evenly with the cheese.
5. Crack 1 egg in each ramekin over cheese.
6. Drizzle with maple syrup and vinegar and then sprinkle with parsley, salt and black pepper.
7. Place the ramekins in an Air Fryer basket.
8. Air Fry for 10 minutes or until desired doneness.
9. Top with mayonnaise and serve.

### Nutrition Values (Per Serving)

- Calories: 245
- Carbohydrate: 10.2g
- Protein: 12.8g
- Fat: 17.1g
- Sugar: 2.7g
- Sodium: 580mg

# Sausage Frittata

**(Yields:** 2 servings / **Prep Time:** 15 minutes / **Cooking Time:** 11 minutes)

## Ingredients

- 1 tablespoon olive oil
- ½ of chorizo sausage, sliced
- ½ cup frozen corn
- 1 large potato, boiled, peeled and cubed
- 3 jumbo eggs
- Salt and freshly ground black pepper, as needed
- 2 tablespoons feta cheese, crumbled
- 1 tablespoon fresh parsley, chopped

## Instructions

1. Set the temperature of Air Fryer to 355 degrees F.
2. In the pan of an Air Fryer, heat the oil and cook the sausage, corn and potato for 5-6 minutes or until golden brown.
3. In a bowl, mix together the eggs, salt, and black pepper.
4. Now, pour the eggs over the sausage mixture and top with cheese and parsley.
5. Air Fry for about 5 minutes or until desired doneness.
6. Serve hot.

## Nutrition Values (Per Serving)

- Calories: 327
- Carbohydrate: 23.3g
- Protein: 15.3g
- Fat: 20.2g
- Sugar: 2.8g
- Sodium: 316mg

---

# Mushroom & Tomato Frittata

**(Yields:** 2 servings / **Prep Time:** 15 minutes / **Cooking Time:** 14 minutes)

## Ingredients

- 1 tablespoon olive oil
- 1 bacon slice, chopped
- 6 cherry tomatoes, halved
- 6 fresh mushrooms, sliced
- Salt and freshly ground black pepper, as needed
- 3 eggs
- 1 tablespoon fresh parsley, chopped
- ½ cup Parmesan cheese, grated

## Instructions

1. Set the temperature of Air Fryer to 390 degrees F.
2. In a baking dish, mix together the bacon, tomatoes, mushrooms, salt, and black pepper.
3. Arrange the baking dish into an Air Fryer basket.
4. Air Fry for about 6 minutes.
5. Add the eggs in a small bowl and beat them well.
6. Add in the parsley and cheese and mix them well.
7. Remove the baking dish from Air Fryer and top the bacon mixture evenly with egg mixture.
8. Return the baking dish in Air Fryer basket.
9. Air Fry for about 8 minutes.
10. Serve hot.

## Nutrition Values (Per Serving)

- Calories: 397
- Carbohydrate: 23.3g
- Protein: 27.3g
- Fat: 26.2g
- Sugar: 11.2g
- Sodium: 693mg

# Trout Frittata

**(Yields:** 4 servings / **Prep Time:** 15 minutes / **Cooking Time:** 25 minutes)

## Ingredients

- 2 tablespoons olive oil
- 1 onion, sliced
- 6 eggs
- ½ tablespoon horseradish sauce
- 2 tablespoons crème fraiche
- 2 hot-smoked trout fillets, chopped
- ¼ cup fresh dill, chopped

## Instructions

1. Set the temperature of air fryer to 320 degrees F.
2. Take a frying pan, heat the oil over medium heat and sauté the onion for about 4-5 minutes.
3. Meanwhile, in a bowl, mix together the eggs, horseradish sauce, and crème fraiche.
4. Now, transfer the onion mixture into a baking dish.
5. Top with the egg mixture, followed by trout.
6. Arrange the baking dish into an air fryer basket.

7. Air fry for about 20 minutes.
8. Serve hot.

## **Nutrition Values (Per Serving)**

- Calories: 342
- Carbohydrate: 21.5g
- Protein: 31.9g
- Fat: 21.6g
- Sugar: 1.8g
- Sodium: 160mg

---

## **Mini Tomato Quiche**

**(Yields:** 2 servings / **Prep Time:** 15 minutes / **Cooking Time:** 30 minutes)

## **Ingredients**

- 4 eggs
- ¼ cup onion, chopped
- ½ cup tomatoes, chopped
- ½ cup milk
- 1 cup Gouda cheese, shredded
- Salt, to taste

## **Instructions**

1. Set the temperature of air fryer to 340 degrees F.
2. In a large ramekin, mix together all the listed ingredients.
3. Arrange the ramekin into an air fryer basket.
4. Air fry for about 30 minutes.
5. Serve hot.

## **Nutrition Values (Per Serving)**

- Calories: 345
- Carbohydrate: 7.9g
- Protein: 26.1g
- Fat: 23.8g
- Sugar: 6.3g
- Sodium: 640mg

# Chicken & Broccoli Quiche

(**Yields:** 8 servings / **Prep Time:** 15 minutes / **Cooking Time:** 12 minutes)

## Ingredients

- 1 frozen ready-made pie crust
- ½ tablespoon olive oil
- 1 egg
- 1/3 cup cheddar cheese, grated
- 3 tablespoons whipping cream
- Salt and freshly ground black pepper, as needed
- ¼ cup boiled broccoli, chopped
- ¼ cup cooked chicken, chopped

## Instructions

1. Set the temperature of Air Fryer to 390 degrees F. Lightly, grease 2 small pie pans with olive oil.
2. Cut 2 (5-inch) rounds from the pie crust.
3. Arrange 1 pie crust round in each pie pan and gently, press in the bottom and sides.
4. In a bowl, mix together the egg, cheese, cream, salt, and black pepper.
5. Pour the egg mixture over dough base.
6. Evenly top with the broccoli and chicken.
7. Arrange the pie pans into an Air Fryer basket.
8. Air Fry for about 12 minutes.
9. Serve hot.

## Nutrition Values (Per Serving)

- Calories: 166
- Carbohydrate: 14.6g
- Protein: 4.2g
- Fat: 10.3g
- Sugar: 8.5g
- Sodium: 186mg

# Potato & Bell Pepper Hash

**(Yields:** 4 servings / **Prep Time:** 20 minutes / **Cooking Time:** 25 minutes)

## Ingredients

- 2 cups water
- 5 russet potatoes, peeled and cubed
- ½ tablespoon extra-virgin olive oil
- ½ of onion, chopped
- ½ jalapeño, chopped
- ½ of red bell pepper, seeded and chopped
- ½ green bell pepper, seeded and chopped
- ¼ tablespoon dried oregano, crushed
- ¼ tablespoon garlic powder
- ¼ tablespoon ground cumin
- ¼ tablespoon red chili powder
- Salt and freshly ground black pepper, as needed

## Instructions

1. In a large bowl, add the water and potatoes and set aside for about 30 minutes.
2. Drain well and pat dry with the paper towels.
3. Set the temperature of Air Fryer to 330 degrees F.
4. Add the potatoes and oil in a bowl and toss to coat well.
5. Place the potatoes into an Air Fryer basket and Air Fry for about 5 minutes.
6. Transfer the potatoes onto a wire rack to cool.
7. In the same bowl, add all the remaining ingredients and toss to coat well.
8. Now, set the temperature of Air Fryer to 390 degrees F.
9. In the bowl of veggie mixture, add in the cooled potatoes and toss to coat well
10. Place the potato mixture in Air Fryer basket and toss well.
11. Air Fry for about 15-20 minutes or until desired doneness.
12. Serve hot.

## Nutrition Values (Per Serving)

- Calories: 220
- Carbohydrate: 46g
- Protein: 5.2g
- Fat: 2.3g
- Sugar: 5.1g
- Sodium: 170mg

# Egg Yolks with Squid

**(Yields:** 4 servings / **Prep Time:** 15 minutes / **Cooking Time:** 20 minutes)

## Ingredients

- ½ cup self-rising flour
- 14 ounces squid flower, cleaned and pat dried
- Salt and freshly ground black pepper
- 1 tablespoon olive oil
- 2 tablespoons butter
- 2 green chilies, seeded and chopped
- 2 curry leaves stalks
- 4 raw salted egg yolks
- ½ cup chicken broth
- 2 tablespoons evaporated milk
- 1 tablespoon sugar

## Instructions

1. Set the temperature of Air Fryer to 355 degrees F. Grease an Air Fryer pan.
2. In a shallow dish, add the flour.
3. Sprinkle the squid flower evenly with salt and black pepper.
4. Coat the squid evenly with flour and then shake off any excess flour.
5. Place the squid into the prepared pan in a single layer.
6. Air Fry for about 9 minutes.
7. Remove from the Air Fryer and set aside
8. Now, heat the oil and butter in a skillet over medium heat and sauté the chilies and curry leaves for about 3 minutes.
9. Add the egg yolks and cook for about 1 minute, stirring continuously.
10. Gradually, add the chicken broth and cook for about 3-5 minutes, stirring continuously.
11. Add in the milk and sugar and mix until well combined.
12. Add the fried squid and toss to coat well.
13. Serve hot.

## Nutrition Values (Per Serving)

- Calories: 311
- Carbohydrate: 19.8g
- Protein: 21g
- Fat: 16.1g
- Sugar: 4.2g
- Sodium: 197mg

# CHAPTER 2 | SNACKS AND APPETIZERS

## Roasted Cashews

**(Yields:** 8 servings / **Prep Time:** 20 minutes / **Cooking Time:** 4 minutes)

### Ingredients

- 2 cups raw cashew nuts
- 1 teaspoon butter, melted
- Salt and freshly ground black pepper, as needed

### Instructions

1. Set the temperature of Air Fryer to 355 degrees F.
2. In a bowl, mix together all the ingredients.
3. Place the cashews nuts in an Air Fryer basket in a single layer. (you can lay a piece of grease-proof baking paper)
4. Air Fry for about 4 minutes, shaking once halfway through.
5. Once done, transfer the hot nuts in a glass bowl and serve.

### Nutrition Values (Per Serving)

- Calories: 201
- Carbohydrate: 11.2g
- Protein: 5.3g
- Fat: 16.4g
- Sugar: 1.7g
- Sodium: 28mg

---

## Roasted Peanuts

**(Yields:** 10 servings / **Prep Time:** 5 minutes / **Cooking Time:** 14 minutes)

### Ingredients

- 2½ cups raw peanuts
- 1 tablespoon olive oil
- Salt, as required

### Instructions

1. Set the temperature of Air Fryer to 320 degrees F.
2. Add the peanuts in an Air Fryer basket in a single layer.
3. Air Fry for about 9 minutes, tossing twice.
4. Remove the peanuts from Air Fryer basket and transfer into a bowl.
5. Add the oil, and salt and toss to coat well.

6. Return the nuts mixture into Air Fryer basket.
7. Air Fry for about 5 minutes.
8. Once done, transfer the hot nuts in a glass or steel bowl and serve.

## Nutrition Values (Per Serving)

- Calories: 219
- Carbohydrate: 5.9g
- Protein: 9.4g
- Fat: 19.4g
- Sugar: 1.5g
- Sodium: 22mg

---

# Roasted Mixed Nuts

**(Yields:** 6 servings / **Prep Time:** 5 minutes / **Cooking Time:** 20 minutes)

## Ingredients

- ½ cup walnuts
- ½ cup pecans
- ½ cup almonds
- 2 tablespoons egg white
- 1 packet stevia
- ½ tablespoon ground cinnamon
- A pinch of cayenne pepper

## Instructions

1. Set the temperature of Air Fryer to 320 degrees F.
2. Take a bowl and mix together all the listed ingredients.
3. Place the nuts in an Air Fryer basket in a single layer. (you can lay a piece of grease-proof baking paper)
4. Air Fry for about 20 minutes, stirring once halfway through.
5. Once done, transfer the hot nuts in a glass or steel bowl and serve.

## Nutrition Values (Per Serving)

- Calories: 190
- Carbohydrate: 4.8g
- Protein: 5.9g
- Fat: 17.9g
- Sugar: 0.9g
- Sodium: 5mg

# Spicy Chickpeas

**(Yields:** 4 servings / **Prep Time:** 5 minutes / **Cooking Time:** 20 minutes)

## Ingredients

- 1 (15-ounces) can chickpeas, rinsed and drained
- 1 tablespoon olive oil
- ½ teaspoon ground cumin
- ½ teaspoon cayenne pepper
- ½ teaspoon smoked paprika
- Salt, to taste

## Instructions

1. Set the temperature of Air Fryer to 390 degrees F.
2. In a bowl, add all the ingredients and toss to coat well.
3. Add the chickpeas in an Air Fryer basket in 2 batches. (you can lay a piece of grease-proof baking paper)
4. Air Fry for about 8-10 minutes.
5. Once done, transfer the hot nuts in a glass or steel bowl and serve.

## Nutrition Values (Per Serving)

- Calories: 251
- Carbohydrate: 36g
- Protein: 11g
- Fat: 7g
- Sugar: 6g
- Sodium: 10mg

---

# Tortilla Chips

**(Yields:** 6 servings / **Prep Time:** 10 minutes / **Cooking Time:** 6 minutes)

## Ingredients

- 8 corn tortillas, cut into triangles
- 1 tablespoon olive oil
- Salt, to taste

## Instructions

1. Set the temperature of Air Fryer to 390 degrees F.
2. Coat the tortilla chips with oil.
3. Sprinkle each side of the tortillas with salt
4. Place them in an Air Fryer basket in a single layer in 2 batches.

5. Air Fry for about 3 minutes.
6. Enjoy with your favorite salsa.

## Nutrition Values (Per Serving)

- Calories: 90
- Carbohydrate: 14.3g
- Protein: 1.8g
- Fat: 3.2g
- Sugar: 0.3g
- Sodium: 42mg

---

# Pineapple Bites

**(Yields:** 4 servings / **Prep Time:** 15 minutes / **Cooking Time:** 10 minutes)

## Ingredients

### For Pineapple Sticks:
- ½ of pineapple
- ¼ cup desiccated coconut

### For Yogurt Dip:
- 1 tablespoon fresh mint leaves, minced
- 1 cup vanilla yogurt

## Instructions

1. With a sharp knife, remove the outer peel of pineapple and then, cut into 1-2 inch thick sticks lengthwise.
2. Add the desiccated coconut in a shallow dish.
3. Coat the pineapple sticks evenly with coconut.
4. Set the temperature of Air Fryer to 390 degrees F.
5. Add the pineapple sticks in an Air Fryer basket in a single layer.
6. Air Fry for about 10 minutes.
7. For dip: in a bowl, mix together the mint, and yogurt.
8. Serve the pineapple sticks with yogurt dip.

## Nutrition Values (Per Serving)

- Calories: 142
- Carbohydrate: 20.7g
- Protein: 4.6g
- Fat: 4.9g
- Sugar: 15.9g
- Sodium: 47mg

# Apple Chips

**(Yields:** 2 servings / **Prep Time:** 10 minutes / **Cooking Time:** 16 minutes)

## Ingredients

- 1 apple, peeled, cored and thinly sliced
- 1 tablespoon sugar
- ½ teaspoon ground cinnamon
- A pinch of ground cardamom
- A pinch of ground ginger
- A pinch of salt

## Instructions

1. Set the temperature of Air Fryer to 390 degrees F.
2. In a bowl, add all the ingredients and toss to coat well.
3. Arrange the apple slices in an Air Fryer basket in a single layer in 2 batches.
4. Air Fry for about 7-8 minutes, flipping once halfway through.
5. Serve.

## Nutrition Values (Per Serving)

- Calories: 72
- Carbohydrate: 19.2g
- Protein: 0.3g
- Fat: 0.2g
- Sugar: 15.5g
- Sodium: 78mg

---

# Banana Chips

**(Yields:** 8 servings / **Prep Time:** 10 minutes / **Cooking Time:** 10 minutes)

## Ingredients

- 2 raw bananas, peeled and sliced
- 2 tablespoons olive oil
- Salt and freshly ground black pepper, as needed

## Instructions

1. Set the temperature of Air Fryer to 355 degrees F.
2. Drizzle the banana slices evenly with oil.
3. Arrange the banana slices in an Air Fryer basket in a single layer.
4. Air Fry for about 10 minutes.
5. Sprinkle with salt and black pepper.
6. Serve.

### Nutrition Values (Per Serving)

- Calories: 56
- Carbohydrate: 6.7g
- Protein: 0.3g
- Fat: 3.6g
- Sugar: 3.6g
- Sodium: 0mg

---

# Kale Chips

**(Yields:** 4 servings / **Prep Time:** 20 minutes / **Cooking Time:** 3 minutes)

## Ingredients

- 1 head fresh kale, stems and ribs removed and cut into 1½ inch pieces
- 1 tablespoon olive oil
- 1 teaspoon soy sauce
- 1/8 teaspoon cayenne pepper
- A pinch of freshly ground black pepper

## Instructions

1. Set the temperature of Air Fryer to 390 degrees F.
2. Take a large bowl and mix together all the ingredients.
3. Place the kale leaves in an Air Fryer basket in a single layer.
4. Air Fry for about 2-3 minutes, tossing once halfway through.
5. Serve.

### Nutrition Values (Per Serving)

- Calories: 143
- Carbohydrate: 23.8g
- Protein: 6.9g
- Fat: 3.5g
- Sugar: 0g
- Sodium: 173mg

---

# Potato Chips

**(Yields:** 6 servings / **Prep Time:** 15 minutes / **Cooking Time:** 30 minutes)

## Ingredients

- 4 small russet potatoes, thinly sliced
- 1 tablespoon olive oil
- 2 tablespoons fresh rosemary, finely chopped
- ¼ teaspoon salt

## Instructions

1. In a large bowl, add the water, and potato slices. Set aside for about 30 minutes, changing the water once halfway through.
2. Drain the potato slices well and pat them dry with the paper towels.
3. Set the temperature of Air Fryer to 350 degrees F.
4. In a bowl, mix together the potato slices, olive oil, rosemary, and salt.
5. Add the potato chips in an Air Fryer basket in a single layer.
6. Air Fry for about 30 minutes.
7. Serve.

## Nutrition Values (Per Serving)

- Calories: 87
- Carbohydrate: 15.9g
- Protein: 1.7g
- Fat: 0.4g
- Sugar: 1.1g
- Sodium: 88mg

---

# Beet Chips

(**Yields:** 6 servings / **Prep Time:** 10 minutes / **Cooking Time:** 15 minutes)

## Ingredients

- 4 medium beetroots, peeled and thinly sliced
- 2 tablespoons olive oil
- ¼ teaspoon smoked paprika
- ½ teaspoon salt

## Instructions

1. Set the temperature of Air Fryer to 325 degrees F.
2. In a bowl, add all the ingredients and toss to coat well.
3. Arrange the beet slices in an Air Fryer basket in a single layer.
4. Air Fry for about 12-15 minutes.
5. Serve.

## Nutrition Values (Per Serving)

- Calories: 60
- Carbohydrate: 5.3g
- Protein: 0.9g
- Fat: 4.8g
- Sugar: 3.7g
- Sodium: 236mg

# Buttered Corn

**(Yields:** 2 servings / **Prep Time:** 5 minutes / **Cooking Time:** 20 minutes)

## Ingredients

- 2 corn on the cob
- Salt and freshly ground black pepper, as needed
- 2 tablespoons butter, softened and divided

## Instructions

1. Set the temperature of Air Fryer to 320 degrees F.
2. Sprinkle the cobs evenly with salt and black pepper.
3. Then, rub with 1 tablespoon of butter.
4. With 1 piece of foil, wrap each cob and place in an Air Fryer basket.
5. Air Fry for about 20 minutes.
6. Top with the remaining butter and serve.

## Nutrition Values (Per Serving)

- Calories: 160
- Carbohydrate: 14.1g
- Protein: 2.1g
- Fat: 12g
- Sugar: 2.3g
- Sodium: 84mg

---

# French Fries

**(Yields:** 8 servings / **Prep Time:** 15 minutes / **Cooking Time:** 30 minutes)

## Ingredients

- 1¾ pounds potatoes, peeled and cut into strips
- ¼ cup olive oil
- 1 teaspoon onion powder
- 1 teaspoon garlic powder
- 2 teaspoons paprika

## Instructions

1. In a large bowl, add the water, and potato strips. Set aside for about 1 hour.
2. Drain the potato strips well and pat them dry with the paper towels.
3. Take a large bowl, add the potato strips and the remaining ingredients. Toss to coat well.
4. Set the temperature of Air Fryer to 375 degrees F.

6. Add the potato strips in an Air Fryer basket in a single layer.
7. Air Fry for about 30 minutes.
8. Serve.

## **Nutrition Values (Per Serving)**

- Calories: 126
- Carbohydrate: 16.4g
- Protein: 1.8g
- Fat: 6.5g
- Sugar: 1.4g
- Sodium: 6mg

---

# **Zucchini Fries**

**(Yields:** 4 servings / **Prep Time:** 10 minutes / **Cooking Time:** 20 minutes)

## **Ingredients**

- 1 pound zucchini, sliced into 2½-inch sticks
- Salt, as required
- 2 tablespoons olive oil
- ¾ cup panko breadcrumbs

## **Instructions**

1. In a colander, add the zucchini and sprinkle with salt. Set aside for about 10 minutes.
2. Set the temperature of Air Fryer to 390 degrees F.
3. Gently pat dry the zucchini sticks with the paper towels and coat with oil.
4. In a shallow dish, add the breadcrumbs.
5. Coat the zucchini sticks evenly with breadcrumbs.
6. Place the zucchini sticks in an Air Fryer basket in a single layer in 2 batches.
7. Now, set the temperature of Air Fryer to 425 degrees F and Air Fry for about 10 minutes.
8. Serve.

## **Nutrition Values (Per Serving)**

- Calories: 158
- Carbohydrate: 18.4g
- Protein: 4.1g
- Fat: 8.3g
- Sugar: 3.2g
- Sodium: 198mg

# Squash Fries

**(Yields:** 2 servings / **Prep Time:** 10 minutes / **Cooking Time:** 35 minutes)

## Ingredients

- 14 ounces butternut squash, peeled, seeded and cut into strips
- 2 teaspoons olive oil
- ½ teaspoon ground cinnamon
- ½ teaspoon red chili powder
- ¼ teaspoon garlic salt
- Salt and freshly ground black pepper, as needed

## Instructions

1. Set the temperature of Air Fryer to 440 degrees F. Line a baking sheet with parchment paper.
2. Take a bowl, add all the listed ingredients and toss to coat well.
3. Place the butternut squash strips onto the prepared baking sheet in a single layer.
4. Arrange the baking sheet in an Air Fryer basket.
5. Air Fry for about 35 minutes.
6. Serve.

## Nutrition Values (Per Serving)

- Calories: 134
- Carbohydrate: 24.3g
- Protein: 2.1g
- Fat: 5g
- Sugar: 4.5g
- Sodium: 92mg

---

# Avocado Fries

**(Yields:** 2 servings / **Prep Time:** 20 minutes / **Cooking Time:** 7 minutes)

## Ingredients

- ¼ cup all-purpose flour
- Salt and freshly ground black pepper, as needed
- 1 egg
- 1 teaspoon water
- ½ cup panko breadcrumbs
- 1 avocado, peeled, pitted and sliced into 8 pieces
- Non-stick cooking spray

## Instructions

1. In a shallow bowl, mix together the flour, salt, and black pepper.
2. In a second bowl, mix well egg and water.
3. In a third bowl, put the breadcrumbs.
4. Coat the avocado slices with flour mixture, then dip into egg mixture and finally, coat evenly with the breadcrumbs.
5. Now, spray the avocado slices evenly with cooking spray.
6. Set the temperature of Air Fryer to 400 degrees F.
7. Place the avocado slices in an Air Fryer basket in a single layer.
8. Air Fry for about 7 minutes, flipping once halfway through.
9. Enjoy!

## Nutrition Values (Per Serving)

- Calories: 363
- Carbohydrate: 35.7g
- Protein: 8.3g
- Fat: 22.4g
- Sugar: 1.2g
- Sodium: 252mg

# Dill Pickle Fries

**(Yields:** 12 servings / **Prep Time:** 15 minutes / **Cooking Time:** 28 minutes)

## Ingredients

- 1½ (16-ounces) jars spicy dill pickle spears, drained and pat dried
- 1 cup all-purpose flour
- ½ teaspoon paprika
- 1 egg, beaten
- ¼ cup milk
- 1 cup panko breadcrumbs
- Nonstick cooking spray

## Instructions

1. In a shallow dish, mix together the flour, and paprika.
2. In a second dish, mix well milk and egg.
3. In a third dish, put the breadcrumbs.
4. Coat the pickle spears with flour mixture, then dip into egg mixture and finally, coat evenly with the breadcrumbs.
5. Now, spray the pickle spears evenly with cooking spray.
6. Set the temperature of Air Fryer to 440 degrees F.

7. Arrange the pickle spears in an Air Fryer basket in a single layer in 2 batches.
8. Air Fry for about 14 minutes, flipping once halfway through.
9. Serve.

## Nutrition Values (Per Serving)
- Calories: 76
- Carbohydrate: 14.8g
- Protein: 2.7g
- Fat: 0.8g
- Sugar: 1.2g
- Sodium: 550mg

---

# Carrot Sticks

(**Yields:** 2 servings / **Prep Time:** 10 minutes / **Cooking Time:** 12 minutes)

## Ingredients
- 1 large carrot, peeled and cut into sticks
- 1 tablespoon fresh rosemary, finely chopped
- 1 tablespoon olive oil
- 2 teaspoons sugar
- ¼ teaspoon cayenne pepper
- Salt and freshly ground black pepper, as needed

## Instructions
1. Set the temperature of Air Fryer to 390 degrees F.
2. In a bowl, add all the ingredients and toss to coat well.
3. Place the carrot sticks in an Air Fryer basket in a single layer.
4. Air Fry for about 12 minutes.
5. Serve.

## Nutrition Values (Per Serving)
- Calories: 96
- Carbohydrate: 8.7g
- Protein: 0.4g
- Fat: 7.3g
- Sugar: 5.8g
- Sodium: 26mg

# Onion Rings

**(Yields:** 4 servings / **Prep Time:** 20 minutes / **Cooking Time:** 10 minutes)

## Ingredients

- 1 large onion, cut into ¼ inch slices
- 1¼ cups all-purpose flour
- 1 teaspoon baking powder
- Salt, as required
- 1 cup milk
- 1 egg
- ¾ cup dry breadcrumbs

## Instructions

1. Separate the onion slices into rings.
2. In a shallow dish, mix together the flour, baking powder, and salt.
3. In a second dish, mix well milk and egg.
4. In a third dish, put the breadcrumbs.
5. Coat each onion ring with flour mixture, then dip into egg mixture and finally, coat evenly with the breadcrumbs.
6. Set the temperature of Air Fryer to 360 degrees F.
7. Place the onion rings in an Air Fryer basket in a single layer.
8. Air Fry for about 7-10 minutes.
9. Serve hot.

## Nutrition Values (Per Serving)

- Calories: 285
- Carbohydrate: 51.6g
- Protein: 10.5g
- Fat: 3.8g
- Sugar: 5.8g
- Sodium: 235mg

---

# Spicy Broccoli Poppers

**(Yields:** 4 servings / **Prep Time:** 15 minutes / **Cooking Time:** 10 minutes)

## Ingredients

- 2 tablespoons plain yogurt
- ½ teaspoon red chili powder
- ¼ teaspoon ground cumin
- ¼ teaspoon ground turmeric
- Salt, to taste
- 1 pound broccoli, cut into small florets
- 2 tablespoons chickpea flour

## Instructions

1. In a bowl, mix together the yogurt, and spices.
2. Add the broccoli and generously coat with marinade.

3. Refrigerate for about 20 minutes.
4. Set the temperature of Air Fryer to 400 degrees F.
5. Sprinkle the broccoli florets with chickpea flour.
6. Add the broccoli florets in an Air Fryer basket in a single layer.
7. Air Fry for about 10 minutes, tossing once halfway through.
8. Serve hot.

## Nutrition Values (Per Serving)
- Calories: 69
- Carbohydrate: 12.2g
- Protein: 4.9g
- Fat: 0.9g
- Sugar: 3.2g
- Sodium: 87mg

# Cheesy Broccoli Bites

**(Yields:** 10 servings / **Prep Time:** 15 minutes / **Cooking Time:** 12 minutes)

## Ingredients
- 2 cups broccoli florets
- 2 eggs, beaten
- 1¼ cups cheddar cheese, grated
- ¼ cup Parmesan cheese, grated
- 1¼ cups panko breadcrumbs
- Salt and freshly ground black pepper, as needed

## Instructions
1. In a food processor, add the broccoli and pulse until finely crumbled.
2. Take a large bowl, mix together the broccoli, and remaining ingredients.
3. Make small equal-sized balls from the mixture.
4. Arrange the balls in a baking sheet and refrigerate for at least 30 minutes.
5. Set the temperature of Air Fryer to 350 degrees F.
6. Put the balls in an Air fryer basket
7. Air Fry for about 12 minutes.
8. Serve.

## Nutrition Values (Per Serving)
- Calories: 136
- Carbohydrate: 11.3g
- Protein: 7.3g
- Fat: 6.8g
- Sugar: 1.1g
- Sodium: 226mg

# Cauliflower Poppers

**(Yields:** 6 servings / **Prep Time:** 10 minutes / **Cooking Time:** 16 minutes)

## Ingredients

- 1 large head cauliflower, cut into bite-sized florets
- 2 tablespoons olive oil
- Salt and freshly ground black pepper, as needed

## Instructions

1. Drizzle the cauliflower florets with oil.
2. Sprinkle with salt and black pepper.
3. Set the temperature of Air Fryer to 390 degrees F.
4. Place the cauliflower florets in a greased Air Fryer basket in a single layer in 2 batches.
5. Air Fry for about 8 minutes, shaking once halfway through.
6. Serve hot.

## Nutrition Values (Per Serving)

- Calories: 51
- Carbohydrate: 2.3g
- Protein: 0.9g
- Fat: 4.7g
- Sugar: 1.1g
- Sodium: 40mg

---

# Crispy Cauliflower Poppers

**(Yields:** 4 servings / **Prep Time:** 10 minutes / **Cooking Time:** 20 minutes)

## Ingredients

- 1 large egg white
- 3 tablespoons ketchup
- 2 tablespoons hot sauce
- ¾ cup panko breadcrumbs
- 4 cups cauliflower florets

## Instructions

1. In a bowl, mix together the egg white, ketchup, and hot sauce.
2. Add the breadcrumbs in another bowl.
3. Dip the cauliflower florets in ketchup mixture and then evenly coat with the breadcrumbs.

4. Set the temperature of Air Fryer to 320 degrees F.
5. Arrange the cauliflower florets in an Air Fryer basket in a single layer.
6. Air Fry for about 20 minutes.
7. Serve.

## Nutrition Values (Per Serving)

- Calories: 94
- Carbohydrate: 19.6g
- Protein: 4.6g
- Fat: 0.5g
- Sugar: 5.5g
- Sodium: 457mg

---

# Crispy Eggplant Slices

**(Yields:** 4 servings / **Prep Time:** 15 minutes / **Cooking Time:** 16 minutes)

## Ingredients

- 1 medium eggplant, peeled and cut into ½-inch round slices
- Salt, as required
- ½ cup all-purpose flour
- 2 eggs, beaten
- 1 cup Italian-style breadcrumbs
- ¼ cup olive oil

## Instructions

1. In a colander, add the eggplant slices and sprinkle with salt.
2. Set aside for about 45 minutes and pat dry the eggplant slices.
3. Add the flour in a shallow dish.
4. Crack the eggs in a second dish and beat well.
5. In a third dish, mix together the oil, and breadcrumbs.
6. Coat each eggplant slice with flour, then dip into beaten eggs and finally, evenly coat with the breadcrumbs mixture.
7. Set the temperature of Air Fryer to 390 degrees F.
8. Arrange the eggplant slices in an Air Fryer basket in a single layer in 2 batches.
9. Air Fry for about 8 minutes.
10. Serve.

## Nutrition Values (Per Serving)

- Calories: 685
- Carbohydrate: 49.1g
- Protein: 42.1g
- Fat: 36.9g
- Sugar: 5.3g
- Sodium: 239mg

# Mixed Veggie Bites

**(Yields:** 10 servings / **Prep Time:** 15 minutes / **Cooking Time:** 10 minutes)

## Ingredients

- 1½ pounds fresh spinach, blanched, drained and chopped
- ½ of onion, chopped
- 1 carrot, peeled and chopped
- 1 garlic clove, minced
- 2 American cheese slices, cut into tiny pieces
- 2 bread slices, toasted and processed into breadcrumbs
- 1 tablespoon corn flour
- 1 teaspoon red chili flakes
- Salt, as required

## Instructions

1. Set the temperature of Air Fryer to 355 degrees F.
2. Add all the listed ingredients except breadcrumbs in a bowl and mix until well combined.
3. Add in the breadcrumbs and gently stir to combine.
4. Make 20 equal-sized balls from the mixture.
5. Now, set the temperature of Air Fryer to 200 degrees F.
6. Place the balls in an Air Fryer basket in a single layer.
7. Air Fry for about 10 minutes.
8. Serve hot.

## Nutrition Values (Per Serving)

- Calories: 43
- Carbohydrate: 5.6g
- Protein: 3.1g
- Fat: 1.5g
- Sugar: 1.2g
- Sodium: 139mg

# Potato Croquettes

**(Yields:** 4 servings / **Prep Time:** 15 minutes / **Cooking Time:** 23 minutes)

## Ingredients

- 2 medium Russet potatoes, peeled and cubed
- 2 tablespoons all-purpose flour
- ½ cup Parmesan cheese, grated
- 1 egg yolk
- 2 tablespoons chives, minced
- A pinch of ground nutmeg
- Salt and freshly ground black pepper, as needed
- 2 eggs
- ½ cup breadcrumbs
- 2 tablespoons vegetable oil

## Instructions

1. Add potatoes in the pan of a boiling water and cook for about 15 minutes.
2. Drain the potatoes well and transfer into a large bowl.
3. With a potato masher, mash the potatoes and set aside to cool completely.
4. In the same bowl of mashed potatoes, add in the flour, Parmesan cheese, egg yolk, chives, nutmeg, salt, and black pepper. Whisk until well combined.
5. Make small equal-sized balls from the mixture.
6. Now, roll each ball into a cylinder shape.
7. In a shallow dish, crack the eggs and beat well.
8. In another dish, mix together the breadcrumbs, and oil.
9. Dip the croquettes in egg mixture and then evenly coat with the breadcrumbs mixture.
10. Set the temperature of Air Fryer to 390 degrees F.
11. Place the croquettes in an Air Fryer basket in a single layer.
12. Air Fry for about 7-8 minutes.
13. Enjoy!

## Nutrition Values (Per Serving)

- Calories: 291
- Carbohydrate: 30.3g
- Protein: 11.9g
- Fat: 14g
- Sugar: 2.3g
- Sodium: 266mg

# Salmon Croquettes

**(Yields:** 16 servings / **Prep Time:** 15 minutes / **Cooking Time:** 14 minutes)

## Ingredients

- 1 large can red salmon, drained
- 2 eggs, lightly beaten
- 2 tablespoons fresh parsley, chopped
- Salt and freshly ground black pepper, as needed
- 1/3 cup vegetable oil
- 1 cup breadcrumbs

## Instructions

1. Set the temperature of Air Fryer to 390 degrees F.
2. In a bowl, add the salmon and mash it completely using a fork.
3. Add the eggs, parsley, salt, and black pepper. Mix until well combined.
4. Make 16 equal-sized croquettes from the mixture.
5. In a shallow dish, mix together the oil, and breadcrumbs.
6. Coat the croquettes evenly with the breadcrumb mixture.
7. Place the croquettes in an Air Fryer basket in a single layer in 2 batches.
8. Air Fry for about 7 minutes.
9. Serve.

## Nutrition Values (Per Serving)

- Calories: 110
- Carbohydrate: 5g
- Protein: 3.8g
- Fat: 7.1g
- Sugar: 0g
- Sodium: 69mg

# Bacon Croquettes

**(Yields:** 6 servings / **Prep Time:** 15 minutes / **Cooking Time:** 8 minutes)

## Ingredients

- 1 pound thin bacon slices
- 1 pound sharp cheddar cheese block, cut into 1-inch rectangular pieces
- 1 cup all-purpose flour
- 3 eggs
- 1 cup breadcrumbs
- Salt, as required
- ¼ cup olive oil

## Instructions

1. Wrap 2 bacon slices around 1 piece of cheddar cheese, covering completely.
2. Repeat with the remaining bacon and cheese pieces.
3. Arrange the croquettes in a baking dish and freeze for about 5 minutes.
4. Add the flour in a shallow dish.
5. In a second dish, crack the eggs and beat well.
6. In a third dish, mix together the breadcrumbs, salt, and oil.
7. Coat the croquettes with flour, then dip into beaten eggs and finally, evenly coat with the breadcrumbs mixture.
8. Set the temperature of Air Fryer to 390 degrees F.
9. Arrange the croquettes in an Air Fryer basket in a single layer.
10. Air Fry for about 7-8 minutes.
11. Serve hot.

## Nutrition Values (Per Serving)

- Calories: 964
- Carbohydrate: 31.1g
- Protein: 54.1g
- Fat: 68.4g
- Sugar: 1.7g
- Sodium: 2000mg

---

# Chicken Nuggets

**(Yields:** 4 servings / **Prep Time:** 15 minutes / **Cooking Time:** 10 minutes)

## Ingredients

- ½ of zucchini, roughly chopped
- ½ of carrot, roughly chopped
- 14 ounces chicken breast, cut into chunks
- ½ tablespoon mustard powder
- 1 tablespoon garlic powder
- 1 tablespoon onion powder
- Salt and freshly ground black pepper, as needed
- 1 cup all-purpose flour
- 2 tablespoons milk
- 1 egg
- 1 cup panko breadcrumbs

## Instructions

1. In a food processor, add the zucchini, and carrot and pulse until finely chopped.

2. Add the chicken, mustard powder, garlic powder, onion powder, salt, and black pepper and pulse until well combined.
3. Put the flour in a shallow dish.
4. In a second dish, mix together the milk, and egg.
5. In a third dish, put the breadcrumbs.
6. Coat the nuggets with flour, then dip into egg mixture and finally, evenly coat with the breadcrumbs.
7. Set the temperature of Air Fryer to 390 degrees F.
8. Arrange the croquettes in an Air Fryer basket in a single layer.
9. Air Fry for about 10 minutes.
10. Serve hot.

## Nutrition Values (Per Serving)

- Calories: 430
- Carbohydrate: 48.7g
- Protein: 41.6g
- Fat: 7g
- Sugar: 4.2g
- Sodium: 341mg

---

# Cod Nuggets

(**Yields:** 4 servings / **Prep Time:** 15 minutes / **Cooking Time:** 10 minutes)

## Ingredients

- 1 cup all-purpose flour
- 2 eggs
- ¾ cup breadcrumbs
- A pinch of salt
- 2 tablespoons olive oil
- 1 pound cod, cut into 1x2½-inch strips

## Instructions

1. Add the flour in a shallow dish.
2. Crack the eggs in a second dish and beat well.
3. In a third dish, mix together the breadcrumbs, salt, and oil.
4. Coat the nuggets with flour, then dip into beaten eggs and finally, evenly coat with the breadcrumbs.
5. Set the temperature of Air Fryer to 390 degrees F.
6. Add the croquettes in an Air Fryer basket in a single layer.
7. Air Fry for about 8-10 minutes.
8. Enjoy!

### Nutrition Values (Per Serving)

- Calories: 404
- Carbohydrate: 36.8g
- Protein: 34.6g
- Fat: 11.6g
- Sugar: 1.5g
- Sodium: 307mg

---

## Mozzarella Sticks

**(Yields:** 4 servings / **Prep Time:** 15 minutes / **Cooking Time:** 24 minutes**)**

### Ingredients

- ¼ cup white flour
- 2 eggs
- 3 tablespoons nonfat milk
- 1 cup plain breadcrumbs
- 1 pound Mozzarella cheese block cut into 3x½-inch sticks

### Instructions

1. Add the flour in a shallow dish.
2. In a second dish, mix together the eggs, and milk.
3. In a third dish, put the breadcrumbs.
4. Coat the Mozzarella sticks with flour, then dip into egg mixture and finally, coat evenly with the breadcrumbs.
5. Arrange the Mozzarella sticks onto a baking sheet and freeze for about 1-2 hours.
6. Set the temperature of Air Fryer to 440 degrees F.
7. Arrange the Mozzarella sticks in an Air Fryer basket in a single layer in 2 batches.
8. Air Fry for about 12 minutes.
9. Enjoy!

### Nutrition Values (Per Serving)

- Calories: 191
- Carbohydrate: 26.4g
- Protein: 9.6g
- Fat: 5g
- Sugar: 2.4g
- Sodium: 177mg

# Polenta Sticks

**(Yields:** 4 servings / **Prep Time:** 10 minutes / **Cooking Time:** 6 minutes)

## Ingredients

- 2½ cups cooked polenta
- Salt, as required
- ¼ cup Parmesan cheese, shredded

## Instructions

1. Add the polenta evenly into a greased baking dish and with the back of a spoon, smooth the top surface.
2. Cover the baking dish and refrigerate for about 1 hour or until set.
3. Remove from the refrigerator and cut down the polenta into the desired size slices.
4. Set the temperature of Air Fryer to 350 degrees F. Grease a baking dish.
5. Arrange the polenta sticks into the prepared baking dish in a single layer and sprinkle with salt.
6. Place the baking dish into an Air Fryer basket.
7. Air Fry for about 5-6 minutes.
8. Top with the cheese and serve.

## Nutrition Values (Per Serving)

- Calories: 367
- Carbohydrate: 76.2g
- Protein: 9.1g
- Fat: 2.2g
- Sugar: 1g
- Sodium: 127mg

---

# Rice Bites

**(Yields:** 4 servings / **Prep Time:** 15 minutes / **Cooking Time:** 20 minutes)

## Ingredients

- 3 cups cooked risotto
- 1/3 cup Parmesan cheese, grated
- 1 egg, beaten
- 3 ounces mozzarella cheese, cubed
- ¾ cup breadcrumbs

## Instructions

1. In a bowl, mix together the risotto, Parmesan cheese, and egg.
2. Make 20 equal-sized balls from the mixture.
3. Insert a mozzarella cube in the center of each ball and using your fingers, smooth the risotto mixture to cover the mozzarella.
4. In a shallow dish, add the breadcrumbs.
5. Coat the balls evenly with breadcrumbs.
6. Set the temperature of Air Fryer to 390 degrees F.
7. Arrange the balls in an Air Fryer basket in a single layer in 2 batches.
8. Air Fry for about 10 minutes or until they turn golden brown.
9. Serve.

## Nutrition Values (Per Serving)

- Calories: 279
- Carbohydrate: 50.7g
- Protein: 9.4g
- Fat: 7.3g
- Sugar: 0.6g
- Sodium: 159mg

---

# Veggie Bread Rolls

**(Yields:** 8 servings / **Prep Time:** 20 minutes / **Cooking Time:** 33 minutes**)**

## Ingredients

- 5 large potatoes, peeled
- 2 tablespoons vegetable oil, divided
- 2 small onions, finely chopped
- 2 green chilies, seeded and chopped
- 2 curry leaves
- ½ teaspoon ground turmeric
- Salt, as required
- 8 bread slices, trimmed

## Instructions

1. In the pan of a boiling water, add the potatoes and cook for about 15-20 minutes.
2. Drain the potatoes well and with a potato masher, mash the potatoes.
3. In a skillet, heat 1 teaspoon of oil over a medium heat and sauté the onion for about 4-5 minutes.
4. Add the green chilies, curry leaves, and turmeric. Sauté for about 1 minute.
5. Add in the mashed potatoes, and salt and mix them well.
6. Once done, remove from the heat and set aside to cool completely.

7. Make 8 equal-sized oval-shaped patties from the mixture.
8. Wet the bread slices completely with water.
9. Using your hands, press each bread slice between your hands to remove the excess water.
10. Place 1 bread slice in your palm and place 1 patty in the center.
11. Roll the bread slice in a spindle shape and seal the edges to secure the filling.
12. Coat the roll with some oil.
13. Repeat with the remaining slices, filling and oil.
14. Set the temperature of Air Fryer to 390 degrees F. Grease the Air Fryer basket with cooking spray.
15. Add rolls into the prepared basket in a single layer.
16. Air Fry for about 12-13 minutes.
17. Serve.

## Nutrition Values (Per Serving)

- Calories: 221
- Carbohydrate: 42.7g
- Protein: 4.8g
- Fat: 4g
- Sugar: 3.9g
- Sodium: 95mg

---

# Spinach Rolls

**(Yields:** 6 servings / **Prep Time:** 20 minutes / **Cooking Time:** 4 minutes)

## Ingredients

- 1 (16-ounces) package frozen spinach, thawed
- 1 red onion, chopped
- 1 cup fresh parsley, chopped
- 1 cup fresh mint leaves, chopped
- 1 egg
- 1 cup feta cheese, crumbled
- ½ cup Romano cheese, grated
- ¼ teaspoon ground cardamom
- Salt and freshly ground black pepper, as needed
- 1 package frozen filo dough, thawed
- 2 tablespoons olive oil

## Instructions

1. Put all the listed ingredients except filo dough and oil in a food processor and pulse until smooth.

2. Place one filo sheet on the cutting board and cut into three rectangular strips.
3. Brush each strip with the oil.
4. Add about one teaspoon of spinach mixture along with the short side of a strip.
5. Roll the dough to secure the filling.
6. Repeat with the remaining filo sheets and spinach mixture.
7. Set the temperature of Air Fryer to 355 degrees F. Grease an Air Fryer basket.
8. Place rolls into the prepared basket in a single layer.
9. Air Fry for about 4 minutes.
10. Enjoy!

## **Nutrition Values (Per Serving)**

- Calories: 320
- Carbohydrate: 31.2g
- Protein: 13.5g
- Fat: 16.6g
- Sugar: 2.4g
- Sodium: 737mg

# **Spring Rolls**

(**Yields:** 6 servings / **Prep Time:** 20 minutes / **Cooking Time:** 15 minutes)

## **Ingredients**

- 2 tablespoons vegetable oil, divided
- 1¾ ounces fresh mushrooms, sliced
- 1 ounce canned water chestnuts, sliced
- 1 teaspoon fresh ginger, finely grated
- 1 ounce bean sprouts
- 1 small carrot, peeled and cut into matchsticks
- 2 scallions (green part), chopped
- 1 tablespoon soy sauce
- 1 teaspoon Chinese five-spice powder
- 3½ ounces cooked shrimps
- 12 spring roll wrappers
- 1 egg, beaten

## **Instructions**

1. Take a skillet, heat one tablespoon of oil over medium heat and sauté the mushrooms, water chestnuts, and ginger for about 2-3 minutes.
2. Add in the beans sprouts, carrot, scallion, soy sauce, and five-spice powder. Sauté for about 1 minute.
3. Stir in the shrimps and remove from heat. Set aside to cool.

4. Divide the veggie mixture evenly between spring rolls.
5. Roll the wrappers around the filling and seal with beaten egg.
6. Coat each roll with the remaining oil.
7. Set the temperature of Air Fryer to 390 degrees F. Grease an Air Fryer basket.
8. Place rolls into the prepared Air Fryer basket in a single layer in 2 batches.
9. Air Fry for about 5 minutes.
10. Serve.

## Nutrition Values (Per Serving)

- Calories: 274
- Carbohydrate: 40.9g
- Protein: 11.8g
- Fat: 6.6g
- Sugar: 0.7g
- Sodium: 575mg

---

# Cheese Sandwich

**(Yields:** 2 servings / **Prep Time:** 10 minutes / **Cooking Time:** 5 minutes)

## Ingredients

- 4 white bread slices
- ½ cup butter, softened
- ½ cup sharp cheddar cheese, grated

## Instructions

1. Set the temperature of Air Fryer to 355 degrees F.
2. Spread the butter evenly over one side of each bread slice.
3. Sprinkle the cheese over buttered side of 2 slices.
4. Top with the remaining slices of bread.
5. Place the sandwiches in an Air Fryer basket in a single layer.
6. Air Fry for about 4-5 minutes.
7. Serve.

## Nutrition Values (Per Serving)

- Calories: 569
- Carbohydrate: 9.5g
- Protein: 89g
- Fat: 56g
- Sugar: 1g
- Sodium: 625mg

# Veggie Sandwich

**(Yields:** 2 servings / **Prep Time:** 15 minutes / **Cooking Time:** 25 minutes)

## Ingredients

### For Barbecue Sauce:
- 1 teaspoon olive oil
- 1 garlic clove, minced
- ¼ of onion, chopped
- ½ cup water
- ½ tablespoon sugar
- ½ tablespoon Worcestershire sauce
- ¼ teaspoon mustard powder
- 1½ tablespoons tomato ketchup
- Salt and ground black pepper, as needed

### For Sandwich:
- 2 tablespoons butter, softened
- 1 cup sweet corn kernels
- 1 roasted green bell pepper, chopped
- 4 bread slices, trimmed and cut horizontally

## Instructions

1. For barbecue sauce: in a medium skillet, heat the oil over medium heat and sauté the garlic, and onion for about 3-5 minutes.
2. Stir in the remaining ingredients and bring to a boil over high heat.
3. Reduce the heat to medium and simmer for about 8-10 minutes or until desired thickness.
4. For the sandwich: in a skillet, melt the butter on medium heat and stir fry the corn for about 1-2 minutes.
5. In a bowl, mix together the barbecue sauce, corn, and bell pepper.
6. Spread the corn mixture on one side of 2 bread slices.
7. Top with the remaining slices.
8. Set the temperature of Air Fryer to 355 degrees F.
9. Place the sandwiches in an Air Fryer basket in a single layer.
10. Air Fry for about 5-6 minutes.
11. Serve.

## Nutrition Values (Per Serving)

- Calories: 286
- Carbohydrate: 36.1g
- Protein: 4.6g
- Fat: 15.8g
- Sugar: 12.6g
- Sodium: 377mg

# Cheese Pastries

**(Yields:** 6 servings / **Prep Time:** 15 minutes / **Cooking Time:** 5 minutes)

## Ingredients

- 1 egg yolk
- 4 ounces feta cheese, crumbled
- 1 scallion, finely chopped
- 2 tablespoons fresh parsley, finely chopped
- Salt and ground black pepper, as needed
- 2 frozen filo pastry sheets, thawed
- 2 tablespoons olive oil

## Instructions

1. In a large bowl, add the egg yolk, and beat well.
2. Add in the feta cheese, scallion, parsley, salt, and black pepper. Mix well.
3. Cut each filo pastry sheet in three strips.
4. Add about 1 teaspoon of feta mixture on the underside of a strip.
5. Fold the tip of sheet over the filling in a zigzag manner to form a triangle.
6. Repeat with the remaining strips and fillings.
7. Set the temperature of Air Fryer to 390 degrees F.
8. Coat each pastry evenly with oil.
9. Place the pastries in an Air Fryer basket in a single layer.
10. Air Fry for about 3 minutes, then air fryer for about 2 minutes on 360 degrees F.
11. Serve.

## Nutrition Values (Per Serving)

- Calories: 135
- Carbohydrate: 8.1g
- Protein: 4.2g
- Fat: 9.8g
- Sugar: 1.1g
- Sodium: 241mg

# Veggie Pastries

**(Yields:** 8 servings / **Prep Time:** 20 minutes / **Cooking Time:** 37 minutes)

## Ingredients

- 2 large potatoes, peeled
- 1 tablespoon olive oil
- ½ cup carrot, peeled and chopped
- ½ cup onion, chopped
- 2 garlic cloves, minced
- 2 tablespoons fresh ginger, minced
- ½ cup green peas, shelled
- Salt and ground black pepper, as needed
- 3 puff pastry sheets

## Instructions

1. In the pan of a boiling water, put the potatoes and cook for about 15-20 minutes.
2. Drain the potatoes well and with a potato masher, mash the potatoes.
3. In a skillet, heat the oil over medium heat and sauté the carrot, onion, ginger, and garlic for about 4-5 minutes.
4. Drain all the fat from the skillet.
5. Stir in the mashed potatoes, peas, salt, and black pepper. Cook for about 1-2 minutes.
6. Once done, remove the potato mixture from heat and set aside to cool completely.
7. Put the puff pastry onto a smooth surface.
8. Cut each puff pastry sheet into four pieces and then cut each piece in a round shape.
9. Add about two tablespoons of veggie filling over each pastry round.
10. Moisten the edges using your wet fingers.
11. Fold each pastry round in half to seal the filling.
12. Using a fork, firmly press the edges.
13. Set the temperature of Air Fryer to 390 degrees F.
14. Add the pastries in an Air Fryer basket in a single layer in 2 batches.
15. Air Fry for about 5 minutes.
16. Serve.

## Nutrition Values (Per Serving)

- Calories: 197
- Carbohydrate: 26.8g
- Protein: 3.7g
- Fat: 8.8g
- Sugar: 2.4g
- Sodium: 56mg

# Fruit Pastries

**(Yields:** 8 servings / **Prep Time:** 15 minutes / **Cooking Time:** 10+10 = 20 minutes)

## Ingredients

- ½ of apple, peeled, cored and chopped
- 1 teaspoon fresh orange zest, finely grated
- ½ tablespoon white sugar
- ½ teaspoon ground cinnamon
- 7.05 ounces prepared frozen puff pastry

## Instructions

1. In a bowl, mix together all the ingredients except puff pastry.
2. Cut the pastry in 16 squares.
3. Using a teaspoon, place apple mixture in the center of each square.
4. Fold each square into a triangle and slightly press the edges with your wet fingers.
5. Then, using a fork, firmly press the edges.
6. Set the temperature of Air Fryer to 390 degrees F.
7. Add the pastries into an Air Fryer basket in a single layer in 2 batches.
8. Air Fry for about 10 minutes.
9. Enjoy!

## Nutrition Values (Per Serving)

- Calories: 147
- Carbohydrate: 13.8g
- Protein: 1.9g
- Fat: 9.5g
- Sugar: 2.1g
- Sodium: 62mg

---

# Crispy Prawns

**(Yields:** 4 servings / **Prep Time:** 15 minutes / **Cooking Time:** 8 minutes)

## Ingredients

- 1 egg
- ½ pound nacho chips, crushed
- 18 prawns, peeled and deveined

## Instructions

1. In a shallow dish, crack the egg, and beat well.
2. Put the crushed nacho chips in another dish.
3. Now, dip the prawn into beaten egg and then, coat with the nacho chips.
4. Set the temperature of Air Fryer to 355 degrees F.
5. Place the prawns in an Air Fryer basket in a single layer.
6. Air Fry for about 8 minutes.
7. Serve hot.

## Nutrition Values (Per Serving)

- Calories: 425
- Carbohydrate: 36.6g
- Protein: 28.6g
- Fat: 17.6g
- Sugar: 2.2g
- Sodium: 606mg

---

# Bacon Wrapped Shrimp

(**Yields:** 6 servings / **Prep Time:** 15 minutes / **Cooking Time:** 7 minutes)

## Ingredients

- 1 pound bacon, thinly sliced
- 1 pound shrimp, peeled and deveined

## Instructions

1. Wrap each shrimp with one bacon slice.
2. Add the shrimp in a baking dish and refrigerate for about 20 minutes.
3. Set the temperature of Air Fryer to 390 degrees F.
4. Add the shrimp in an Air Fryer basket in a single layer.
5. Air Fry for about 5-7 minutes.
6. Serve.

## Nutrition Values (Per Serving)

- Calories: 499
- Carbohydrate: 2.2g
- Protein: 45.2g
- Fat: 32.6g
- Sugar: 0g
- Sodium: 1930mg

# Chocolate Cookie Dough Balls

**(Yields:** 6 servings / **Prep Time:** 15 minutes / **Cooking Time:** 20 minutes)

## Ingredients

- 16½ ounces store-bought chilled chocolate chip cookie dough
- ¼ cup butter, melted
- ½ cup chocolate cookie crumbs
- 2 tablespoons sugar

## Instructions

1. Cut the cookie dough into 12 equal-sized pieces and then, shape each into a ball.
2. Add the melted butter in a shallow dish.
3. In another dish, mix together the cookie crumbs, and sugar.
4. Dip each cookie ball in the melted butter and then evenly coat with the cookie crumbs.
5. In the bottom of a baking sheet, place the coated cookie balls and freeze for at least 2 hours.
6. Preheat the air fryer to 350 degrees F.
7. Line the air fryer basket with a piece of foil.
8. Place the cookies balls in an Air Fryer basket in a single layer in 2 batches.
9. Air Fry for about 10 minutes.
10. Enjoy!

## Nutrition Values (Per Serving)

- Calories: 286
- Carbohydrate: 35.2g
- Protein: 4.2g
- Fat: 13.6g
- Sugar: 21.9g
- Sodium: 190mg

# Buttermilk Biscuits

**(Yields:** 4 servings / **Prep Time:** 15 minutes / **Cooking Time:** 8 minutes)

## Ingredients

- ½ cup cake flour
- 1¼ cups all-purpose flour
- ¼ teaspoon baking soda
- ½ teaspoon baking powder
- 1 teaspoon granulated sugar
- Salt, as required
- ¼ cup cold unsalted butter, cut into cubes
- ¾ cup buttermilk
- 2 tablespoons butter, melted

## Instructions

1. In a large bowl, sift together the flours, baking soda, baking powder, sugar, and salt.
2. Using two forks, cut in the butter until coarse crumb forms.
3. Slowly, add in the buttermilk and mix until a smooth dough forms.
4. Then, take out the dough from bowl and put onto a floured surface. Using your hands, press it into ½ inch thickness.
5. With a 1¾-inch round cookie cutter, cut the biscuits.
6. Cut out the remaining biscuits from dough.
7. Set the temperature of Air Fryer to 400 degrees F.
8. Place the biscuits in a pie pan in a single layer and coat with butter.
9. Put the pie pan in an Air Fryer basket.
10. Air Fry for about 8 minutes.
11. Serve.

## Nutrition Values (Per Serving)

- Calories: 374
- Carbohydrate: 45.2g
- Protein: 7.3g
- Fat: 18.2g
- Sugar: 3.4g
- Sodium: 291mg

# Lemon Biscuits

**(Yields:** 10 servings / **Prep Time:** 15 minutes / **Cooking Time:** 5 minutes**)**

## Ingredients

- 8½ ounces self-rising flour
- 3½ ounces caster sugar
- 3½ ounces cold butter
- 1 small egg
- 1 teaspoon fresh lemon zest, finely grated
- 2 tablespoons fresh lemon juice
- 1 teaspoon vanilla extract

## Instructions

1. In a bowl, mix together the flour, and sugar.
2. Using two forks, cut in the butter until coarse crumb forms.
3. Add in the egg, vanilla extract, lemon juice, and zest. Mix until a soft dough forms.
4. Then, take out the dough from bowl and put onto a floured surface.
5. Now, roll it into an even thickness. (½ inch)
6. Cut the dough into medium-sized biscuits using a cookie cutter.
7. Set the temperature of Air Fryer to 355 degrees F.
8. Place the biscuits in a baking sheet in a single layer.

9. Put the baking sheet in an Air Fryer basket.
10. Air Fry for about 5 minutes or until golden brown.
11. Enjoy!

## Nutrition Values (Per Serving)

- Calories: 203
- Carbohydrate: 28.5g
- Protein: 3.1g
- Fat: 8.7g
- Sugar: 10.2g
- Sodium: 63mg

---

# Coconut Cookies

(**Yields:** 8 servings / **Prep Time:** 15 minutes / **Cooking Time:** 12 minutes)

## Ingredients

- 2¼ ounces caster sugar
- 3½ ounces butter
- 1 small egg
- 1 teaspoon vanilla extract
- 5 ounces self-rising flour
- 1¼ ounces white chocolate, chopped
- 3 tablespoons desiccated coconut

## Instructions

1. In a large bowl, add the sugar, and butter and beat until fluffy and light.
2. Add the egg, and vanilla extract and whisk until well combined.
3. Now, add the flour, and chocolate and mix well.
4. In a shallow bowl, place the coconut.
5. With your hands, make small balls from the mixture and roll evenly into the coconut.
6. Place the balls onto an ungreased baking sheet about 1- inch apart and gently, press each ball.
7. Set the temperature of air fryer to 355 degrees F.
8. Place baking sheet into the air fryer basket.
9. Air fry for about 8 minutes and then, another 4 minutes at 320 degrees F.
10. Remove from air fryer and place the baking sheet onto a wire rack to cool for about 5 minutes.
11. Now, invert the cookies onto wire rack to cool completely before serving.
12. Serve.

## Nutrition Values (Per Serving)

- Calories: 222
- Carbohydrate: 24.5g
- Protein: 2.8g
- Fat: 12.7g
- Sugar: 10.9g
- Sodium: 83mg

# Cheese Cookies

**(Yields:** 10 servings / **Prep Time:** 15 minutes / **Cooking Time:** 12 minutes)

## Ingredients

**For Dough:**
- 3.38 fluid ounces cream
- 5.30 ounces margarine
- 6.35 ounces Gruyere cheese, grated
- 1 teaspoon paprika
- Salt, as required
- 5.30 ounces flour, sifted
- ½ teaspoon baking powder

**For Topping:**
- 1 tablespoon milk
- 2 egg yolks, beaten
- 2 tablespoons poppy seeds

## Instructions

1. For cookies: in a bowl, mix together the cream, margarine, cheese, paprika, and salt.
2. Place the flour, and baking powder onto a smooth surface. Mix them well.
3. Using your hands, create a well in the center of flour.
4. Add the cheese mixture and knead until a soft dough forms.
5. Roll the dough into 1-1½-inch thickness.
6. Cut the cookies using a cookie cutter.
7. In another bowl, mix together the milk, and egg yolks.
8. Coat the cookies with milk mixture and then, sprinkle with poppy seeds.
9. Set the temperature of Air Fryer to 340 degrees F.
10. Place cookies onto the grill pan of an Air Fryer in a single layer.
11. Air Fry for about 12 minutes.
12. Serve.

## Nutrition Values (Per Serving)

- Calories: 264
- Carbohydrate: 12.8g
- Protein: 8.1g
- Fat: 20.3g
- Sugar: 0.6g
- Sodium: 224mg

# CHAPTER 3 | CHICKEN AND POULTRY

## Cornish Game Hens

(**Yields:** 4 servings / **Prep Time:** 20 minutes / **Cooking Time:** 16 minutes)

### Ingredients

- ½ cup olive oil
- 1 teaspoon fresh rosemary, chopped
- 1 teaspoon fresh thyme, chopped
- 1 teaspoon fresh lemon zest, finely grated
- ¼ teaspoon sugar
- ¼ teaspoon red pepper flakes, crushed
- Salt and ground black pepper, as required
- 2 pounds Cornish game hen, backbone removed and halved

### Instructions

1. In a bowl, mix together oil, herbs, lemon zest, sugar, and spices.
2. Add the hen portions and generously coat with the marinade.
3. Cover and refrigerate for about 24 hours.
4. In a strainer, place the hen portions and set aside to drain any liquid.
5. Set the temperature of Air Fryer to 390 degrees F. Grease an Air Fryer basket.
6. Place hen portions into the prepared Air fryer basket.
7. Air Fry for about 14-16 minutes.
8. Remove from the Air Fryer and transfer the hen portions onto serving plates and serve.

### Nutrition Values (Per Serving)

- Calories: 523
- Carbohydrate: 0.8g
- Protein: 52.9g
- Fat: 34.1g
- Sugar: 0.6g
- Sodium: 143mg

(**Note:** If your air fryer does not have the exact temperature setting mentioned in the recipe, consult your manual for suggested temperature settings).

## Roasted Chicken with Potatoes

**(Yields:** 2 servings / **Prep Time:** 15 minutes / **Cooking Time:** 1 hour)

### Ingredients

- 1 (1½-pounds) whole chicken
- Salt and ground black pepper, as required
- 1 tablespoon olive oil
- ½ pound small potatoes

### Instructions

1. Set the temperature of Air Fryer to 390 degrees F. Grease an Air Fryer basket.
2. Season the chicken with salt and black pepper.
3. Place chicken into the prepared Air Fryer basket.
4. Air Fry for about 35-40 minutes or until done completely.
5. Transfer the chicken onto a platter and cover with a piece of foil to keep warm.
6. In a bowl, add the potatoes, oil, salt, and black pepper and toss to coat well.
7. Again, set the temperature of Air Fryer to 390 degrees F. Grease an Air Fryer basket.
8. Place potatoes into the prepared Air Fryer basket.
9. Air Fry for about 20 minutes or until golden brown.
10. Remove from the Air Fryer and transfer potatoes into a bowl.
11. Cut the chicken into desired size pieces using a sharp knife and serve alongside the potatoes.

### Nutrition Values (Per Serving)

- Calories: 431
- Carbohydrate: 178g
- Protein: 511g
- Fat: 16.2g
- Sugar: 1.3g
- Sodium: 153mg

## Herbed Roasted Chicken

**(Yields:** 7 servings / **Prep Time:** 15 minutes / **Cooking Time:** 1 hour)

### Ingredients

- 3 garlic cloves, minced
- 1 teaspoon fresh lemon zest, finely grated
- 1 teaspoon dried thyme, crushed
- 1 teaspoon dried oregano, crushed

- 1 teaspoon dried rosemary, crushed
- 1 teaspoon smoked paprika
- Salt and ground black pepper, as required
- 2 tablespoons fresh lemon juice
- 2 tablespoons olive oil
- 1 (5-pounds) whole chicken

## Instructions

1. In a bowl, mix together the garlic, lemon zest, herbs and spices.
2. Rub the chicken evenly with herb mixture.
3. Drizzle the chicken with lemon juice and oil.
4. Set aside at the room temperature for about 2 hours.
5. Set the temperature of Air Fryer to 360 degrees F. Grease an Air Fryer basket.
6. Place chicken into the prepared Air Fryer basket, breast side down.
7. Air Fry for about 50 minutes.
8. Flip the chicken and Air Fry for about 10 more minutes.
9. Remove from the Air Fryer and place chicken onto a cutting board for about 10 minutes before carving.
10. With a knife, slice the chicken into desired size pieces and serve.

## Nutrition Values (Per Serving)

- Calories: 860
- Carbohydrate: 1.3g
- Protein: 71.1g
- Fat: 50g
- Sugar: 0.2g
- Sodium: 299mg

---

# Spiced Roasted Chicken

(**Yields:** 6 servings / **Prep Time:** 15 minutes / **Cooking Time:** 1 hour)

## Ingredients

- 2 teaspoons dried thyme
- 2 teaspoons paprika
- 1 teaspoon cayenne pepper
- 1 teaspoon ground white pepper
- 1 teaspoon onion powder
- 1 teaspoon garlic powder
- Salt and ground black pepper, as required
- 3 tablespoons oil
- 1 (5-pounds) whole chicken, necks and giblets removed

## Instructions

1. In a bowl, mix together the thyme and spices.
2. Generously, coat the chicken with oil and then rub it with spice mixture.
3. Set the temperature of Air Fryer to 350 degrees F. Grease an Air Fryer basket.
4. Place chicken into the prepared Air Fryer basket, breast side down.
5. Air Fry for about 30 minutes.
6. Flip the chicken and Air Fry for about 30 more minutes.
7. Remove from the Air Fryer and place chicken onto a cutting board for about 10 minutes before carving.
8. Slice the chicken into desired size pieces using a sharp knife and serve.

## Nutrition Values (Per Serving)

- Calories: 871
- Carbohydrate: 1.7g
- Protein: 70.6g
- Fat: 60g
- Sugar: 0.4g
- Sodium: 296mg

# Spicy Chicken Legs

**(Yields:** 3 servings / **Prep Time:** 15 minutes / **Cooking Time:** 25 minutes)

## Ingredients

- 3 (8-ounces) chicken legs
- 1 cup buttermilk
- 2 cups white flour
- 1 teaspoon garlic powder
- 1 teaspoon onion powder
- 1 teaspoon ground cumin
- 1 teaspoon paprika
- Salt and ground black pepper, as required
- 1 tablespoon olive oil

## Instructions

1. In a bowl, put the chicken legs, and buttermilk. Refrigerate for about 2 hours.
2. In another bowl, mix together the flour and spices.
3. Remove the chicken from buttermilk.
4. Coat the chicken legs with flour mixture, then dip into buttermilk and finally, coat with the flour mixture again.
5. Set the temperature of Air Fryer to 360 degrees F. Grease an Air Fryer basket.
6. Arrange chicken legs into the prepared Air Fryer basket and drizzle with the oil

7. Air Fry for about 20-25 minutes.
8. Remove from the Air Fryer and transfer chicken legs onto a serving platter.
9. Serve hot.

## Nutrition Values (Per Serving)

- Calories: 781
- Carbohydrate: 69.5g
- Protein: 55.9g
- Fat: 7.6g
- Sugar: 4.7g
- Sodium: 288mg

---

# Tandoori Chicken Legs

**(Yields:** 4 servings / **Prep Time:** 15 minutes / **Cooking Time:** 20 minutes)

## Ingredients

- 4 chicken legs
- 3 tablespoons fresh lemon juice
- 3 teaspoons ginger paste
- 3 teaspoons garlic paste
- Salt, as required
- 4 tablespoons hung curd*
- 2 tablespoons tandoori masala powder
- 2 teaspoons red chili powder
- 1 teaspoon garam masala powder
- 1 teaspoon ground cumin
- 1 teaspoon ground coriander
- 1 teaspoon ground turmeric
- Ground black pepper, as required
- Pinch of orange food color

## Instructions

1. In a bowl, mix well chicken legs, lemon juice, ginger paste, garlic paste, and salt.
2. Set aside for about 15 minutes.
3. Meanwhile, in another bowl, mix together the curd, spices, and food color.
4. Add the chicken legs into bowl and generously coat with the spice mixture.
5. Cover the bowl of chicken and refrigerate for at least 10-12 hours.
6. Set the temperature of air fryer to 445 degrees F. Line an air fryer basket with a piece of foil.
7. Arrange chicken legs into the prepared air fryer basket.

8. Air fry for about 18-20 minutes.
9. Remove from air fryer and transfer the chicken legs onto serving plates.
10. Serve hot.

## Nutrition Values (Per Serving)
- Calories: 356
- Carbohydrate: 3.7g
- Protein: 51.5g
- Fat: 13.9g
- Sugar: 0.5g
- Sodium: 259mg

(**Note: Hung curd\*** - Hung curd is nothing but yogurt drained of all its water. It can be made very easily at home.)

---

# Gingered Chicken Drumsticks

(**Yields:** 3 servings / **Prep Time:** 10 minutes / **Cooking Time:** 25 minutes)

## Ingredients
- ¼ cup full-fat coconut milk
- 2 teaspoons fresh ginger, minced
- 2 teaspoons galangal, minced
- 2 teaspoons ground turmeric
- Salt, to taste
- 3 (6-ounces) chicken drumsticks

## Instructions
1. In a bowl, mix together the coconut milk, galangal, ginger, and spices.
2. Add the chicken drumsticks and generously coat with the marinade.
3. Refrigerate to marinate for at least 6-8 hours.
4. Set the temperature of Air Fryer to 375 degrees F. Grease an Air Fryer basket.
5. Place chicken drumsticks into the prepared Air Fryer basket in a single layer.
6. Air Fry for about 20-25 minutes.
7. Remove from Air Fryer and transfer the chicken drumsticks onto a serving platter.
8. Serve hot.

## Nutrition Values (Per Serving)
- Calories: 338
- Carbohydrate: 2.6g
- Protein: 47.4g
- Fat: 13.9g
- Sugar: 0.4g
- Sodium: 192mg

# Sweet & Spicy Chicken Drumsticks

**(Yields:** 4 servings / **Prep Time:** 15 minutes / **Cooking Time:** 20 minutes)

## Ingredients

- 1 garlic clove, crushed
- 1 tablespoon mustard
- 2 teaspoons brown sugar
- 1 teaspoon cayenne pepper
- 1 teaspoon red chili powder
- Salt and ground black pepper, as required
- 1 tablespoon vegetable oil
- 4 (6-ounces) chicken drumsticks

## Instructions

1. In a bowl, mix together garlic, mustard, brown sugar, oil, and spices
2. Rub the chicken drumsticks with marinade and refrigerate to marinate for about 20-30 minutes.
3. Set the temperature of Air Fryer to 390 degrees F. Grease an Air Fryer basket.
4. Arrange drumsticks into the prepared Air Fryer basket in a single layer.
5. Air Fry for about 10 minutes and then 10 more minutes at 300 degrees F.
6. Remove from Air Fryer and transfer the chicken drumsticks onto a serving platter.
7. Serve hot.

## Nutrition Values (Per Serving)

- Calories: 341
- Carbohydrate: 3.3g
- Protein: 47.7g
- Fat: 14.1g
- Sugar: 1.8g
- Sodium: 182mg

---

# Honey Glazed Chicken Drumsticks

**(Yields:** 4 servings / **Prep Time:** 15 minutes / **Cooking Time:** 22 minutes)

## Ingredients

- ¼ cup Dijon mustard
- 1 tablespoon honey
- 2 tablespoons olive oil
- ½ tablespoon fresh rosemary, minced

- 1 tablespoon fresh thyme, minced
- Salt and ground black pepper, as required
- 4 (6-ounces) boneless chicken drumsticks

## Instructions

1. In a bowl, mix well the mustard, honey, oil, herbs, salt, and black pepper.
2. Add the drumsticks and generously coat with the mixture.
3. Cover and refrigerate to marinate overnight.
4. Set the temperature of Air Fryer to 320 degrees F. Grease an Air Fryer basket.
5. Arrange the chicken drumsticks into the prepared Air Fryer basket in a single layer.
6. Air Fry for about 12 minutes.
7. Now, set the temperature of Air Fryer to 355 degrees F.
8. Air Fry for 5-10 more minutes.
9. Remove from Air Fryer and transfer the chicken drumsticks onto a serving platter.
10. Serve hot.

## Nutrition Values (Per Serving)

- Calories: 377
- Carbohydrate: 5.9g
- Protein: 47.6g
- Fat: 3.6g
- Sugar: 4.5g
- Sodium: 353mg

# Chinese Chicken Drumsticks

**(Yields:** 4 servings / **Prep Time:** 15 minutes / **Cooking Time:** 20 minutes)

## Ingredients

- 1 tablespoon oyster sauce
- 1 teaspoon light soy sauce
- ½ teaspoon sesame oil
- 1 teaspoon Chinese five spice powder
- Salt and ground white pepper, as required
- 4 (6-ounces) chicken drumsticks
- 1 cup corn flour

## Instructions

1. In a bowl, mix together the sauces, oil, five spice powder, salt, and black pepper.
2. Add the chicken drumsticks and generously coat with the marinade.

3. Refrigerate for at least 30-40 minutes.
4. In a shallow dish, place the corn flour.
5. Remove the chicken from marinade and lightly coat with corn flour.
6. Set the temperature of Air Fryer to 390 degrees F. Grease an Air Fryer basket.
7. Arrange chicken drumsticks into the prepared Air Fryer basket in a single layer.
8. Air Fry for about 20 minutes.
9. Remove from Air Fryer and transfer the chicken drumsticks onto a serving platter.
10. Serve hot.

## Nutrition Values (Per Serving)

- Calories: 400
- Carbohydrate: 22.7g
- Protein: 48.9g
- Fat: 11.4g
- Sugar: 0.2g
- Sodium: 279mg

---

# Crispy Chicken Drumsticks

**(Yields:** 2 servings / **Prep Time:** 15 minutes / **Cooking Time:** 20 minutes)

## Ingredients

- 4 (4-ounces) chicken drumsticks
- ½ cup buttermilk
- ½ cup all-purpose flour
- ½ cup panko breadcrumbs
- ¼ teaspoon baking powder
- ¼ teaspoon dried oregano
- ¼ teaspoon dried thyme
- ¼ teaspoon celery salt
- ¼ teaspoon garlic powder
- ¼ teaspoon ground ginger
- ¼ teaspoon cayenne pepper
- ¼ teaspoon paprika
- Salt and ground black pepper, as required
- 3 tablespoons butter, melted

## Instructions

1. Place the chicken drumsticks and buttermilk in a resealable plastic bag.
2. Squeeze the air out and seal the bag tightly.
3. Refrigerate for about 2-3 hours.

4. In a shallow bowl, mix well flour, breadcrumbs, baking powder, herbs and spices.
5. Remove the chicken drumsticks from bag and shake off the excess buttermilk.
6. Coat chicken drumsticks evenly with the seasoned flour mixture.
7. Set the temperature of air fryer to 390 degrees F. Line an air fryer basket with a piece of foil.
8. Arrange chicken drumsticks into the prepared air fryer basket.
9. Air fry for about 20 minutes, flipping once and coating with the melted butter.
10. Remove from air fryer and transfer the chicken drumsticks onto serving plates.
11. Serve hot.

## **Nutrition Values (Per Serving)**

- Calories: 771
- Carbohydrate: 32.1g
- Protein: 68.7g
- Fat: 33.1g
- Sugar: 3.2g
- Sodium: 449mg

# **Sweet & Sour Chicken Thighs**

**(Yields:** 2 servings / **Prep Time:** 15 minutes / **Cooking Time:** 20 minutes**)**

## **Ingredients**

- 1 scallion, finely chopped
- 1 garlic clove, minced
- ½ tablespoon soy sauce
- ½ tablespoon rice vinegar
- 1 teaspoon sugar
- Salt and ground black pepper, as required
- 2 (4-ounces) skinless, boneless chicken thighs
- ½ cup corn flour

## **Instructions**

1. Mix together all the ingredients except chicken, and corn flour in a bowl.
2. Add the chicken thighs and generously coat with marinade.
3. Add the corn flour in another bowl.
4. Remove the chicken thighs from marinade and coat with corn flour.
5. Set the temperature of Air Fryer to 390 degrees F. Grease an Air Fryer basket.
6. Arrange chicken thighs into the prepared Air Fryer basket, skin side down.
7. Air Fry for about 10 minutes and then another 10 minutes at 355 degrees F.
8. Remove from Air Fryer and transfer the chicken thighs onto a serving platter.
9. Serve hot.

### Nutrition Values (Per Serving)

- Calories: 264
- Carbohydrate: 25.3g
- Protein: 27.8g
- Fat: 5.2g
- Sugar: 2.8g
- Sodium: 347mg

---

## Crispy Chicken Thighs

**(Yields:** 4 servings / **Prep Time:** 15 minutes / **Cooking Time:** 25 minutes)

### Ingredients

- ½ cup all-purpose flour
- 1½ tablespoons Cajun seasoning
- 1 teaspoon seasoning salt
- 1 egg
- 4 (4-ounces) skin-on chicken thighs

### Instructions

1. Mix together the flour, Cajun seasoning, and salt in a shallow bowl.
2. In another bowl, crack the egg and beat well.
3. Coat each chicken thigh with the flour mixture, then dip into beaten egg and finally, coat with the flour mixture again.
4. Shake off the excess flour thoroughly.
5. Set the temperature of Air Fryer to 390 degrees F. Grease an Air Fryer basket.
6. Arrange chicken thighs into the prepared Air Fryer basket, skin side down.
7. Air Fry for about 25 minutes.
8. Remove from Air Fryer and transfer the chicken thighs onto a serving platter.
9. Serve hot.

### Nutrition Values (Per Serving)

- Calories: 353
- Carbohydrate: 12g
- Protein: 31.5g
- Fat: 18.8g
- Sugar: 0.1g
- Sodium: 749mg

# Cheesy Chicken Cutlets

**(Yields:** 4 servings / **Prep Time:** 15 minutes / **Cooking Time:** 30 minutes)

## Ingredients

- ¾ cup all-purpose flour
- 2 large eggs
- 1½ cups panko breadcrumbs
- ¼ cup Parmesan cheese, grated
- 1 tablespoon mustard powder
- Salt and ground black pepper, as required
- 4 (6-ounces) (¼-inch thick) skinless, boneless chicken cutlets
- 1 lemon, cut into slices

## Instructions

1. In a shallow bowl, add the flour.
2. In a second bowl, crack the eggs and beat well.
3. In a third bowl, mix together the breadcrumbs, cheese, mustard powder, salt, and black pepper.
4. Season the chicken with salt, and black pepper.
5. Coat the chicken with flour, then dip into beaten eggs and finally coat with the breadcrumbs mixture.
6. Set the temperature of Air Fryer to 355 degrees F. Grease an Air Fryer basket.
7. Arrange chicken cutlets into the prepared Air Fryer basket in a single layer.
8. Air Fry for about 30 minutes.
9. Remove from Air Fryer and transfer the chicken cutlets onto a serving platter.
10. Serve hot with the topping of lemon slices.

## Nutrition Values (Per Serving)

- Calories: 503
- Carbohydrate: 42g
- Protein: 49.3g
- Fat: 42.3g
- Sugar: 1.3g
- Sodium: 226mg

---

# Breaded Chicken Tenderloins

**(Yields:** 4 servings / **Prep Time:** 15 minutes / **Cooking Time:** 15 minutes)

## Ingredients

- 1 egg, beaten
- 2 tablespoons vegetable oil
- ½ cup breadcrumbs
- 8 skinless, boneless chicken tenderloins

## Instructions

1. In a shallow dish, beat the egg.
2. In another dish, add the oil and breadcrumbs and mix until a crumbly mixture forms.
3. Dip the chicken tenderloins into beaten egg and then coat with the breadcrumbs mixture.
4. Shake off the excess coating.
5. Set the temperature of Air Fryer to 355 degrees F. Grease an Air Fryer basket.
6. Arrange chicken tenderloins into the prepared Air Fryer basket in a single layer.
7. Air Fry for about 12-15 minutes.
8. Remove from Air Fryer and transfer the chicken thighs onto a serving platter.
9. Serve hot.

## Nutrition Values (Per Serving)

- Calories: 271
- Carbohydrate: 12g
- Protein: 30.4g
- Fat: 11.5g
- Sugar: 0.9g
- Sodium: 113mg

---

# Oats Crusted Chicken Breasts

**(Yields:** 2 servings / **Prep Time:** 20 minutes / **Cooking Time:** 12 minutes)

## Ingredients

- 2 (6-ounces) chicken breasts
- Salt and ground black pepper, as required
- ¾ cup oats
- 2 tablespoons mustard powder
- 1 tablespoon fresh parsley
- 2 medium eggs

## Instructions

1. Put the chicken breasts onto a cutting board and with a meat mallet, flatten each into even thickness.
2. Then, cut each breast in half.
3. Sprinkle the chicken pieces with salt and black pepper and set aside.
4. In a blender, add the oats, mustard powder, parsley, salt and black pepper. Pulse until a coarse breadcrumb like mixture is formed.
5. Transfer the oat mixture into a shallow bowl.
6. In another bowl, crack the eggs and beat well.

7. Coat the chicken with oats mixture and then, dip into beaten eggs and again, coat with the oats mixture.
8. Set the temperature of Air Fryer to 350 °F. Grease a grill pan of Air Fryer.
9. Arrange chicken breasts into the prepared grill pan in a single layer.
10. Air Fry for about 12 minutes, flipping once halfway through.
11. Remove from Air Fryer and transfer the chicken breasts onto a serving platter.
12. Serve hot.

## Nutrition Values (Per Serving)

- Calories: 556
- Carbohydrate: 25.1g
- Protein: 61.6g
- Fat: 22.2g
- Sugar: 1.4g
- Sodium: 289mg

---

# Spiced Chicken Breasts

**(Yields:** 4 servings / **Prep Time:** 20 minutes / **Cooking Time:** 23 minutes)

## Ingredients

- 2 tablespoons butter, melted
- ¼ teaspoon garlic powder
- ¼ teaspoon onion powder
- ¼ teaspoon smoked paprika
- Salt and ground black pepper, as required
- 4 (6-ounces) boneless, skinless chicken breasts

## Instructions

1. In a bowl, mix together butter, and spices.
2. Coat the chicken breasts evenly with the butter mixture.
3. Set the temperature of Air Fryer to 350 degrees F. Grease an Air Fryer basket.
4. Arrange chicken breasts into the prepared Air Fryer basket in a single layer.
5. Air Fry for about 15 minutes.
6. Flip the chicken breasts and Air Fry for 5-8 more minutes.
7. Remove from Air Fryer and transfer the chicken breasts onto a serving platter.
8. Serve hot.

## Nutrition Values (Per Serving)

- Calories: 376
- Carbohydrate: 0.3g
- Protein: 49.3g
- Fat: 18.4g
- Sugar: 0.1g
- Sodium: 226mg

(**Note:** We can avoid the chicken breasts from touching each other by placing the chicken pieces against the sides of air fryer basket.)

# Cheesy Chicken Breasts

**(Yields:** 2 servings / **Prep Time:** 20 minutes / **Cooking Time:** 22 minutes)

## Ingredients

- 2 (6-ounces) chicken breasts
- 1 egg, beaten
- 4 ounces' breadcrumbs
- 1 tablespoon fresh basil
- 2 tablespoons vegetable oil
- ¼ cup pasta sauce
- ¼ cup Parmesan cheese, grated

## Instructions

1. In a shallow bowl, beat the egg.
2. In another bowl, add the oil, breadcrumbs, and basil and mix until a crumbly mixture forms.
3. Now, dip each chicken breast into the beaten egg and then, coat with the breadcrumb mixture.
4. Set the temperature of Air Fryer to 350 degrees F. Grease an Air Fryer basket.
5. Arrange chicken breasts into the prepared basket
6. Air Fry for about 15 minutes.
7. Spoon the pasta sauce evenly over chicken breast and sprinkle with cheese.
8. Air Fry for about 5-7 more minutes.
9. Remove from Air Fryer and transfer the chicken breasts onto a serving platter.
10. Serve hot.

## Nutrition Values (Per Serving)

- Calories: 623
- Carbohydrate: 44.3g
- Protein: 51g
- Fat: 25.8g
- Sugar: 6.2g
- Sodium: 739mg

---

# Sausage Stuffed Chicken Breasts

**(Yields:** 4 servings / **Prep Time:** 15 minutes / **Cooking Time:** 15 minutes)

## Ingredients

- 4 (4-ounces) skinless, boneless chicken breasts
- 4 sausages, casing removed

## Instructions

1. Place the chicken breasts onto a smooth surface and with a meat mallet, pound each into an even thickness.
2. Place 1 sausage over each chicken breast.
3. Roll each breast around the sausage and secure with toothpicks.
4. Set the temperature of Air Fryer to 375 degrees F. Grease an Air Fryer basket.
5. Arrange chicken breasts into the prepared Air Fryer basket.
6. Air Fry for about 15 minutes.
7. Remove from Air Fryer and transfer the chicken breasts onto a serving platter.
8. Serve hot.

## Nutrition Values (Per Serving)

- Calories: 345
- Carbohydrate: 0g
- Protein: 37g
- Fat: 21.1g
- Sugar: 0g
- Sodium: 490mg

---

# Spinach Stuffed Chicken Breasts

**(Yields:** 2 servings / **Prep Time:** 15 minutes / **Cooking Time:** 30 minutes**)**

## Ingredients

- 1 tablespoon olive oil
- 1¾ ounces fresh spinach
- ¼ cup ricotta cheese, shredded
- 2 (4-ounces) skinless, boneless chicken breasts
- Salt and ground black pepper, as required
- 2 tablespoons cheddar cheese, grated
- ¼ teaspoon paprika

## Instructions

1. In a medium skillet, add the oil over medium heat and cook until heated.
2. Add the spinach and cook for about 3-4 minutes.
3. Stir in the ricotta and cook for about 40-60 seconds.
4. Remove the skillet from heat and set aside to cool.
5. Cut slits into the chicken breasts about ¼-inch apart but not all the way through.
6. Stuff each chicken breast with the spinach mixture.
7. Sprinkle each chicken breast evenly with salt and black pepper and then with cheddar cheese and paprika.

8. Set the temperature of Air Fryer to 390 degrees F. Grease an Air Fryer basket.
9. Arrange chicken breasts into the prepared basket in a single layer.
10. Air Fry for about 20-25 minutes.
11. Remove from Air Fryer and transfer the chicken breasts onto a serving platter.
12. Serve hot.

## Nutrition Values (Per Serving)

- Calories: 279
- Carbohydrate: 2.7g
- Protein: 31.4g
- Fat: 16g
- Sugar: 0.3g
- Sodium: 220mg

# Cheese Stuffed Chicken Breasts

**(Yields:** 4 servings / **Prep Time:** 15 minutes / **Cooking Time:** 15 minutes)

## Ingredients

- 2 (8-ounces) skinless, boneless chicken breast fillets
- Salt and ground black pepper, as required
- 4 Brie cheese slices
- 1 tablespoon fresh chive, minced
- 4 cured ham slices

## Instructions

1. Cut each chicken fillet in 2 equal-sized pieces.
2. Carefully, make a slit in each chicken piece horizontally about ¼-inch from the edge.
3. Open each chicken piece and season with the salt and black pepper.
4. Place 1 cheese slice in the open area of each chicken piece and sprinkle with chives.
5. Close the chicken pieces and wrap each one with a ham slice.
6. Set the temperature of Air Fryer to 355 degrees F. Grease an Air Fryer basket.
7. Arrange the wrapped chicken pieces into the prepared Air Fryer basket.
8. Air Fry for about 15 minutes.
9. Remove from Air Fryer and transfer the chicken fillets onto a serving platter.
10. Serve hot.

## Nutrition Values (Per Serving)

- Calories: 376
- Carbohydrate: 1.5g
- Protein: 44.5g
- Fat: 20.2g
- Sugar: 0g
- Sodium: 639mg

# Bacon Wrapped Chicken Breasts

**(Yields:** 4 servings / **Prep Time:** 20 minutes / **Cooking Time:** 23 minutes)

## Ingredients

- 1 tablespoon palm sugar
- 6-7 Fresh basil leaves
- 2 tablespoons fish sauce
- 2 tablespoons water
- 2 (8-ounces) chicken breasts, cut each breast in half horizontally
- Salt and ground black pepper, as required
- 12 bacon strips
- 1½ teaspoon honey

## Instructions

1. In a small heavy-bottomed pan, add palm sugar over medium-low heat and cook for about 2-3 minutes or until caramelized, stirring continuously.
2. Add the basil, fish sauce and water and stir to combine.
3. Remove from heat and transfer the sugar mixture into a large bowl.
4. Sprinkle each chicken breast with salt and black pepper.
5. Add the chicken pieces in sugar mixture and coat generously.
6. Refrigerate to marinate for about 4-6 hours.
7. Set the temperature of Air Fryer to 365 degrees F. Grease an Air Fryer basket.
8. Wrap each chicken piece with 3 bacon strips.
9. Coat each piece slightly with honey.
10. Arrange chicken pieces into the prepared Air Fryer basket.
11. Air Fry for about 20 minutes, flipping once halfway through.
12. Remove from Air Fryer and transfer the chicken pieces onto a serving platter.
13. Serve hot.

## Nutrition Values (Per Serving)

- Calories: 365
- Carbohydrate: 2.7g
- Protein: 30.2g
- Fat: 24.8g
- Sugar: 2.1g
- Sodium: 1300mg

# Buffalo Chicken Tenders

**(Yields:** 3 servings / **Prep Time:** 20 minutes / **Cooking Time:** 12 minutes)

## Ingredients

- 1 tablespoon water
- 1 large egg
- 16 ounces boneless, skinless chicken breasts, sliced into tenders
- ½ cup pork rinds, crushed
- ½ cup unflavored whey protein powder
- ½ teaspoon garlic powder
- Salt and ground black pepper, as required
- 2 tablespoons butter, melted
- ¼ cup buffalo wing sauce

## Instructions

1. In a large bowl, add the water, and egg. Beat until well combined.
2. Add the chicken and generously coat with egg mixture.
3. Place the chicken in a colander to drain completely.
4. In a shallow bowl, mix together the pork rinds, protein powder, garlic powder, salt, and black pepper.
5. Coat chicken tenders with the pork rinds mixture.
6. Set the temperature of Air Fryer to 400 degrees F. Grease an Air Fryer basket.
7. Arrange chicken tenders into the prepared Air Fryer basket and drizzle with the melted butter.
8. Air Fry for about 10-12 minutes.
9. Remove from Air Fryer and transfer the chicken tenders into a bowl.
10. Place with the buffalo sauce and toss to coat well.
11. Serve immediately.

## Nutrition Values (Per Serving)

- Calories: 292
- Carbohydrate: 0.9g
- Protein: 43.6g
- Fat: 12.9g
- Sugar: 0.2g
- Sodium: 261mg

# **Crispy Chicken Tenders**

**(Yields:** 3 servings / **Prep Time:** 20 minutes / **Cooking Time:** 15+15 = 30 minutes)

## Ingredients

- 2 (6-ounces) boneless, skinless chicken breasts, pounded into ½-inch thickness and cut into tenders
- ¾ cup buttermilk
- 1½ teaspoons Worcestershire sauce, divided
- ½ teaspoon smoked paprika, divided
- Salt and ground black pepper, as required
- ½ cup all-purpose flour
- 1½ cups panko breadcrumbs
- ¼ cup Parmesan cheese, finely grated
- 2 tablespoons butter, melted
- 2 large eggs

## Instructions

1. In a large bowl, mix together buttermilk, ¾ teaspoon of Worcestershire sauce, ¼ teaspoon of paprika, salt, and black pepper.
2. Add in the chicken tenders and refrigerate overnight.
3. In another bowl, mix together the flour, remaining paprika, salt, and black pepper.
4. Place the remaining Worcestershire sauce and eggs in a third bowl and beat until well combined.
5. Mix well the panko, Parmesan, and butter in a fourth bowl.
6. Remove the chicken tenders from bowl and discard the buttermilk.
7. Coat the chicken tenders with flour mixture, then dip into egg mixture and finally coat with the panko mixture.
8. Set the temperature of air fryer to 400 degrees F. Grease an air fryer basket.
9. Arrange chicken tenders into the prepared air fryer basket in 2 batches in a single layer.
10. Air fry for about 13-15 minutes, flipping once halfway through.
11. Remove from air fryer and transfer the chicken tenders onto a serving platter.
12. Serve hot.

## Nutrition Values (Per Serving)

- Calories: 654
- Carbohydrate: 28g
- Protein: 454g
- Fat: 25.5g
- Sugar: 3.9g
- Sodium: 399mg

# Simple Chicken Wings

**(Yields:** 2 servings / **Prep Time:** 10 minutes / **Cooking Time:** 25 minutes)

## Ingredients

- 1 pound chicken wings
- Salt and ground black pepper, as required

## Instructions

1. Set the temperature of Air Fryer to 380 degrees F. Generously, grease an Air Fryer basket.
2. Sprinkle the chicken wings evenly with salt and black pepper.
3. Arrange chicken wings into the prepared Air Fryer basket in a single layer.
4. Air Fry for about 25 minutes, flip the wings once halfway through.
5. Remove from Air Fryer and transfer the chicken wings onto a serving platter.
6. Serve hot.

## Nutrition Values (Per Serving)

- Calories: 431
- Carbohydrate: 0g
- Protein: 65.6g
- Fat: 16.8g
- Sugar: 0g
- Sodium: 273mg

---

# Crispy Chicken Wings

**(Yields:** 2 servings / **Prep Time:** 20 minutes / **Cooking Time:** 25 minutes)

## Ingredients

- 2 lemongrass stalk (white portion), minced
- 1 onion, finely chopped
- 1 tablespoon soy sauce
- 1½ tablespoons honey
- Salt and ground white pepper, as required
- 1 pound chicken wings, rinsed and trimmed
- ½ cup cornstarch

## Instructions

1. In a bowl, mix together the lemongrass, onion, soy sauce, honey, salt, and white pepper.
2. Add the wings and generously coat with marinade.

3. Cover and refrigerate to marinate overnight.
4. Set the temperature of Air Fryer to 355 degrees F. Grease an Air Fryer basket.
5. Remove the chicken wings from marinade and coat with the cornstarch.
6. Arrange chicken wings into the prepared Air Fryer basket in a single layer.
7. Air Fry for about 25 minutes, flipping once halfway through.
8. Remove from Air Fryer and transfer the chicken wings onto a serving platter.
9. Serve hot.

## Nutrition Values (Per Serving)

- Calories: 724
- Carbohydrate: 56.9g
- Protein: 43.5g
- Fat: 36.2g
- Sugar: 15.4g
- Sodium: 702mg

---

# BBQ Chicken Wings

**(Yields:** 4 servings / **Prep Time:** 10 minutes / **Cooking Time:** 30 minutes)

## Ingredients

- 2 pounds chicken wings, cut into drumettes and flats
- ½ cup BBQ sauce

## Instructions

1. Set the temperature of Air Fryer to 380 degrees F. Grease an Air Fryer basket.
2. Arrange chicken wings into the prepared Air Fryer basket in a single layer.
3. Air Fry for about 24 minutes, flipping once halfway through.
4. Now, set the temperature of Air Fryer to 400 degrees F.
5. Air Fry for about 6 minutes.
6. Remove from Air Fryer and transfer the chicken wings into a bowl.
7. Drizzle with the BBQ sauce and toss to coat well.
8. Serve immediately.

## Nutrition Values (Per Serving)

- Calories: 478
- Carbohydrate: 11.3g
- Protein: 65.6g
- Fat: 16.9g
- Sugar: 8.1g
- Sodium: 545mg

# Buffalo Chicken Wings

**(Yields:** 6 servings / **Prep Time:** 20 minutes / **Cooking Time:** 22 minutes)

## Ingredients

- 2 pounds chicken wings, cut into drumettes and flats
- 1 teaspoon chicken seasoning
- 1 teaspoon garlic powder
- Ground black pepper, to taste
- 1 tablespoon olive oil
- ¼ cup red hot sauce
- 2 tablespoons low-sodium soy sauce

## Instructions

1. Set the temperature of Air Fryer to 400 degrees F. Grease an Air Fryer basket.
2. Sprinkle each chicken wing evenly with chicken seasoning, garlic powder, and black pepper.
3. Arrange chicken wings into the prepared Air Fryer basket in a single layer and drizzle with oil.
4. Air Fry for about 10 minutes, shaking the basket once halfway through.
5. Remove from Air Fryer and transfer the chicken wings into a bowl.
6. Drizzle with the red hot sauce, oil, and soy sauce. Toss to coat well.
7. Place chicken wings for the second time into the Air Fryer basket in a single layer.
8. Air Fry for about 7-12 minutes at the same temperature.
9. Remove from Air Fryer and transfer the chicken wings onto a serving platter.
10. Serve hot.

## Nutrition Values (Per Serving)

- Calories: 311
- Carbohydrate: 0.6g
- Protein: 44g
- Fat: 13.6g
- Sugar: 0.3g
- Sodium: 491mg

(**Note: Buffalo Chicken Wings** – When red hot sauce is used with chicken wings, it's called Buffalo Chicken Wings.)

# Sweet Chicken Kabobs

**(Yields:** 3 servings / **Prep Time:** 20 minutes / **Cooking Time:** 14 minutes)

## Ingredients

- 4 scallions, chopped
- 1 tablespoon fresh ginger, finely grated
- 4 garlic cloves, minced
- ½ cup pineapple juice
- ½ cup soy sauce
- ¼ cup sesame oil
- 2 teaspoons sesame seeds, toasted
- A pinch of black pepper
- 1 pound chicken tenders

## Instructions

1. In a large baking dish, mix together the scallion, ginger, garlic, pineapple juice, soy sauce, oil, sesame seeds, and black pepper.
2. Thread chicken tenders onto the pre-soaked wooden skewers.
3. Add the skewers into the baking dish and evenly coat with marinade.
4. Cover and refrigerate for about 2 hours or overnight.
5. Set the temperature of Air Fryer to 390 degrees F. Grease an Air Fryer basket.
6. Place chicken skewers into the prepared Air Fryer basket in 2 batches.
7. Air Fry for about 5-7 minutes.
8. Remove from Air Fryer and transfer the chicken skewers onto a serving platter.
9. Serve hot.

## Nutrition Values (Per Serving)

- Calories: 392
- Carbohydrate: 9.9g
- Protein: 35.8g
- Fat: 23g
- Sugar: 4.1g
- Sodium: 1800mg

# Chicken & Scallion Kabobs

**(Yields:** 4 servings / **Prep Time:** 20 minutes / **Cooking Time:** 24 minutes)

## Ingredients

- ¼ cup light soy sauce
- 1 tablespoon mirin
- 1 teaspoon garlic salt
- 1 teaspoon sugar
- 4 (4-ounces) skinless, boneless chicken thighs, cubed into 1-inch size
- 5 scallions, cut into 1-inch pieces lengthwise

### Instructions

1. In a baking dish, mix together the soy sauce, mirin, garlic salt, and sugar.
2. Thread chicken and scallions onto pre-soaked wooden skewers.
3. Place skewers into the baking dish and generously coat with marinade.
4. Cover and refrigerate for about 3 hours.
5. Set the temperature of Air Fryer to 355 degrees F. Grease an Air Fryer basket.
6. Arrange skewers into the prepared Air Fryer basket in 2 batches in a single layer.
7. Air Fry for about 10-12 minutes.
8. Once done, remove from Air Fryer and transfer the chicken skewers onto a serving platter.
9. Serve hot.

### Nutrition Values (Per Serving)

- Calories: 161
- Carbohydrate: 6.9g
- Protein: 26.2g
- Fat: 4.1g
- Sugar: 4g
- Sodium: 781mg

## Chicken & Veggie Kabobs

(**Yields:** 3 servings / **Prep Time:** 20 minutes / **Cooking Time:** 30 minutes)

### Ingredients

- 1 lb. skinless, boneless chicken thighs, cut into cubes
- ½ cup plain Greek yogurt
- 1 tablespoon olive oil
- 2 teaspoons curry powder
- ½ teaspoon smoked paprika
- ¼ teaspoon cayenne pepper
- Salt, to taste
- 2 small bell peppers, seeded and cut into large chunks
- 1 large red onion, cut into large chunks

### Instructions

1. In a bowl, add the chicken, oil, yogurt, and spices and mix until well combined
2. Refrigerate to marinate for about 2 hours.
3. Thread the chicken cubes, bell pepper and onion onto pre-soaked wooden skewers.
4. Set the temperature of Air Fryer to 360 degrees F. Grease an Air Fryer basket.
5. Arrange chicken skewers into the prepared Air Fryer basket in 2 batches.
6. Air Fry for about 15 minutes.

7. Remove from Air Fryer and transfer the chicken skewers onto a serving platter.
8. Serve hot.

## Nutrition Values (Per Serving)
- Calories: 222
- Carbohydrate: 8.7g
- Protein: 27.9g
- Fat: 8.2g
- Sugar: 5.3g
- Sodium: 104mg

---

# Jerk Chicken, Pineapple & Veggie Kabobs

**(Yields:** 8 servings / **Prep Time:** 20 minutes / **Cooking Time:** 18 minutes**)**

## Ingredients
- 8 (4-ounces) boneless, skinless chicken thigh fillets, trimmed and cut into cubes
- 1 tablespoon jerk seasoning
- 2 large zucchini, sliced
- 8 ounces white mushrooms, stems removed
- Salt and ground black pepper, as required
- 1 (20-ounces) can pineapple chunks, drained
- 1 tablespoon jerk sauce

## Instructions
1. In a bowl, mix together the chicken cubes and jerk seasoning.
2. Cover the bowl and refrigerate overnight.
3. Sprinkle the zucchini slices, and mushrooms evenly with salt and black pepper.
4. Thread the chicken, vegetables and pineapple onto greased metal skewers.
5. Set the temperature of Air Fryer to 370 degrees F. Grease an Air Fryer basket.
6. Arrange skewers into the prepared Air Fryer basket in 2 batches.
7. Air Fry for about 8-9 minutes, flipping and coating with jerk sauce once halfway through.
8. Remove from Air Fryer and transfer the chicken skewers onto a serving platter.
9. Serve hot.

## Nutrition Values (Per Serving)
- Calories: 274
- Carbohydrate: 14.1g
- Protein: 35.1g
- Fat: 8.7g
- Sugar: 9.9g
- Sodium: 150mg

# **Curried Chicken**

**(Yields:** 3 servings / **Prep Time:** 15 minutes / **Cooking Time:** 18 minutes)

## **Ingredients**

- 1 pound boneless chicken, cubed
- 1 tablespoon light soy sauce
- ½ tablespoon cornstarch
- 1 egg
- 2 tablespoons olive oil
- 1 medium yellow onion, thinly sliced
- 1 green chili, chopped
- 3 teaspoons garlic, minced
- 1 teaspoon fresh ginger, grated
- 5 curry leaves
- 1 teaspoon curry powder
- 1 tablespoon chili sauce
- 1 teaspoon sugar
- Salt and ground black pepper, as required
- ½ cup evaporated milk

## **Instructions**

1. In a bowl, add the chicken cubes, soy sauce, cornstarch, and egg and mix until well combined.
2. Cover the bowl and place at room temperature for about 1 hour.
3. Remove chicken cubes from the bowl and with paper towels, pat them dry.
4. Set the temperature of Air Fryer to 390 degrees F. Grease an Air Fryer basket.
5. Arrange chicken cubes into the prepared Air Fryer basket.
6. Air Fry for about 10 minutes.
7. Remove chicken cubes from the Air fryer and set aside.
8. In a medium skillet, add the oil over medium heat and cook until heated.
9. Add the onion, green chili, garlic, ginger, and curry leaves. Sauté for about 3-4 minutes.
10. Add the chicken cubes, curry powder, chili sauce, sugar, salt, and black pepper and mix until well combined.
11. Stir in the evaporated milk and cook for about 3-4 minutes.
12. Remove from heat and transfer the chicken mixture into a serving bowl.
13. Serve hot.

## **Nutrition Values (Per Serving)**

- Calories: 363
- Carbohydrate: 10g
- Protein: 37.1g
- Fat: 19g
- Sugar: 0.8g
- Sodium: 789mg

# Chicken with Apple

**(Yields:** 2 servings / **Prep Time:** 20 minutes / **Cooking Time:** 20 minutes)

## Ingredients

- 1 shallot, thinly sliced
- 1 tablespoon fresh ginger, finely grated
- 1 teaspoon fresh thyme, minced
- ½ cup apple cider
- 2 tablespoons maple syrup
- Salt and ground black pepper, as required
- 2 (4-ounces) boneless, skinless chicken thighs, sliced into chunks
- 1 large apple, cored and cubed

## Instructions

1. In a bowl, mix together the shallot, ginger, thyme, apple cider, maple syrup, salt, and black pepper.
2. Add the chicken pieces and generously mix with the marinade.
3. Refrigerate to marinate for about 6-8 hours.
4. Set the temperature of Air Fryer to 390 degrees F. Grease an Air Fryer basket.
5. Place the chicken pieces and cubed apple into the prepared Air Fryer basket.
6. Air Fry for about 20 minutes, flipping once halfway.
7. Remove from Air Fryer and transfer the chicken mixture onto a serving platter.
8. Serve hot.

## Nutrition Values (Per Serving)

- Calories: 299
- Carbohydrate: 39.9g
- Protein: 26.2g
- Fat: 4.6g
- Sugar: 30.4g
- Sodium: 125mg

# Chicken with Carrots

**(Yields:** 2 servings / **Prep Time:** 15 minutes / **Cooking Time:** 25 minutes)

## Ingredients

- 1 carrot, peeled and thinly sliced
- Salt and ground black pepper, as required
- 2 tablespoons butter
- 2 (4-ounces) chicken breast halves
- 1 tablespoon fresh rosemary, chopped
- 2 tablespoons fresh lemon juice

## Instructions

1. Arrange 2 square-shaped parchment papers onto a smooth surface.
2. Place carrot slices evenly in the center of each parchment paper.
3. Place ½ tablespoon of butter over carrot slices and sprinkle with salt and black pepper.
4. Arrange 1 chicken breast over carrot slices in each parcel.
5. Top each chicken breast evenly with rosemary and drizzle with lemon juice.
6. Top with the remaining butter.
7. Seal each parchment paper by folding all four corners.
8. Set the temperature of Air Fryer to 375 degrees F.
9. Arrange the chicken parcels into an Air Fryer basket.
10. Air Fry for about 20-25 minutes.
11. Remove from Air Fryer and transfer the chicken mixture onto a serving platter.
12. Serve hot.

## Nutrition Values (Per Serving)

- Calories: 339
- Carbohydrate: 4.4g
- Protein: 33.4g
- Fat: 20.3g
- Sugar: 18g
- Sodium: 282mg

# Chicken with Veggies

**(Yields:** 2 servings / **Prep Time:** 20 minutes / **Cooking Time:** 45 minutes)

## Ingredients

- 2 garlic cloves, minced
- 2 tablespoons chicken broth
- 2 tablespoons red wine vinegar
- 2 tablespoons olive oil
- 1 tablespoon Dijon mustard
- 1/8 teaspoon dried thyme
- 1/8 teaspoon dried basil
- 4 small artichoke hearts, quartered
- 4 fresh large button mushrooms, quartered
- ½ small onion, cut in large chunks
- Salt and ground black pepper, as required
- 2 skinless, boneless chicken breasts
- 2 tablespoons fresh parsley, chopped

## Instructions

1. Grease a small baking dish that will fit in the cooking basket of Air Fryer.
2. In a small bowl, mix together the garlic, broth, vinegar, olive oil, mustard, thyme, and basil.
3. In the prepared baking dish, add the artichokes, mushrooms, onions, salt, and black pepper and mix well
4. Now, place the chicken breasts on top of veggie mixture in a single layer.
5. Spread half of the mustard mixture evenly over chicken breasts.
6. Set the temperature of Air Fryer to 350 degrees F.
7. Arrange the baking dish into an Air Fryer cooking basket.
8. Air Fry for about 23 minutes.
9. Coat the chicken breasts with the remaining mustard mixture and flip the side.
10. Air Fry for about 22 minutes.
11. Remove from Air Fryer and transfer the chicken mixture onto a serving platter.
12. Garnish with parsley and serve hot.

## Nutrition Values (Per Serving)

- Calories: 448
- Carbohydrate: 39.1g
- Protein: 38.5g
- Fat: 19.1g
- Sugar: 5g
- Sodium: 566mg

(**Note:** If you want your chicken to be crispy, then set the temperature of air fryer to 375 degrees F).

# Chicken Chilaquiles

**(Yields:** 3 servings / **Prep Time:** 20 minutes / **Cooking Time:** 50 minutes)

## Ingredients

- 1 (8-ounces) skinless, boneless chicken breast
- 2 bay leaves
- 1 small yellow onion, chopped
- 3 garlic cloves, chopped
- ½ of poblano pepper
- 1 (14½-ounce) can diced tomatoes
- 1 (10-ounces) can Rotel tomatoes
- Salt, to taste
- 10 corn tortillas, cut into diamond slices
- 1 tablespoon olive oil
- 4 tablespoons feta cheese, crumbled
- ¼ cup sour cream
- 2 red onions, sliced

## Instructions

1. In a pan of water, add the chicken, and bay leaves and cook for about 20 minutes.
2. With a slotted spoon, transfer chicken breasts into a bowl and set aside to cool.
3. Shred the chicken using 2 forks.
4. In a food processor, add the onion, garlic, poblano pepper, and both cans of tomatoes and pulse until smooth.
5. Transfer the sauce into a skillet over medium-high heat and bring to a boil.
6. Reduce the heat to medium-low and cook for about 10 minutes.
7. Season with salt and remove from the heat.
8. Set the temperature of Air Fryer to 400 degrees F. Grease an Air Fryer basket.
9. In a bowl, add the tortilla slices, oil and salt and toss to coat well.
10. Arrange tortilla slices into the prepared Air Fryer basket in 2 batches in a single layer.
11. Air Fry for about 10 minutes.
12. Transfer the tortilla slices into the serving bowl.
13. Add the sauce, cheese, and sour cream and mix well.
14. Top with the chicken, and red onions and serve.

## Nutrition Values (Per Serving)

- Calories: 375
- Carbohydrate: 42.8g
- Protein: 25.9g
- Fat: 12.7g
- Sugar: 7g
- Sodium: 536mg

# Chicken with Broccoli & Rice

**(Yields:** 6 servings / **Prep Time:** 20 minutes / **Cooking Time:** 15 minutes)

## Ingredients

- 3 tablespoons dried parsley, crushed
- 1 tablespoon onion powder
- 1 tablespoon garlic powder
- ½ teaspoon red chili powder
- ½ teaspoon paprika
- 2 pounds boneless, skinless chicken breasts, sliced
- 3 cups instant white rice
- ¾ cup cream soup
- 3 cups small broccoli florets
- 1/3 cup butter
- 3 cups water

## Instructions

1. Mix together the parsley and spices in a large bowl.
2. Add the chicken slices and generously coat with spice mixture.
3. Arrange 6 large pieces of foil onto a smooth surface.
4. Place ½ cup of rice over each foil piece, followed by 1/6 of chicken, 2 tablespoons of cream soup, ½ cup of broccoli, 1 tablespoon of butter, and ½ cup of water.
5. Fold the foil tightly to seal the rice mixture.
6. Set the temperature of Air Fryer to 390 degrees F.
7. Arrange the foil packets into an Air Fryer basket.
8. Air Fry for about 15 minutes.
9. Remove from Air Fryer and carefully, transfer the rice mixture onto serving plates.
10. Serve hot.

## Nutrition Values (Per Serving)

- Calories: 583
- Carbohydrate: 65.6g
- Protein: 42.7g
- Fat: 23.1g
- Sugar: 1.6g
- Sodium: 374mg

---

# Chicken with Veggies & Rice

**(Yields:** 3 servings / **Prep Time:** 15 minutes / **Cooking Time:** 20 minutes)

## Ingredients

- 3 cups cold boiled white rice
- 6 tablespoons soy sauce

- 1 tablespoon vegetable oil
- 1 cup cooked chicken, diced
- ½ cup frozen carrots
- ½ cup frozen peas
- ½ cup onion, chopped

## Instructions

1. In a large bowl, add the rice, soy sauce, and oil and mix thoroughly.
2. Add the remaining ingredients and mix until well combined.
3. Transfer the rice mixture into a 7" nonstick pan.
4. Arrange the pan into an Air Fryer basket.
5. Set the temperature of Air Fryer to 360 degrees F.
6. Air Fry for about 20 minutes.
7. Remove the pan from Air Fryer and transfer the rice mixture onto serving plates.
8. Serve immediately.

## Nutrition Values (Per Serving)

- Calories: 405
- Carbohydrate: 63g
- Protein: 21.7g
- Fat: 6.4g
- Sugar: 3.5g
- Sodium: 1500mg

---

# Crispy Chicken Burgers

**(Yields:** 4 servings / **Prep Time:** 20 minutes / **Cooking Time:** 30 minutes)

## Ingredients

- 6 boneless, skinless chicken breasts
- 1 teaspoon mustard powder
- ½ teaspoon paprika
- 1 teaspoon Worcestershire sauce
- 1¾ ounces plain flour
- 1 small egg
- 6¾ tablespoons breadcrumbs
- ¼ teaspoon dried parsley
- ¼ teaspoon dried tarragon
- ¼ teaspoon dried oregano
- 1 teaspoon dried garlic
- 1 teaspoon chicken seasoning
- ½ teaspoon cayenne pepper
- Salt and ground black pepper, as required
- 4 hamburger buns, split and toasted
- 4 lettuce leaves
- 4 mozzarella cheese slices

## Instructions

1. In a food processor, add the chicken breasts and pulse until minced.
2. Add the mustard, paprika, Worcester sauce, salt, and black pepper and pulse until well combined.
3. Make 4 equal-sized patties from the mixture.
4. In a shallow bowl, place the flour.
5. In a second bowl, crack the egg and beat well.
6. In a third bowl, mix well breadcrumbs, dried herbs, and spices.
7. Coat each chicken patty with flour, then dip into egg and finally, coat with breadcrumb mixture.
8. Set the temperature of air fryer to 355 degrees F. Grease an air fryer basket.
9. Arrange chicken patties into the prepared air fryer basket in a single layer.
10. Air fry for about 15 minutes per side.
11. Remove from air fryer and place the patties onto a plate.
12. Place one lettuce leaf over bottom half of each bun, followed by one patty and cheese slice.
13. Cover with bun top and serve.

## Nutrition Values (Per Serving)

- Calories: 677
- Carbohydrate: 50.1g
- Protein: 66.6g
- Fat: 21.7g
- Sugar: 1.3g
- Sodium: 720mg

# Simple Turkey Breast

**(Yields:** 10 servings / **Prep Time:** 20 minutes / **Cooking Time:** 45 minutes)

## Ingredients

- 1 (8-pounds) bone-in turkey breast
- Salt and ground black pepper, as required
- 2 tablespoons olive oil

## Instructions

1. Set the temperature of Air Fryer to 360 degrees F. Grease an Air Fryer basket.
2. Sprinkle the turkey breast with salt and black pepper and drizzle with oil.
3. Arrange turkey breast into the prepared Air Fryer basket, skin side down.
4. Air Fry for about 20 minutes.
5. Flip the side and cook for another 20-25 minutes.
6. Remove from Air Fryer and place the turkey breast onto a cutting board for about 10 minutes before slicing.
7. With a sharp knife, cut the turkey breast into desired size slices and serve.

### Nutrition Values (Per Serving)

- Calories: 719
- Carbohydrate: 0g
- Protein: 97.2g
- Fat: 35.9g
- Sugar: 0g
- Sodium: 386mg

(**Note:** Make sure the height of turkey breast is below the top of basket before you start cooking).

---

## Herbed Turkey Breast

(**Yields:** 3 servings / **Prep Time:** 15 minutes / **Cooking Time:** 35 minutes)

### Ingredients

- 1 teaspoon dried thyme, crushed
- 1 teaspoon dried rosemary, crushed
- ½ teaspoon dried sage, crushed
- ½ teaspoon dark brown sugar
- ½ teaspoon garlic powder
- ½ teaspoon paprika
- 1 (2½-pounds) bone-in, skin-on turkey breast
- 1 tablespoon olive oil

### Instructions

1. In a bowl, mix together the herbs, brown sugar, and spices.
2. Coat the turkey breast evenly with oil and then, generously rub with the herb mixture.
3. Set the temperature of Air Fryer to 360 degrees F. Grease an Air Fryer basket.
4. Arrange turkey breast into the prepared Air Fryer basket, skin-side down.
5. Air Fry for about 35 minutes, flipping once halfway through.
6. Remove from Air Fryer and place the turkey breast onto a cutting board for about 10 minutes before slicing.
7. With a sharp knife, cut the turkey breast into desired size slices and serve.

### Nutrition Values (Per Serving)

- Calories: 688
- Carbohydrate: 1.6g
- Protein: 81.2g
- Fat: 31.8g
- Sugar: 0.8g
- Sodium: 473mg

# Glazed Turkey Breast

**(Yields:** 8 servings / **Prep Time:** 15 minutes / **Cooking Time:** 55 minutes)

## Ingredients

- 1 teaspoon dried thyme, crushed
- ½ teaspoon dried sage, crushed
- ½ teaspoon smoked paprika
- Salt and ground black pepper, as required
- 1 (5-pounds) boneless turkey breast
- 2 teaspoons olive oil
- ¼ cup maple syrup
- 2 tablespoons Dijon mustard
- 1 tablespoon butter, softened

## Instructions

1. In a bowl, mix together the herbs, paprika, salt, and black pepper.
2. Coat the turkey breast evenly with oil.
3. Now, coat the outer side of turkey breast with herb mixture.
4. Set the temperature of Air Fryer to 350 degrees F. Grease an Air Fryer basket.
5. Place turkey breast into the prepared Air Fryer basket.
6. Air Fry for about 25 minutes.
7. Flip the side and Air Fry for another 12 minutes.
8. Again flip the side and Air Fry for 13 more minutes.
9. Meanwhile, in a bowl, mix together the maple syrup, mustard, and butter.
10. Coat the turkey evenly with glaze.
11. Air Fry for about 5 more minutes.
12. Remove from Air Fryer and place the turkey breast onto a cutting board for about 10 minutes before slicing.
13. With a sharp knife, cut the turkey breast into desired size slices and serve.

## Nutrition Values (Per Serving)

- Calories: 302
- Carbohydrate: 5.6g
- Protein: 56.2g
- Fat: 3.3g
- Sugar: 4.7g
- Sodium: 170mg

---

# Turkey Legs

**(Yields:** 2 servings / **Prep Time:** 15 minutes / **Cooking Time:** 30 minutes)

## Ingredients

- 2 garlic cloves, minced
- 1 tablespoon fresh rosemary, minced

- 1 teaspoon fresh lime zest, finely grated
- 2 tablespoons olive oil
- 1 tablespoon fresh lime juice
- Salt and ground black pepper, as required
- 2 turkey legs

## Instructions

1. Mix together the garlic, rosemary, lime zest, oil, lime juice, salt, and black pepper in a large bowl.
2. Add the turkey legs and generously coat with marinade.
3. Refrigerate to marinate for about 6-8 hours.
4. Set the temperature of Air Fryer to 350 degrees F. Grease an Air Fryer basket.
5. Place turkey legs into the prepared Air Fryer basket.
6. Air Fry for about 30 minutes, flipping once halfway through.
7. Remove from Air Fryer and place the turkey legs onto the serving plates.
8. Serve hot.

## Nutrition Values (Per Serving)

- Calories: 458
- Carbohydrate: 2.3g
- Protein: 44.6g
- Fat: 29.5g
- Sugar: 0.1g
- Sodium: 247mg

# Buttermilk Brined Turkey Breast

(**Yields:** 8 servings / **Prep Time:** 15 minutes / **Cooking Time:** 20 minutes)

## Ingredients

- ¾ cup brine from a can of olives
- ½ cup buttermilk
- 3½ pounds boneless, skinless turkey breast
- 2 fresh thyme sprigs
- 1 fresh rosemary sprig

## Instructions

1. In a bowl, add the olive brine, and buttermilk and beat until well combined.
2. In a resealable plastic bag, place the turkey breast, buttermilk mixture and herb sprigs
3. Seal the bag and refrigerate for about 8 hours.
4. Remove the turkey breast from bag and set aside until it reaches room temperature.
5. Set the temperature of air fryer to 350 degrees F. Grease an air fryer basket.

6. Arrange turkey breast into the prepared air fryer basket.
7. Air fry for about 20 minutes, flipping once after 15 minutes.
8. Remove from air fryer and place the turkey breast onto a platter.
9. Cover the turkey breast loosely with a piece of foil for about 10-15 minutes before slicing.
10. Cut the turkey into desired size slices and serve.

## Nutrition Values (Per Serving)
- Calories: 215
- Carbohydrate: 9.4g
- Protein: 34.4g
- Fat: 3.5g
- Sugar: 7.7g
- Sodium: 2000mg

# Turkey Wings

**(Yields:** 4 servings / **Prep Time:** 10 minutes / **Cooking Time:** 26 minutes)

## Ingredients
- 2 pounds turkey wings
- 4 tablespoons chicken rub
- 3 tablespoons olive oil

## Instructions
1. In a large bowl, mix together the turkey wings, chicken rub, and oil using your hands.
2. Set the temperature of Air Fryer to 380 degrees F. Grease an Air Fryer basket.
3. Arrange turkey wings into the prepared Air Fryer basket.
4. Air Fry for about 26 minutes, flipping once halfway through.
5. Remove from Air Fryer and place the turkey wings onto the serving plates.
6. Serve hot.

## Nutrition Values (Per Serving)
- Calories: 204
- Carbohydrate: 3g
- Protein: 12g
- Fat: 15.5g
- Sugar: 0g
- Sodium: 465mg

# Turkey Rolls

**(Yields:** 3 servings / **Prep Time:** 20 minutes / **Cooking Time:** 40 minutes)

## Ingredients

- 1 pound turkey breast fillet
- 1 garlic clove, crushed
- 1½ teaspoons ground cumin
- 1 teaspoon ground cinnamon
- ½ teaspoon red chili powder
- Salt, to taste
- 2 tablespoons olive oil
- 3 tablespoons fresh parsley, finely chopped
- 1 small red onion, finely chopped

## Instructions

1. Place the turkey fillet on a cutting board.
2. Carefully, cut horizontally along the length about 1/3 of way from the top, stopping about ¼-inch from the edge.
3. Open this part to have a long piece of fillet.
4. In a bowl, mix together the garlic, spices, and oil.
5. In a small cup, reserve about 1 tablespoon of oil mixture.
6. In the remaining oil mixture, add the parsley, and onion and mix well.
7. Set the temperature of Air Fryer to 355 degrees F. Grease an Air Fryer basket.
8. Coat the open side of fillet with onion mixture.
9. Roll the fillet tightly from the short side.
10. With a kitchen string, tie the roll at 1-1½-inch intervals.
11. Coat the outer side of roll with the reserved oil mixture.
12. Arrange roll into the prepared Air Fryer basket.
13. Air Fry for about 40 minutes.
14. Remove from Air Fryer and place the turkey roll onto a cutting board for about 5-10 minutes before slicing.
15. With a sharp knife, cut the turkey roll into desired size slices and serve.

## Nutrition Values (Per Serving)

- Calories: 239
- Carbohydrate: 3.2g
- Protein: 37.5g
- Fat: 8.2g
- Sugar: 0.9g
- Sodium: 46mg

# Turkey Meatloaf

(**Yields:** 4 servings / **Prep Time:** 20 minutes / **Cooking Time:** 20 minutes)

## Ingredients

- 1 pound ground turkey
- 1 cup kale leaves, trimmed and finely chopped
- 1 cup onion, chopped
- 1 (4-ounces) can chopped green chilies
- 2 garlic cloves, minced
- 1 egg, beaten
- ½ cup fresh breadcrumbs
- 1 cup Monterey Jack cheese, grated
- ¼ cup salsa verde
- 3 tablespoons chopped fresh cilantro
- 1 teaspoon red chili powder
- ½ teaspoon ground cumin
- ½ teaspoon dried oregano, crushed
- Salt and ground black pepper, as required

## Instructions

1. In a deep bowl, put all the ingredients and with your hands, mix until well combined.
2. Divide the turkey mixture into 4 equal-sized portions and shape each into a mini loaf.
3. Set the temperature of air fryer to 400 degrees F. Grease an air fryer basket.
4. Arrange loaves into the prepared air fryer basket.
5. Air fry for about 20 minutes.
6. Remove from air fryer and place the loaves onto plates for about 5 minutes before serving.
7. Serve warm.

## Nutrition Values (Per Serving)

- Calories: 435
- Carbohydrate: 18.1g
- Protein: 42.2g
- Fat: 23.1g
- Sugar: 3.6g
- Sodium: 641mg

# Buttered Duck Breasts

**(Yields:** 4 servings / **Prep Time:** 15 minutes / **Cooking Time:** 22 minutes)

## Ingredients

- 2 (12-ounces) duck breasts
- Salt and ground black pepper, as required
- 3 tablespoons unsalted butter, melted
- ½ teaspoon dried thyme, crushed
- ¼ teaspoon star anise powder

## Instructions

1. With a sharp knife, score the fat of duck breasts several times.
2. Season the duck breasts generously with salt and black pepper.
3. Set the temperature of Air Fryer to 390 degrees F. Grease an Air Fryer basket.
4. Arrange duck breasts into the prepared Air Fryer basket.
5. Air Fry for about 10 minutes.
6. Remove duck breasts from the basket and coat with melted butter and sprinkle with thyme and star anise powder.
7. Place duck breasts into the Air Fryer basket for the second time.
8. Air Fry for about 12 more minutes.
9. Remove from Air Fryer and place the duck breasts onto a cutting board for about 5-10 minutes before slicing.
10. Using a sharp knife, cut each duck breast into desired size slices and serve.

## Nutrition Values (Per Serving)

- Calories: 296
- Carbohydrate: 0.1g
- Protein: 37.5g
- Fat: 15.5g
- Sugar: 0g
- Sodium: 100mg

# Beer Coated Duck Breast

**(Yields:** 2 servings / **Prep Time:** 15 minutes / **Cooking Time:** 20 minutes)

## Ingredients

- 1 tablespoon olive oil
- 1 teaspoon mustard
- 1 tablespoon fresh thyme, chopped
- 1 cup beer
- Salt and ground black pepper, as required
- 1 (10½-ounces) duck breast
- 6 cherry tomatoes
- 1 tablespoon balsamic vinegar

## Instructions

1. In a bowl, mix together the oil, mustard, thyme, beer, salt, and black pepper.
2. Add the duck breast and generously coat with marinade.
3. Cover and refrigerate for about 4 hours.
4. Set the temperature of Air Fryer to 390 degrees F.
5. With a piece of foil, cover the duck breast and arrange into an Air Fryer basket.
6. Air Fry for about 15 minutes.
7. Remove the foil from breast.
8. Now, set the temperature of Air Fryer to 355 degrees F. Grease the Air Fryer basket.
9. Place duck breast and tomatoes into the prepared Air Fryer basket.
10. Air Fry for about 5 minutes.
11. Remove from Air Fryer and place the duck breast onto a cutting board for about 5 minutes before slicing.
12. With a sharp knife, cut the duck breast into desired size slices and transfer onto serving plates.
13. Drizzle with vinegar and serve alongside the cherry tomatoes.

## Nutrition Values (Per Serving)

- Calories: 332
- Carbohydrate: 9.2g
- Protein: 34.6g
- Fat: 13.7g
- Sugar: 2.5g
- Sodium: 88mg

# Duck Breast with Figs

**(Yields:** 2 servings / **Prep Time:** 20 minutes / **Cooking Time:** 45 minutes)

## Ingredients

- 2 cups fresh pomegranate juice
- 2 tablespoons lemon juice
- 3 tablespoons brown sugar
- 1 pound boneless duck breast
- 6 fresh figs, halved
- 1 teaspoon olive oil
- Salt and ground black pepper, as required
- 1 tablespoon fresh thyme, chopped

## Instructions

1. In a medium saucepan, add the pomegranate juice, lemon juice, and brown sugar over medium heat and bring to a boil.
2. Now, lower the heat to low and cook for about 25 minutes until the mixture becomes thick.
3. Remove the pan from heat and let it cool slightly.
4. Set the temperature of Air Fryer to 400 degrees F. Grease an Air Fryer basket.
5. Score the fat of duck breasts several times using a sharp knife.
6. Sprinkle the duck breast with salt and black pepper.
7. Arrange duck breast into the prepared Air Fryer basket, skin side up.
8. Air Fry for about 14 minutes, flipping once halfway through.
9. Remove from Air Fryer and place the duck breast onto a cutting board for about 5-10 minutes.
10. Meanwhile, in a bowl, add the figs, oil, salt, and black pepper and toss to coat well.
11. Once again, set the temperature of Air Fryer to 400 degrees F. Grease the Air Fryer basket.
12. Arrange figs into the prepared basket in a single layer.
13. Air Fry for about 5 minutes.
14. Using a sharp knife, cut the duck breast into desired size slices and transfer onto serving plates alongside the roasted figs.
15. Drizzle with warm pomegranate juice mixture and serve with the garnishing of fresh thyme.

## Nutrition Values (Per Serving)

- Calories: 669
- Carbohydrate: 90g
- Protein: 519g
- Fat: 12.1g
- Sugar: 74g
- Sodium: 110mg

# Herbed Duck Legs

(**Yields:** 2 servings / **Prep Time:** 10 minutes / **Cooking Time:** 30 minutes)

## Ingredients

- 1 garlic clove, minced
- ½ tablespoon fresh thyme, chopped
- ½ tablespoon fresh parsley, chopped
- 1 teaspoon five spice powder
- Salt and ground black pepper, as required
- 2 duck legs

## Instructions

1. Set the temperature of air fryer to 340 degrees F. Grease an air fryer basket.
2. In a bowl, mix together the garlic, herbs, five spice powder, salt, and black pepper.
3. Generously rub the duck legs with garlic mixture.
4. Arrange duck legs into the prepared air fryer basket.
5. Air fry for about 25 minutes and then 5 more minutes at 390 degrees F.
6. Remove from air fryer and place the duck legs onto the serving platter.
7. Serve hot.

## Nutrition Values (Per Serving)

- Calories: 138
- Carbohydrate: 1g
- Protein: 25g
- Fat: 4.5g
- Sugar: 0g
- Sodium: 82mg

# CHAPTER 4 | BEEF, PORK AND LAMB

## Easy Rib Eye Steak

**(Yields:** 4 servings / **Prep Time:** 10 minutes / **Cooking Time:** 14 minutes)

### Ingredients

- 2 lbs. rib eye steak
- 1 tablespoon olive oil
- 1 tablespoon steak rub*

### Instructions

1. Set the temperature of air fryer to 400 degrees F. Grease an air fryer basket.
2. Coat the steak with oil and then, generously rub with steak rub.
3. Place steak into the prepared air fryer basket.
4. Air fry for about 14 minutes, flipping once halfway through.
5. Remove from air fryer and place the steak onto a cutting board for about 10 minutes before slicing.
6. Cut the steak into desired size slices and transfer onto serving plates.
7. Serve immediately.

### Nutrition Values (Per Serving)

- Calories: 438
- Carbohydrate: 0g
- Protein: 26.88g
- Fat: 35.8g
- Sugar: 0g
- Sodium: 157mg

(**Note: To prepare the Steak Rub*** - You can buy in your local store or on Amazon. You can also prepare at your home:

2 tbsp fresh cracked black pepper

2 tbsp kosher salt

2 tbsp paprika

1 tbsp crushed red pepper flakes

1 tbsp crushed coriander seeds (not ground)

1 tbsp garlic powder

1 tbsp onion powder

2 tsp cayenne pepper

Mix all ingredients in a medium bowl and stir well to combine.)

# Buttered Striploin Steak

**(Yields:** 2 servings / **Prep Time:** 10 minutes / **Cooking Time:** 12 minutes)

## Ingredients

- 2 (7-ounces) striploin steak
- 1½ tablespoons butter, softened
- Salt and ground black pepper, as required

## Instructions

1. Coat each steak evenly with butter and then, season with salt and black pepper.
2. Set the temperature of air fryer to 392 degrees F. Grease an air fryer basket.
3. Arrange steaks into the prepared air fryer basket.
4. Air fry for about 8-12 minutes.
5. Remove from air fryer and transfer the steaks onto serving plates.
6. Serve hot.

## Nutrition Values (Per Serving)

- Calories: 595
- Carbohydrate: 0g
- Protein: 58.1g
- Fat: 37.6g
- Sugar: 0g
- Sodium: 452mg

---

# Simple New York Strip Steak

**(Yields:** 2 servings / **Prep Time:** 10 minutes / **Cooking Time:** 8 minutes)

## Ingredients

- 1 (9½-ounces) New York strip steak
- Kosher salt and ground black pepper, as required
- 1 teaspoon olive oil

## Instructions

1. Set the temperature of air fryer to 400 degrees F. Grease an air fryer basket.
2. Coat the steak with oil and then, generously season with salt and black pepper.
3. Place steak into the prepared air fryer basket.
4. Air fry for about 7-8 minutes or until desired doneness.
5. Remove from air fryer and place the steak onto a cutting board for about 10 minutes before slicing.
6. Cut the steak into desired size slices and transfer onto serving plates.
7. Serve immediately.

### Nutrition Values (Per Serving)
- Calories: 186
- Carbohydrate: 0g
- Protein: 30.2g
- Fat: 7g
- Sugar: 0g
- Sodium: 177mg

---

## Crispy Sirloin Steak

**(Yields:** 2 servings / **Prep Time:** 15 minutes / **Cooking Time:** 10 minutes)

### Ingredients
- 1 cup white flour
- 2 eggs
- 1 cup panko breadcrumbs
- 1 teaspoon garlic powder
- 1 teaspoon onion powder
- Salt and ground black pepper, as required
- 2 (6-ounces) sirloin steaks, pounded

### Instructions
1. In a shallow bowl, place the flour.
2. Crack the eggs in a second bowl and beat well.
3. In a third bowl, mix together the panko and spices.
4. Coat each steak with the white flour, then dip into beaten eggs and finally, coat with panko mixture.
5. Set the temperature of air fryer to 360 degrees F. Grease an air fryer basket.
6. Arrange steaks into the prepared air fryer basket.
7. Air fry for about 10 minutes.
8. Remove from air fryer and transfer the steaks onto the serving plates.
9. Serve immediately.

### Nutrition Values (Per Serving)
- Calories: 561
- Carbohydrate: 6.1g
- Protein: 31.9g
- Fat: 50.3g
- Sugar: 0.6g
- Sodium: 100mg

# Spiced & Herbed Skirt Steak

(**Yields:** 4 servings / **Prep Time:** 15 minutes / **Cooking Time:** 10 minutes)

## Ingredients

- 3 garlic cloves, minced
- 1 cup fresh parsley leaves, finely chopped
- 3 tablespoons fresh oregano, finely chopped
- 3 tablespoons fresh mint leaves, finely chopped
- 1 tablespoon ground cumin
- 2 teaspoons smoked paprika
- 1 teaspoon cayenne pepper
- 1 teaspoon red pepper flakes, crushed
- Salt and ground black pepper, as required
- ¾ cup olive oil
- 3 tablespoons red wine vinegar
- 2 (8-ounces) skirt steaks

## Instructions

1. In a bowl, mix together the garlic, herbs, spices, oil, and vinegar.
2. In a resealable bag, place ¼ cup of the herb mixture and steaks.
3. Seal the bag and shake to coat well.
4. Refrigerate for about 24 hours.
5. Reserve the remaining herb mixture in refrigerator.
6. Take out the steaks from fridge and place at room temperature for about 30 minutes.
7. Set the temperature of air fryer to 390 degrees F. Grease an air fryer basket.
8. Arrange steaks into the prepared air fryer basket.
9. Air fry for about 8-10 minutes.
10. Remove from air fryer and place the steaks onto a cutting board for about 10 minutes before slicing.
11. Cut each steak into desired size slices and transfer onto serving platter.
12. Top with reserved herb mixture and serve.

## Nutrition Values (Per Serving)

- Calories: 561
- Carbohydrate: 6.1g
- Protein: 31.9g
- Fat: 50.3g
- Sugar: 0.6g
- Sodium: 100mg

# Skirt Steak with Veggies

**(Yields:** 4 servings / **Prep Time:** 15 minutes / **Cooking Time:** 6 minutes)

## Ingredients

- ¼ cup olive oil, divided
- 2 tablespoons soy sauce
- 2 tablespoons honey
- 1 (12-ounces) skirt steak, cut into thin strips
- ½ pound fresh mushrooms, quartered
- 6 ounces snow peas
- 1 onion, cut into half rings
- Salt and ground black pepper, as required

## Instructions

1. In a bowl, mix together 2 tablespoons of oil, soy sauce, and honey.
2. Add the steak strips and generously coat with the oil mixture.
3. In another bowl, add the vegetables, remaining oil, salt, and black pepper. Toss to coat well.
4. Set the temperature of air fryer to 390 degrees F. Grease an air fryer basket.
5. Arrange steak strips and vegetables into the prepared air fryer basket.
6. Air fry for about 5-6 minutes or until desired doneness.
7. Remove from air fryer and place the steak onto a cutting board for about 10 minutes before slicing.
8. Cut each steak into desired size slices and transfer onto serving plates.
9. Serve immediately alongside the veggies.

## Nutrition Values (Per Serving)

- Calories: 360
- Carbohydrate: 16.7g
- Protein: 26.7g
- Fat: 21.5g
- Sugar: 12.6g
- Sodium: 522mg

# Steak with Bell Peppers

**(Yields:** 4 servings / **Prep Time:** 20 minutes / **Cooking Time:** 22 minutes)

## Ingredients

- 1 teaspoon dried oregano, crushed
- 1 teaspoon onion powder
- 1 teaspoon garlic powder
- 1 teaspoon red chili powder
- 1 teaspoon paprika
- Salt, to taste
- 1¼ pounds beef steak, cut into thin strips
- 2 green bell peppers, seeded and cubed
- 1 red bell pepper, seeded and cubed
- 1 red onion, sliced
- 2 tablespoons olive oil

## Instructions

1. In a large bowl, mix together the oregano and spices.
2. Add the beef strips, bell peppers, onion, and oil. Mix until well combined.
3. Set the temperature of air fryer to 390 degrees F. Grease an air fryer basket.
4. Arrange steak strips mixture into the prepared Air Fryer basket in 2 batches.
5. Air Fry for about 10-11 minutes or until done completely.
6. Remove from air fryer and transfer the steak mixture onto serving plates.
7. Serve immediately.

## Nutrition Values (Per Serving)

- Calories: 372
- Carbohydrate: 11.2g
- Protein: 44.6g
- Fat: 16.3g
- Sugar: 6.2g
- Sodium: 143mg

# Buttered Filet Mignon

**(Yields:** 4 servings / **Prep Time:** 10 minutes / **Cooking Time:** 14 minutes**)**

## Ingredients

- 2 (6-ounces) filet mignon steaks
- 1 tablespoon butter, softened
- Salt and ground black pepper, as required

## Instructions

1. Coat each steak evenly with butter and then, season with salt and black pepper.
2. Set the temperature of air fryer to 390 degrees F. Grease an air fryer basket.
3. Arrange steaks into the prepared air fryer basket.
4. Air fry for about 14 minutes, flipping once halfway through.
5. Remove from the air fryer and transfer onto serving plates.
6. Serve hot.

## Nutrition Values (Per Serving)

- Calories: 403
- Carbohydrate: 0g
- Protein: 48.7g
- Fat: 22g
- Sugar: 0g
- Sodium: 228mg

# Bacon Wrapped Filet Mignon

**(Yields:** 2 servings / **Prep Time:** 15 minutes / **Cooking Time:** 15 minutes**)**

## Ingredients

- 2 bacon slices
- 2 (6-ounces) filet mignon steaks
- Salt and ground black pepper, as required
- 1 teaspoon avocado oil

## Instructions

1. Wrap 1 bacon slice around each mignon steak and secure with a toothpick.
2. Season the steak evenly with salt and black pepper.
3. Then, coat each steak with avocado oil.
4. Set the temperature of air fryer to 375 degrees F. Grease an air fryer basket.
5. Arrange steaks into the prepared air fryer basket.
6. Air fry for about 15 minutes, flipping once halfway through.

7. Remove from air fryer and transfer the steaks onto serving plates.
8. Serve hot.

## Nutrition Values (Per Serving)
- Calories: 512
- Carbohydrate: 0.5g
- Protein: 59.4g
- Fat: 28.6g
- Sugar: 0g
- Sodium: 857mg

## Beef Short Ribs

**(Yields:** 8 servings / **Prep Time:** 15 minutes / **Cooking Time:** 16 minutes)

## Ingredients
- 4 pounds bone-in beef short ribs
- 1/3 cup scallions, chopped
- 1 tablespoon fresh ginger, finely grated
- 1 cup low-sodium soy sauce
- ½ cup rice vinegar
- 1 tablespoon Sriracha
- 2 tablespoons brown sugar
- 1 teaspoon ground black pepper

## Instructions
1. In a resealable bag, put the ribs and all the above ingredients.
2. Seal the bag and shake to coat well.
3. Refrigerate overnight.
4. Set the temperature of air fryer to 380 degrees F. Grease an air fryer basket.
5. Take out the short ribs from resealable bag and arrange into the prepared air fryer basket in 2 batches in a single layer.
6. Air Fry for about 8 minutes, flipping once halfway through.
7. Remove from air fryer and transfer onto a serving platter.
8. Serve hot.

## Nutrition Values (Per Serving)
- Calories: 507
- Carbohydrate: 6.3g
- Protein: 67.3g
- Fat: 20.5g
- Sugar: 2.8g
- Sodium: 1200mg

# Herbed Beef Roast

**(Yields:** 5 servings / **Prep Time:** 10 minutes / **Cooking Time:** 45 minutes)

## Ingredients

- 2 pounds beef roast
- 1 tablespoon olive oil
- 1 teaspoon dried rosemary, crushed
- 1 teaspoon dried thyme, crushed
- Salt, as required

## Instructions

1. In a bowl, mix together the oil, herbs, and salt.
2. Generously coat the roast with herb mixture.
3. Set the temperature of air fryer to 360 degrees F. Grease an air fryer basket.
4. Arrange roast into the prepared air fryer basket.
5. Air fry for about 45 minutes.
6. Remove from air fryer and transfer the roast onto a platter.
7. With a piece of foil, cover the roast for about 10 minutes before slicing.
8. Cut the roast into desired size slices and serve.

## Nutrition Values (Per Serving)

- Calories: 362
- Carbohydrate: 0.3g
- Protein: 55.1g
- Fat: 14.2g
- Sugar: 0g
- Sodium: 151mg

---

# Beef Roast

**(Yields:** 6 servings / **Prep Time:** 10 minutes / **Cooking Time:** 50 minutes)

## Ingredients

- 2½ pounds beef eye of round roast, trimmed
- 2 tablespoons olive oil
- ½ teaspoon onion powder
- ½ teaspoon garlic powder
- ½ teaspoon cayenne pepper
- ½ teaspoon ground black pepper
- Salt, to taste

## Instructions

1. In a bowl, mix together the oil, and spices.
2. Generously coat the roast with spice mixture.
3. Set the temperature of air fryer to 360 degrees F. Grease an air fryer basket.
4. Arrange roast into the prepared air fryer basket.
5. Air fry for about 50 minutes.
6. Remove from air fryer and transfer the roast onto a platter.
7. With a piece of foil, cover the roast for about 10 minutes before slicing.
8. Cut the roast into desired size slices and serve.

## Nutrition Values (Per Serving)

- Calories: 397
- Carbohydrate: 0.5g
- Protein: 55.5g
- Fat: 12.4g
- Sugar: 0.2g
- Sodium: 99mg

---

# Beef Tips with Onion

**(Yields:** 2 servings / **Prep Time:** 15 minutes / **Cooking Time:** 10 minutes)

## Ingredients

- 1 pound top round beef, cut into 1½-inch cubes
- ½ yellow onion, chopped
- 2 tablespoons Worcestershire sauce
- 1 tablespoon avocado oil
- 1 teaspoon onion powder
- 1 teaspoon garlic powder
- Salt and ground black pepper, as required

## Instructions

1. In a bowl, mix together the beef tips, onion, Worcestershire sauce, oil, and spices.
2. Set the temperature of Air Fryer to 360 degrees F. Grease an Air Fryer basket.
3. Arrange beef mixture into the prepared Air Fryer basket.
4. Air Fry for about 8-10 minutes.
5. Remove from Air Fryer and transfer the steak mixture onto serving plates.
6. Serve hot.

## Nutrition Values (Per Serving)

- Calories: 266
- Carbohydrate: 4g
- Protein: 36.3g
- Fat: 10.5g
- Sugar: 2.5g
- Sodium: 192mg

# Buttered Rib Eye Steak

**(Yields:** 2 servings / **Prep Time:** 20 minutes / **Cooking Time:** 14 minutes)

## Ingredients

- ½ cup unsalted butter, softened
- 2 tablespoons fresh parsley, chopped
- 2 teaspoons garlic, minced
- 1 teaspoon Worcestershire sauce
- Salt, as required
- 2 (8-ounces) rib eye steak
- Ground black pepper, as required
- 1 tablespoon olive oil

## Instructions

1. In a bowl, add the butter, parsley, garlic, Worcestershire sauce, and salt. Mix until well combined.
2. Place the butter mixture onto a parchment paper and roll into a log.
3. Refrigerate until using.
4. Coat the steak evenly with oil and then, sprinkle with salt and black pepper.
5. Set the temperature of air fryer to 400 degrees F. Grease an air fryer basket.
6. Arrange steaks into the prepared air fryer basket.
7. Air fry for about 14 minutes, flipping once halfway through.
8. Remove from air fryer and place the steaks onto a platter for about 5 minutes.
9. Cut each steak into desired size slices and divide onto serving plates.
10. Now, cut the butter log into slices.
11. Top each steak with butter slices and serve.

## Nutrition Values (Per Serving)

- Calories: 731
- Carbohydrate: 1.2g
- Protein: 27.3g
- Fat: 68.8g
- Sugar: 0.4g
- Sodium: 375mg

# Beef Jerky

**(Yields:** 3 servings / **Prep Time:** 20 minutes / **Cooking Time:** 1 hour)

## Ingredients

- ½ cup dark brown sugar
- ½ cup soy sauce
- ¼ cup Worcestershire sauce
- 1 tablespoon chili pepper sauce
- 1 tablespoon hickory liquid smoke
- 1 teaspoon garlic powder
- 1 teaspoon onion powder
- 1 teaspoon cayenne pepper
- ½ teaspoon smoked paprika
- ½ teaspoon ground black pepper
- 1 pound bottom round beef, cut into thin strips

## Instructions

1. In a large bowl, mix together the brown sugar, all sauces, liquid smoke, and spices.
2. Add the beef strips and generously coat with marinade.
3. Cover the bowl and marinate overnight.
4. Set the temperature of Air Fryer to 180 degrees F. Lightly, grease an Air Fryer basket.
5. Remove the beef strips from fridge and with paper towels, pat them dry.
6. Arrange half of the beef strips in the bottom of prepared Air Fryer basket in a single layer.
7. Now, arrange a cooking rack over the strips.
8. Place the remaining beef strips on top of the rack in a single layer.
9. Air Fry for about 1 hour.
10. Remove from Air Fryer and arrange the strips onto a paper towel-lined baking sheet to cool completely before serving.

## Nutrition Values (Per Serving)

- Calories: 471
- Carbohydrate: 33.1g
- Protein: 48.7g
- Fat: 14.8g
- Sugar: 28.8g
- Sodium: 2000mg

# Beef & Veggie Kebabs

(**Yields:** 4 servings / **Prep Time:** 20 minutes / **Cooking Time:** 12 minutes)

## Ingredients

- ¼ cup soy sauce
- ¼ cup olive oil
- 1 tablespoon garlic, minced
- 1 teaspoon brown sugar
- ½ teaspoon ground cumin
- Salt and ground black pepper, as required
- 1 pound sirloin steak, cut into-inch chunks
- 8 ounces baby Bella mushrooms, stems removed
- 1 large bell pepper, seeded and cut into 1-inch pieces
- 1 red onion, cut into 1-inch pieces

## Instructions

1. In a bowl, mix together the soy sauce, oil, garlic, brown sugar, cumin, salt, and black pepper.
2. Add the steak cubes and generously coat with marinade.
3. Refrigerate to marinate for about 30 minutes.
4. Thread the steak cubes, mushrooms, bell pepper, and onion onto metal skewers.
5. Set the temperature of Air Fryer to 390 degrees F. Grease an Air Fryer basket.
6. Arrange skewers into the prepared Air Fryer basket.
7. Air Fry for about 10-12 minutes, flipping once halfway through.
8. Remove from Air Fryer and transfer the kebabs onto a platter.
9. Serve hot.

## Nutrition Values (Per Serving)

- Calories: 369
- Carbohydrate: 10.5g
- Protein: 37.6g
- Fat: 20g
- Sugar: 4.7g
- Sodium: 1018mg

# Beef Stuffed Bell Peppers

(**Yields:** 4 servings / **Prep Time:** 20 minutes / **Cooking Time:** 26 minutes)

## Ingredients

- 1 teaspoon olive oil
- ½ medium onion, chopped
- 2 garlic cloves, minced
- 1 pound lean ground beef
- 1 teaspoon dried basil, crushed
- 1 teaspoon garlic salt
- ½ teaspoon red chili powder
- Ground black pepper, as required
- ½ cup cooked jasmine rice
- 2/3 cup light Mexican cheese, shredded and divided
- 8 ounces tomato sauce, divided
- 2 teaspoons Worcestershire sauce
- 4 bell peppers, tops removed and seeded

## Instructions

1. In a medium-sized skillet, heat oil over medium heat and sauté the onion and garlic for about 3-5 minutes or until cooked thoroughly.
2. Add the ground beef, basil, and spices. Cook for about 8-10 minutes.
3. Remove the skillet from heat and drain off the excess grease from skillet.
4. Add the rice, half of the cheese, 2/3 of the tomato sauce and Worcestershire sauce and mix until well combined.
5. Stuff each bell pepper evenly with beef mixture.
6. Set the temperature of air fryer to 400 degrees F. Grease an air fryer basket.
7. Arrange bell peppers into the prepared air fryer basket.
8. Air fry for about 7 minutes.
9. Remove from air fryer and top each bell pepper with the remaining tomato sauce and cheese.
10. Air fry for about 4 more minutes.
11. Remove from air fryer and transfer the bell peppers onto a platter.
12. Serve warm.

## Nutrition Values (Per Serving)

- Calories: 439
- Carbohydrate: 34.4g
- Protein: 11.3g
- Fat: 3.1g
- Sugar: 1.6g
- Sodium: 160mg

# Smoky Beef Burgers

**(Yields:** 4 servings / **Prep Time:** 20 minutes / **Cooking Time:** 10 minutes)

## Ingredients

- 1 pound ground beef
- 1 tablespoon Worcestershire sauce
- 1 teaspoon Maggi seasoning sauce*
- 3-4 drops liquid smoke
- 1 teaspoon dried parsley
- ½ teaspoon garlic powder
- ½ teaspoon onion powder
- Salt and ground black pepper, as required
- Olive oil cooking spray
- 4 whole-wheat hamburger buns, split and toasted

## Instructions

1. In a large bowl, mix together the beef, sauces, liquid smoke, parsley, and spices.
2. Make 4 equal-sized patties from the mixture.
3. Set the temperature of Air Fryer to 350 degrees F. Grease an Air Fryer pan.
4. Arrange patties into the prepared pan in a single layer.
5. Using your thumb, make an indent in the center of each patty and spray with cooking spray.
6. Air Fry for about 10 minutes.
7. Remove patties from the Air Fryer.
8. Serve hot on a bun with your favorite side dishes.

## Nutrition Values (Per Serving)

- Calories: 316
- Carbohydrate: 20.4g
- Protein: 37.8g
- Fat: 8.8g
- Sugar: 4.4g
- Sodium: 384mg

(**Note: Maggi Seasoning Sauce*** - The ingredients in the Swiss version are: Water, salt, hydrolysed soya protein, Sodium glutamate, Disodium inosinate (E631), Yeast extract, Citric acid, acetic acid, wheat and "aroma."

Maggi seasoning sauce can be substituted with equal parts dark soy sauce and Worcestershire sauce.)

# Beef Cheeseburgers

**(Yields:** 2 servings / **Prep Time:** 15 minutes / **Cooking Time:** 12 minutes)

## Ingredients

- ½ pound ground beef
- 1 garlic clove, minced
- 2 tablespoons fresh cilantro, minced
- Salt and ground black pepper, as required
- 2 slices cheddar cheese
- 2 salad leaves
- 2 dinner rolls, cut into half

## Instructions

1. In a bowl, mix together the beef, garlic, cilantro, salt, and black pepper.
2. Make 2 (4-inch) patties from the mixture.
3. Set the temperature of air fryer to 390 degrees F. Grease an air fryer pan.
4. Arrange patties into the prepared pan in a single layer.
5. Air fry for about 10-11 minutes.
6. Place 1 cheese slice over each patty and air fry for about 1 more minute.
7. Remove patties from the air fryer.
8. Arrange salad leaf between each dinner roll and top with 1 patty.
9. Serve immediately.

## Nutrition Values (Per Serving)

- Calories: 773
- Carbohydrate: 45g
- Protein: 50.8g
- Fat: 42.9g
- Sugar: 4.9g
- Sodium: 710mg

---

# Cheesy Beef Meatballs

**(Yields:** 8 servings / **Prep Time:** 20 minutes / **Cooking Time:** 34 minutes)

## Ingredients

- 2 pounds ground beef
- 1¼ cups breadcrumbs
- ¼ cup Parmigiana-Reggiano cheese, grated
- 2 large eggs
- ¼ cup fresh parsley, chopped
- 1 small garlic clove, chopped
- 1 teaspoon dried oregano, crushed
- Salt and ground black pepper, as required

## Instructions

1. Add all the ingredients in a bowl and with your hands, mix until well combined.
2. Gently shape the mixture into 2-inches balls.
3. Set the temperature of Air Fryer to 350 degrees F. Line an Air Fryer basket with greased paper towels.
4. Arrange meatballs into the prepared Air Fryer basket in a single layer in 2 batches.
5. Air Fry for about 10-12 minutes.
6. Flip the side and Air Fry for extra 4-5 minutes.
7. Remove from Air Fryer and transfer the meatballs onto a serving platter.
8. Serve warm.

## Nutrition Values (Per Serving)

- Calories: 307
- Carbohydrate: 12.4g
- Protein: 39.3g
- Fat: 10.4g
- Sugar: 1.2g
- Sodium: 251mg

---

# Beef & Mushroom Meatloaf

(**Yields:** 4 servings / **Prep Time:** 15 minutes / **Cooking Time:** 25 minutes)

## Ingredients

- 1 pound lean ground beef
- 1 small onion, finely chopped
- 1 tablespoon fresh thyme, finely chopped
- 3 tablespoons dry breadcrumbs
- 1 egg, lightly beaten
- Salt and ground black pepper, as required
- 2 mushrooms, thickly sliced
- 1 tablespoon olive oil

## Instructions

1. In a bowl, add the beef, onion, thyme, breadcrumbs, egg, salt, and black pepper. With your hands, mix until well combined.
2. Put the beef mixture into a lightly greased baking pan and with the back of spoon, smooth the top surface.
3. Arrange the mushroom slices on top and gently, press each inside the meatloaf.
4. Coat the meatloaf with oil.
5. Set the temperature of Air Fryer to 392 degrees F.
6. Arrange the pan of meatloaf into the Air Fryer basket.

7. Air Fry for about 25 minutes or until meatloaf becomes golden brown.
8. Remove from Air Fryer and place the pan onto a wire rack for about 10 minutes before serving.
9. Cut into desired size wedges and serve.

## Nutrition Values (Per Serving)

- Calories: 267
- Carbohydrate: 6.1g
- Protein: 37g
- Fat: 12g
- Sugar: 1.3g
- Sodium: 167mg

---

# Beef Taco Wraps

**(Yields:** 6 servings / **Prep Time:** 15 minutes / **Cooking Time:** 4 minutes)

## Ingredients

- 6 (12-inch) flour tortillas
- 2 pounds cooked ground beef
- 12 ounces nacho cheese
- 6 tostadas
- 2 cups sour cream
- 2 cups Bibb lettuce, shredded
- 3 Roma tomatoes, sliced
- 2 cups Mexican blend cheese, shredded
- Olive oil cooking spray

## Instructions

1. Arrange the tortillas onto a smooth surface.
2. Divide each ingredient into 6 portions.
3. Place 1 portion of beef in the center of each tortilla, followed by the nacho cheese, tostada, sour cream, lettuce, tomato slices and Mexican cheese.
4. Bring the edges of each tortilla up, over the center to look like a pinwheel.
5. Set the temperature of Air Fryer to 400 degrees F. Grease an Air Fryer basket.
6. Arrange taco wraps into the prepared Air Fryer basket, seam side down and spray each with cooking spray.
7. Air Fry for about 2 minutes.
8. Carefully flip the wraps and spray each with cooking spray again.
9. Air Fry for about 2 more minutes.
10. Remove from Air Fryer and transfer the wraps onto a platter.
11. Serve warm.

## Nutrition Values (Per Serving)

- Calories: 930
- Carbohydrate: 41.6g
- Protein: 66.4g
- Fat: 55.6g
- Sugar: 4.6g
- Sodium: 1200mg

# Breaded Pork Chops

**(Yields:** 2 servings / **Prep Time:** 15 minutes / **Cooking Time:** 15 minutes)

## Ingredients

- 2 (6-ounces) pork chops
- Salt and ground black pepper, as required
- ¼ cup plain flour
- 1 egg
- 4 ounces breadcrumbs
- 1 tablespoon vegetable oil

## Instructions

1. Season each pork chop evenly with salt and pepper.
2. In a shallow bowl, place the flour
3. Crack the egg in a second bowl and beat well.
4. Add the breadcrumbs, and oil in a third bowl and mix until a crumbly mixture forms.
5. Coat the pork chop with flour, then dip into beaten egg and finally, coat with the breadcrumbs mixture.
6. Set the temperature of air fryer to 400 degrees F. Grease an air fryer basket.
7. Arrange chops into the prepared air fryer basket in a single layer.
8. Air fry for about 15 minutes, flipping once halfway through.
9. Remove from air fryer and transfer the chops onto plates.
10. Serve hot.

## Nutrition Values (Per Serving)

- Calories: 621
- Carbohydrate: 53.3g
- Protein: 43.9g
- Fat: 26.1g
- Sugar: 3.7g
- Sodium: 963mg

---

# Sweet & Sour Pork Chops

**(Yields:** 6 servings / **Prep Time:** 15 minutes / **Cooking Time:** 16 minutes)

## Ingredients

- 6 pork loin chops
- Salt and ground black pepper, as required
- 2 garlic cloves, minced
- 2 tablespoons honey
- 2 tablespoons soy sauce
- 1 tablespoon balsamic vinegar
- ¼ teaspoon ground ginger

## Instructions

1. With a meat tenderizer, tenderize the chops completely and then, sprinkle each with salt and black pepper.
2. In a large bowl, mix the remaining ingredients.
3. Add the chops and generously coat with marinade.
4. Cover and refrigerate for about 2-8 hours.
5. Set the temperature of air fryer to 355 degrees F. Grease an air fryer basket.
6. Arrange chops into the prepared air fryer basket in a single layer.
7. Air fry for about 6-8 minutes per side.
8. Remove from air fryer and transfer the chops onto plates.
9. Serve hot.

## Nutrition Values (Per Serving)

- Calories: 282
- Carbohydrate: 6.6g
- Protein: 18.4g
- Fat: 19.9g
- Sugar: 5.9g
- Sodium: 357mg

# Herbed Pork Chops

(**Yields:** 4 servings / **Prep Time:** 15 minutes / **Cooking Time:** 12 minutes)

## Ingredients

- 2 garlic cloves, minced
- ½ tablespoon fresh cilantro, chopped
- ½ tablespoon fresh rosemary, chopped
- ½ tablespoon fresh parsley, chopped
- 2 tablespoons olive oil
- ¾ tablespoon Dijon mustard
- 1 tablespoon ground coriander
- 1 teaspoon sugar
- Salt, to taste
- 2 (6-ounces) (1-inch thick) pork chops

## Instructions

1. In a bowl, mix together the garlic, herbs, oil, mustard, coriander, sugar, and salt.
2. Add the pork chops and generously coat with marinade.
3. Cover and refrigerate for about 2-3 hours.
4. Remove chops from the refrigerator and set aside at room temperature for about 30 minutes.
5. Set the temperature of air fryer to 390 degrees F. Grease an air fryer basket.
6. Arrange chops into the prepared air fryer basket in a single layer.
7. Air fry for about 10-12 minutes.

8. Remove from air fryer and transfer the chops onto plates.
9. Serve hot.

## **Nutrition Values (Per Serving)**

- Calories: 683
- Carbohydrate: 3.9g
- Protein: 38.8g
- Fat: 50.7g
- Sugar: 2.1g
- Sodium: 256mg

---

# **Pork Chops with Peanut Sauce**

(**Yields:** 4 servings / **Prep Time:** 20 minutes / **Cooking Time:** 12 minutes)

## **Ingredients**

**For Chops:**

- 1 teaspoon fresh ginger, minced
- 1 garlic clove, minced
- 2 tablespoons soy sauce
- 1 tablespoon olive oil
- 1 teaspoon hot pepper sauce
- 1-pound boneless pork chop, cubed into 1-inch size

**For Peanut Sauce:**

- 1 tablespoon olive oil
- 1 shallot, finely chopped
- 1 garlic clove, minced
- 1 teaspoon ground coriander
- ¾ cup ground peanuts
- 1 teaspoon hot pepper sauce
- ¾ cup coconut milk

## **Instructions**

1. For pork: in a bowl, mix together the ginger, garlic, soy sauce, oil, and hot pepper sauce.
2. Add the pork chops and generously coat with mixture.
3. Place at the room temperature for about 15 minutes.
4. Set the temperature of air fryer to 390 degrees F. Grease an air fryer basket.
5. Arrange chops into the prepared air fryer basket in a single layer.
6. Air fry for about 12 minutes.
7. Meanwhile, for the sauce: in a pan, heat oil over medium heat and sauté the shallot and garlic for about 2-3 minutes.
8. Add the coriander and sauté for about 1 minute.
9. Stir in the remaining ingredients and cook for about 5 minutes, stirring continuously.
10. Remove the pan of sauce from heat and let it cool slightly.
11. Remove the chops from air fryer and transfer onto serving plates.
12. Serve immediately with the topping of peanut sauce.

### Nutrition Values (Per Serving)

- Calories: 725
- Carbohydrate: 9.5g
- Protein: 34.4g
- Fat: 62.9g
- Sugar: 2.8g
- Sodium: 543mg

---

## Pork Spare Ribs

**(Yields:** 6 servings / **Prep Time:** 15 minutes / **Cooking Time:** 20 minutes)

### Ingredients

- 5-6 garlic cloves, minced
- ½ cup rice vinegar
- 2 tablespoons soy sauce
- Salt and ground black pepper, as required
- 12 (1-inch) pork spare ribs
- ½ cup cornstarch
- 2 tablespoons olive oil

### Instructions

1. In a large bowl, mix together the garlic, vinegar, soy sauce, salt, and black pepper.
2. Add the ribs and generously coat with mixture.
3. Refrigerate to marinate overnight.
4. In a shallow bowl, place the cornstarch.
5. Coat the ribs evenly with cornstarch and then, drizzle with oil.
6. Set the temperature of air fryer to 390 degrees F. Grease an air fryer basket.
7. Arrange ribs into the prepared air fryer basket in a single layer.
8. Air fry for about 10 minutes per side.
9. Remove from air fryer and transfer the ribs onto serving plates.
10. Serve immediately.

### Nutrition Values (Per Serving)

- Calories: 557
- Carbohydrate: 11g
- Protein: 35g
- Fat: 51.3g
- Sugar: 0.1g
- Sodium: 997mg

# BBQ Pork Ribs

**(Yields:** 4 servings / **Prep Time:** 15 minutes / **Cooking Time:** 26 minutes)

## Ingredients

- ¼ cup honey, divided
- ¾ cup BBQ sauce
- 2 tablespoons tomato ketchup
- 1 tablespoon Worcestershire sauce*
- 1 tablespoon soy sauce
- ½ teaspoon garlic powder
- Freshly ground white pepper, to taste
- 1¾ pounds pork ribs

## Instructions

1. In a bowl, mix together 3 tablespoons of honey and the remaining ingredients except pork ribs.
2. Add the pork ribs and generously coat with the mixture.
3. Refrigerate to marinate for about 20 minutes.
4. Set the temperature of air fryer to 355 degrees F. Grease an air fryer basket
5. Arrange ribs into the prepared air fryer basket in a single layer.
6. Air fry for about 13 minutes per side.
7. Remove from air fryer and transfer the ribs onto plates.
8. Drizzle with the remaining honey and serve immediately.

## Nutrition Values (Per Serving)

- Calories: 691
- Carbohydrate: 37.7g
- Protein: 53.1g
- Fat: 31.3g
- Sugar: 32.2g
- Sodium: 991mg

(**Note - Worcestershire sauce*** - The other ingredients that make up this savory sauce usually include onions, molasses, high fructose corn syrup (depending on the country of production), salt, garlic, tamarind, cloves, chili pepper extract, water and natural flavorings.)

# Glazed Pork Shoulder

**(Yields:** 5 servings / **Prep Time:** 15 minutes / **Cooking Time:** 18 minutes)

## Ingredients

- 1/3 cup soy sauce
- 2 tablespoons sugar
- 1 tablespoon honey
- 2 pounds pork shoulder, cut into 1½-inch thick slices

## Instructions

1. In a bowl, mix together all the soy sauce, sugar, and honey.
2. Add the pork and generously coat with marinade.
3. Cover and refrigerate to marinate for about 4-6 hours.
4. Set the temperature of air fryer to 335 degrees F. Grease an air fryer basket.
5. Place pork shoulder into the prepared air fryer basket.
6. Air fry for about 10 minutes and then, another 6-8 minutes at 390 degrees F.
7. Remove from air fryer and transfer the pork shoulder onto a platter.
8. With a piece of foil, cover the pork for about 10 minutes before serving.
9. Enjoy!

## Nutrition Values (Per Serving)

- Calories: 475
- Carbohydrate: 8g
- Protein: 36.1g
- Fat: 32.4g
- Sugar: 7.1g
- Sodium: 165mg

---

# Pork Shoulder with Pineapple Sauce

**(Yields:** 3 servings / **Prep Time:** 20 minutes / **Cooking Time:** 24 minutes)

## Ingredients

### For Pork:

- 10½ ounces pork shoulder, cut into bite-sized pieces
- 2 pinches of Maggi seasoning
- 1 teaspoon light soy sauce
- Dash of sesame oil
- 1 egg
- ¼ cup plain flour

### For Sauce:

- 1 teaspoon olive oil
- 1 medium onion, sliced
- 1 tablespoon garlic, minced
- 1 large pineapple slice, cubed
- 1 medium tomato, chopped
- 2 tablespoons tomato sauce
- 2 tablespoons oyster sauce
- 1 tablespoon Worcestershire sauce
- 1 teaspoon sugar
- 1 tablespoon water
- ½ tablespoon corn flour

## Instructions

1. For pork: in a large bowl, mix together the Maggi seasoning, soy sauce, and sesame oil.
2. Add the pork cubes and generously mix with the mixture.
3. Refrigerate to marinate for about 4-6 hours.
4. In a shallow dish, beat the egg.
5. In another dish, place the plain flour.
6. Dip the cubed pork in beaten egg and then, coat evenly with the flour.
7. Set the temperature of air fryer to 248 degrees F. Grease an air fryer basket.
8. Arrange pork cubes into the prepared air fryer basket in a single layer.
9. Air fry for about 20 minutes.
10. Meanwhile, for the sauce: in a skillet, heat oil over medium heat and sauté the onion and garlic for about 1 minute.
11. Add the pineapple, and tomato and cook for about 1 minute.
12. Add the tomato sauce, oyster sauce, Worcestershire sauce, and sugar and stir to combine.
13. Meanwhile, in a bowl, mix together the water and corn flour.
14. Add the corn flour mixture into the sauce, stirring continuously.
15. Cook until the sauce is thicken enough, stirring continuously.
16. Remove pork cubes from air fryer and add into the sauce.
17. Cook for about 1-2 minutes or until coated completely.
18. Remove from the heat and serve hot.

## Nutrition Values (Per Serving)

- Calories: 557
- Carbohydrate: 57.5g
- Protein: 28.8g
- Fat: 25.1g
- Sugar: 35.1g
- Sodium: 544mg

(**Note:** If you don't have fresh pineapple in hands, then you can use canned pineapple. But remember to skip sugar from the sauce).

# Bacon Wrapped Pork tenderloin

**(Yields:** 4 servings / **Prep Time:** 15 minutes / **Cooking Time:** 30 minutes)

## Ingredients

- 1 (1½ pound) pork tenderloins
- 4 bacon strips
- 2 tablespoons Dijon mustard

## Instructions

1. Coat the tenderloin evenly with mustard.
2. Wrap the tenderloin with bacon strips.
3. Set the temperature of air fryer to 360 degrees F. Grease an air fryer basket.
4. Arrange pork tenderloin into the prepared air fryer basket.
5. Air fry for about 15 minutes.
6. Flip and air fry for another 10-15 minutes.
7. Remove from air fryer and transfer the pork tenderloin onto a platter, wait for about 5 minutes before slicing.
8. Cut the tenderloin into desired size slices and serve.

## Nutrition Values (Per Serving)

- Calories: 504
- Carbohydrate: 0.8g
- Protein: 61.9
- Fat: 26.2g
- Sugar: 9.1g
- Sodium: 867mg

---

# Pork Tenderloin with Bell Peppers

**(Yields:** 3 servings / **Prep Time:** 20 minutes / **Cooking Time:** 15 minutes)

## Ingredients

- 1 large red bell pepper, seeded and cut into thin strips
- 1 red onion, thinly sliced
- 2 teaspoons Herbs de Provence
- Salt and ground black pepper, as required
- 1 tablespoon olive oil
- 10½-ounces pork tenderloin, cut into 4 pieces
- ½ tablespoon Dijon mustard

### Instructions

1. In a bowl, add the bell pepper, onion, Herbs de Provence, salt, black pepper, and ½ tablespoon of oil and toss to coat well.
2. Rub the pork pieces with mustard, salt, and black pepper.
3. Drizzle with the remaining oil.
4. Set the temperature of air fryer to 390 degrees F. Grease an air fryer pan.
5. Place bell pepper mixture into the prepared Air Fryer pan and top with the pork pieces.
6. Air fry for about 15 minutes, flipping once halfway through.
7. Remove from air fryer and transfer the pork mixture onto serving plates.
8. Serve hot.

### Nutrition Values (Per Serving)

- Calories: 218
- Carbohydrate: 7.1g
- Protein: 27.7g
- Fat: 8.8g
- Sugar: 3.7g
- Sodium: 110mg

## Pork Tenderloin with Bacon & Veggies

(**Yields:** 3 servings / **Prep Time:** 20 minutes / **Cooking Time:** 28 minutes)

### Ingredients

- 3 potatoes
- ¾ pound frozen green beans
- 6 bacon slices
- 3 (6-ounces) pork tenderloins
- 2 tablespoons olive oil

### Instructions

1. Set the temperature of air fryer to 390 degrees F. Grease an air fryer basket.
2. With a fork, pierce the potatoes.
3. Place potatoes into the prepared air fryer basket and air fry for about 15 minutes.
4. Wrap one bacon slice around 4-6 green beans.
5. Coat the pork tenderloins with oil.
6. After 15 minutes, add the pork tenderloins into air fryer basket with potatoes and air fry for about 5-6 minutes.
7. Remove the pork tenderloins from basket.
8. Place bean rolls into the basket and top with the pork tenderloins.
9. Air fry for another 7 minutes.
10. Remove from air fryer and transfer the pork tenderloins onto a platter.
11. Cut each tenderloin into desired size slices.
12. Serve alongside the potatoes and green beans rolls.

### Nutrition Values (Per Serving)
- Calories: 918
- Carbohydrate: 42.4g
- Protein: 77.9g
- Fat: 47.7g
- Sugar: 4g
- Sodium: 1400mg

---

## Pork Loin with Potatoes

**(Yields:** 5 servings / **Prep Time:** 15 minutes / **Cooking Time:** 25 minutes)

### Ingredients
- 2 pounds pork loin
- 3 tablespoons olive oil, divided
- 1 teaspoon fresh parsley, chopped
- Salt and ground black pepper, as required
- 3 large red potatoes, chopped
- ½ teaspoon garlic powder
- ½ teaspoon red pepper flakes, crushed

### Instructions
1. Coat the pork loin with oil and then, season evenly with parsley, salt, and black pepper.
2. In a large bowl, add the potatoes, remaining oil, garlic powder, red pepper flakes, salt, and black pepper and toss to coat well.
3. Set the temperature of air fryer to 325 degrees F. Grease an air fryer basket.
4. Place loin into the prepared air fryer basket.
5. Arrange potato pieces around the pork loin.
6. Air fry for about 25 minutes.
7. Remove from air fryer and transfer the pork loin onto a platter, wait for about 5 minutes before slicing.
8. Cut the pork loin into desired size slices and serve alongside the potatoes.

### Nutrition Values (Per Serving)
- Calories: 556
- Carbohydrate: 29.6g
- Protein: 44.9g
- Fat: 28.3g
- Sugar: 1.9g
- Sodium: 132mg

# Pork Rolls

**(Yields:** 4 servings / **Prep Time:** 20 minutes / **Cooking Time:** 15 minutes)

## Ingredients

- 1 scallion, chopped
- ¼ cup sun-dried tomatoes, finely chopped
- 2 tablespoons fresh parsley, chopped
- Salt and ground black pepper, as required
- 4 (6-ounces) pork cutlets, pounded slightly
- 2 teaspoons paprika
- ½ tablespoon olive oil

## Instructions

1. In a bowl, mix well scallion, tomatoes, parsley, salt, and black pepper.
2. Spread the tomato mixture over each pork cutlet.
3. Roll each cutlet and secure with cocktail sticks.
4. Rub the outer part of rolls with paprika, salt and black pepper.
5. Coat the rolls evenly with oil.
6. Set the temperature of air fryer to 390 degrees F. Grease an air fryer basket.
7. Arrange pork rolls into the prepared air fryer basket in a single layer.
8. Air fry for about 15 minutes.
9. Remove from air fryer and transfer the pork rolls onto serving plates.
10. Serve hot.

## Nutrition Values (Per Serving)

- Calories: 244
- Carbohydrate: 14.5g
- Protein: 20.1g
- Fat: 8.2g
- Sugar: 1.7g
- Sodium: 708mg

---

# Pork Sausage Casserole

**(Yields:** 4 servings / **Prep Time:** 15 minutes / **Cooking Time:** 30 minutes)

## Ingredients

- 6 ounces flour, sifted
- 2 eggs
- 1 red onion, thinly sliced
- 1 garlic clove, minced
- Salt and ground black pepper, as required
- ¾ cup milk
- 2/3 cup cold water
- 8 small sausages
- 8 fresh rosemary sprigs

## Instructions

1. In a bowl, mix together the flour, and eggs.
2. Add the onion, garlic, salt, and black pepper. Mix them well.
3. Gently, add in the milk, and water and mix until well combined.
4. In each sausage, pierce 1 rosemary sprig.
5. Set the temperature of air fryer to 320 degrees F. Grease a baking dish.
6. Arrange sausages into the prepared baking dish and top evenly with the flour mixture.
7. Air fry for about 30 minutes.
8. Remove from the air fryer and serve warm.

## Nutrition Values (Per Serving)

- Calories: 334
- Carbohydrate: 37.7g
- Protein: 14g
- Fat: 14g
- Sugar: 3.5g
- Sodium: 250mg

---

# Pork Neck Salad

(**Yields:** 2 servings / **Prep Time:** 20 minutes / **Cooking Time:** 12 minutes)

## Ingredients

**For Pork:**

- 1 tablespoon soy sauce
- 1 tablespoon fish sauce
- ½ tablespoon oyster sauce
- ½ pound pork neck

**For Dressing:**

- 3 tablespoons fish sauce
- 2 tablespoons olive oil
- 1 teaspoon apple cider vinegar
- 1 tablespoon palm sugar
- 1 bird eye chili
- 1 tablespoon garlic, minced

**For Salad:**

- 1 ripe tomato, thickly sliced
- 1 red onion, sliced
- 1 scallion, chopped
- 1 bunch fresh basil leaves
- 1 bunch fresh cilantro leaves

### Instructions

1. For pork: in a bowl, mix together all the sauces.
2. Add the pork neck and generously coat with marinade.
3. Refrigerate for about 2-3 hours.
4. Set the temperature of air fryer to 340 degrees F. Grease an air fryer basket.
5. Place pork neck into the prepared basket.
6. Air fry for about 12 minutes.
7. Meanwhile, for the salad: in a serving bowl, mix together all the ingredients.
8. For dressing: in another bowl, add all the ingredients and beat until well combined.
9. Remove pork neck from air fryer and cut into desired size slices.
10. Place the pork slices over salad.
11. Add the dressing and toss to coat well.
12. Serve.

### Nutrition Values (Per Serving)

- Calories: 448
- Carbohydrate: 15.2g
- Protein: 20.5g
- Fat: 39.7g
- Sugar: 8.5g
- Sodium: 2000mg

---

# Glazed Ham

**(Yields:** 4 servings / **Prep Time:** 15 minutes / **Cooking Time:** 40 minutes)

### Ingredients

- 1 pound 10½ ounces ham
- 1 cup whiskey
- 2 tablespoons French mustard
- 2 tablespoons honey

### Instructions

1. Place the ham at room temperature for about 30 minutes before cooking.
2. In a bowl, mix together the whiskey, mustard, and honey.
3. Place the ham in a baking dish that fits in the air fryer.
4. Top with half of the honey mixture and coat well.
5. Set the temperature of air fryer to 320 degrees F. Place the baking dish into the air fryer.
6. Air fry for about 15 minutes.
7. Flip the side of ham and top with the remaining honey mixture.

8. Air fry for about 25 more minutes.
9. Remove from air fryer and place the ham onto a platter for about 10 minutes before slicing.
10. Cut the ham into desired size slices and serve.

## **Nutrition Values (Per Serving)**

- Calories: 558
- Carbohydrate: 18.6g
- Protein: 43g
- Fat: 22.2g
- Sugar: 8.7g
- Sodium: 3000mg

# **Simple Lamb Chops**

**(Yields:** 2 servings / **Prep Time:** 10 minutes / **Cooking Time:** 6 minutes)

## **Ingredients**

- 1 tablespoon olive oil
- Salt and ground black pepper, as required
- 4 (4-ounces) lamb chops

## **Instructions**

1. In a large bowl, mix together the oil, salt, and black pepper.
2. Add the chops and coat evenly with the mixture.
3. Set the temperature of air fryer to 390 degrees F. Grease an air fryer basket.
4. Arrange chops into the prepared air fryer basket in a single layer.
5. Air fry for about 5-6 minutes.
6. Remove from air fryer and transfer the chops onto plates.
7. Serve hot.

## **Nutrition Values (Per Serving)**

- Calories: 486
- Carbohydrate: 0.8g
- Protein: 63.8g
- Fat: 31.7g
- Sugar: 0g
- Sodium: 250mg

# Lamb Loin Chops with Lemon

**(Yields:** 4 servings / **Prep Time:** 15 minutes / **Cooking Time:** 30 minutes)

## Ingredients

- 2 tablespoons Dijon mustard
- 1 tablespoon fresh lemon juice
- ½ teaspoon olive oil
- 1 teaspoon dried tarragon
- Salt and ground black pepper, as required
- 8 (4-ounces) lamb loin chops

## Instructions

1. In a large bowl, mix together the mustard, lemon juice, oil, tarragon, salt, and black pepper.
2. Add chops and generously coat with the mixture.
3. Set the temperature of air fryer to 390 degrees F. Grease an air fryer basket.
4. Arrange chops into the prepared air fryer basket in a single layer in 2 batches.
5. Air fry for about 15 minutes, flipping once halfway through.
6. Remove the chops from air fryer and transfer onto serving plates.
7. Serve hot.

## Nutrition Values (Per Serving)

- Calories: 433
- Carbohydrate: 0.6g
- Protein: 64.1g
- Fat: 17.6g
- Sugar: 0.2g
- Sodium: 201mg

---

# Herbed Lamb Chops

**(Yields:** 2 servings / **Prep Time:** 10 minutes / **Cooking Time:** 7 minutes)

## Ingredients

- 1 tablespoon fresh lemon juice
- 1 tablespoon olive oil
- 1 teaspoon dried rosemary
- 1 teaspoon dried thyme
- 1 teaspoon dried oregano
- ½ teaspoon ground cumin
- ½ teaspoon ground coriander
- Salt and ground black pepper, as required
- 4 (4-ounces) lamb chops

## Instructions

1. In a large bowl, mix together the lemon juice, oil, herbs, and spices.
2. Add the chops and coat evenly with the herb mixture.

3. Refrigerate to marinate for about 1 hour
4. Set the temperature of air fryer to 390 degrees F. Grease an air fryer basket.
5. Arrange chops into the prepared air fryer basket in a single layer.
6. Air fry for about 7 minutes, flipping once halfway through.
7. Remove from air fryer and transfer the chops onto plates.
8. Serve hot.

## Nutrition Values (Per Serving)

- Calories: 491
- Carbohydrate: 1.6g
- Protein: 64g
- Fat: 24g
- Sugar: 0.2g
- Sodium: 253mg

# Lamb Loin Chops with Garlic

**(Yields:** 4 servings / **Prep Time:** 10 minutes / **Cooking Time:** 30 minutes)

## Ingredients

- 3 garlic cloves, crushed
- 1 tablespoon fresh lemon juice
- 1 teaspoon olive oil
- 1 tablespoon Za'atar*
- Kosher salt and ground black pepper, as required
- 8 (3½-ounces) bone-in lamb loin chops, trimmed

## Instructions

1. In a large bowl, mix together the garlic, lemon juice, oil, Za'atar, salt, and black pepper.
2. Add chops and generously coat with the mixture.
3. Set the temperature of air fryer to 400 degrees F. Grease an air fryer basket.
4. Arrange chops into the prepared air fryer basket in a single layer in 2 batches.
5. Air Fry for about 15 minutes, flipping once after 4-5 minutes per side.
6. Remove from air fryer and transfer the chops onto plates.
7. Serve hot.

## Nutrition Values (Per Serving)

- Calories: 433
- Carbohydrate: 0.6g
- Protein: 64.1g
- Fat: 17.6g
- Sugar: 0.2g
- Sodium: 201mg

(**Note: Za'atar\*** - Za'atar is generally made with ground dried thyme, oregano, marjoram, or some combination thereof, mixed with toasted sesame seeds, and salt, though other spices such as sumac might also be added. Some commercial varieties also include roasted flour.)

---

# Lamb Chops with Veggies

(**Yields:** 4 servings / **Prep Time:** 20 minutes / **Cooking Time:** 8 minutes)

## Ingredients

- 2 tablespoons fresh rosemary, minced
- 2 tablespoons fresh mint leaves, minced
- 1 garlic clove, minced
- 3 tablespoons olive oil
- Salt and ground black pepper, as required
- 4 (6-ounces) lamb chops
- 1 purple carrot, peeled and cubed
- 1 yellow carrot, peeled and cubed
- 1 parsnip, peeled and cubed
- 1 fennel bulb, cubed

## Instructions

1. In a large bowl, mix together the herbs, garlic, oil, salt, and black pepper.
2. Add the chops and generously coat with mixture.
3. Refrigerate to marinate for about 3 hours.
4. In a large pan of water, soak the vegetables for about 15 minutes.
5. Drain the vegetables completely.
6. Set the temperature of air fryer to 390 degrees F. Grease an air fryer basket.
7. Arrange chops into the prepared air fryer basket in a single layer.
8. Air Fry for about 2 minutes.
9. Remove chops from the air fryer.
10. Place vegetables into the air fryer basket and top with the chops in a single layer.
11. Air Fry for about 6 minutes.
12. Remove from air fryer and transfer the chops and vegetables onto serving plates.
13. Serve hot.

## Nutrition Values (Per Serving)

- Calories: 470
- Carbohydrate: 14.8g
- Protein: 49.4g
- Fat: 23.5g
- Sugar: 3.1g
- Sodium: 186mg

# Nut Crusted Rack of Lamb

**(Yields:** 5 servings / **Prep Time:** 15 minutes / **Cooking Time:** 35 minutes)

## Ingredients

- 1 tablespoon olive oil
- 1 garlic clove, minced
- Salt and ground black pepper, as required
- 1¾ pounds rack of lamb
- 1 egg
- 1 tablespoon breadcrumbs
- 3 ounces almonds, finely chopped

## Instructions

1. In a bowl, mix together the oil, garlic, salt, and black pepper.
2. Coat the rack of lamb evenly with oil mixture.
3. Crack the egg in a shallow bowl and beat well.
4. In another bowl, mix together the breadcrumbs and almonds.
5. Dip the rack of lamb in beaten egg and then, coat with almond mixture.
6. Set the temperature of air fryer to 220 degrees F. Grease an air fryer basket.
7. Place rack of lamb into the prepared air fryer basket.
8. Air fry for about 30 minutes and then 5 more minutes at 390 degrees F.
9. Remove from air fryer and place the rack of lamb onto a cutting board for about 5 minutes
10. With a sharp knife, cut the rack of lamb into individual chops and serve.

## Nutrition Values (Per Serving)

- Calories: 340
- Carbohydrate: 4.1g
- Protein: 31g
- Fat: 21.9g
- Sugar: 0.7g
- Sodium: 140mg

---

# Herbs Crumbed Rack of Lamb

**(Yields:** 5 servings / **Prep Time:** 20 minutes / **Cooking Time:** 30 minutes)

## Ingredients

- 1 tablespoon butter, melted
- 1 garlic clove, finely chopped
- 1¾ pounds rack of lamb
- Salt and ground black pepper, as required
- 1 egg
- ½ cup panko breadcrumbs
- 1 tablespoon fresh thyme, minced
- 1 tablespoon fresh rosemary, minced

## Instructions

1. In a bowl, mix together the butter, garlic, salt, and black pepper.
2. Coat the rack of lamb evenly with garlic mixture.
3. In a shallow dish, beat the egg.
4. In another dish, mix together the breadcrumbs and herbs.
5. Dip the rack of lamb in beaten egg and then, coat with breadcrumbs mixture.
6. Set the temperature of air fryer to 212 degrees F. Grease an air fryer basket.
7. Place rack of lamb into the prepared air fryer basket.
8. Air Fry for about 25 minutes and then 5 more minutes at 390 degrees F.
9. Remove from air fryer and place the rack of lamb onto a cutting board for about 5 minutes
10. With a sharp knife, cut the rack of lamb into individual chops and serve.

## Nutrition Values (Per Serving)

- Calories: 277
- Carbohydrate: 5.9g
- Protein: 28.6g
- Fat: 14.6g
- Sugar: 0.2g
- Sodium: 191mg

---

# Pesto Coated Rack of Lamb

**(Yields:** 4 servings / **Prep Time:** 15 minutes / **Cooking Time:** 15 minutes)

## Ingredients

- ½ bunch fresh mint
- 1 garlic clove
- ¼ cup extra-virgin olive oil
- ½ tablespoon honey
- Salt and ground black pepper, as required
- 1 (1½-pounds) rack of lamb

## Instructions

1. For pesto: in a blender, add the mint, garlic, oil, honey, salt, and black pepper and pulse until smooth.
2. Coat the rack of lamb evenly with some pesto.
3. Set the temperature of air fryer to 200 degrees F. Grease an air fryer basket.
4. Place rack of lamb into the prepared air fryer basket.
5. Air fry for about 15 minutes, coating with the remaining pesto after every 5 minutes.
6. Remove from air fryer and place the rack of lamb onto a cutting board for about 5 minutes
7. Cut the rack into individual chops and serve.

### Nutrition Values (Per Serving)

- Calories: 406
- Carbohydrate: 2.9g
- Protein: 34.9g
- Fat: 27.7g
- Sugar: 2.2g
- Sodium: 161mg

---

## Spiced Lamb Steaks

(**Yields:** 3 servings / **Prep Time:** 15 minutes / **Cooking Time:** 15 minutes)

### Ingredients

- ½ onion, roughly chopped
- 5 garlic cloves, peeled
- 1 tablespoon fresh ginger, peeled
- 1 teaspoon garam masala
- 1 teaspoon ground fennel
- ½ teaspoon ground cumin
- ½ teaspoon ground cinnamon
- ½ teaspoon cayenne pepper
- Salt and ground black pepper, as required
- 1½ pounds boneless lamb sirloin steaks

### Instructions

1. In a blender, add the onion, garlic, ginger, and spices and pulse until smooth.
2. Transfer the mixture into a large bowl.
3. Add the lamb steaks and generously coat with the mixture.
4. Refrigerate to marinate for about 24 hours.
5. Set the temperature of air fryer to 330 degrees F. Grease an air fryer basket.
6. Arrange steaks into the prepared air fryer basket in a single layer.
7. Air fry for about 15 minutes, flipping once halfway through.
8. Once done, remove the steaks from air fryer and serve.

### Nutrition Values (Per Serving)

- Calories: 252406
- Carbohydrate: 4.2g
- Protein: 21.7g
- Fat: 16.7g
- Sugar: 0.7g
- Sodium: 42mg

# Herbed Leg of Lamb

(**Yields:** 5 servings / **Prep Time:** 10 minutes / **Cooking Time:** 75 minutes)

## Ingredients

- 2 pounds bone-in leg of lamb
- 2 tablespoons olive oil
- Salt and ground black pepper, as required
- 2 fresh rosemary sprigs
- 2 fresh thyme sprigs

## Instructions

1. Coat the leg of lamb with oil and sprinkle with salt and black pepper.
2. Wrap the leg of lamb with herb sprigs.
3. Set the temperature of air fryer to 300 degrees F. Grease an air fryer basket.
4. Place leg of lamb into the prepared air fryer basket.
5. Air fry for about 75 minutes.
6. Remove from air fryer and transfer the leg of lamb onto a platter.
7. With a piece of foil, cover the leg of lamb for about 10 minutes before slicing.
8. Cut the leg of lamb into desired size pieces and serve.

## Nutrition Values (Per Serving)

- Calories: 534
- Carbohydrate: 2.4g
- Protein: 69.8g
- Fat: 25.8g
- Sugar: 0g
- Sodium: 190mg

# Leg of Lamb with Brussels Sprout

(**Yields:** 6 servings / **Prep Time:** 20 minutes / **Cooking Time:** 90 minutes)

## Ingredients

- 2¼ pounds leg of lamb
- 3 tablespoons olive oil, divided
- 1 tablespoon fresh rosemary, minced
- 1 tablespoon fresh lemon thyme
- 1 garlic clove, minced
- Salt and ground black pepper, as required
- 1½ pounds Brussels sprouts, trimmed
- 2 tablespoons honey

## Instructions

1. With a sharp knife, score the leg of lamb at several places.
2. In a bowl, mix together 2 tablespoons of oil, herbs, garlic, salt, and black pepper.
3. Generously coat the leg of lamb with oil mixture.
4. Set the temperature of air fryer to 300 degrees F. Grease an air fryer basket.
5. Place leg of lamb into the prepared air fryer basket.
6. Air fry for about 75 minutes.
7. Meanwhile, coat the Brussels sprout evenly with the remaining oil and honey.
8. Now, set the temperature of air fryer to 392 degrees F.
9. Arrange Brussels sprout into the air fryer basket with leg of lamb.
10. Air Fry for about 15 minutes.
11. Remove from air Fryer and transfer the leg of lamb onto a platter.
12. With a piece of foil, cover the leg of lamb for about 10 minutes before slicing.
13. Cut the leg of lamb into desired size pieces and serve alongside the Brussels sprout.

## Nutrition Values (Per Serving)

- Calories: 449
- Carbohydrate: 16.6g
- Protein: 51.7g
- Fat: 19.9g
- Sugar: 8.2g
- Sodium: 185mg

# Garlic Lamb Roast

(**Yields:** 6 servings / **Prep Time:** 20 minutes / **Cooking Time:** 1½ hours)

## Ingredients

- 2¾ pounds half lamb leg roast
- 3 garlic cloves, cut into thin slices
- 2 tablespoons extra-virgin olive oil
- 1 tablespoon dried rosemary, crushed
- Salt and ground black pepper, as required

## Instructions

1. In a small bowl, mix together the oil, rosemary, salt, and black pepper.
2. With the tip of a sharp knife, make deep slits on the top of lamb roast fat.
3. Insert the garlic slices into the slits.
4. Coat the lamb roast evenly with oil mixture.
5. Set the temperature of air fryer to 390 degrees F. Grease an air fryer basket.
6. Arrange lamb into the prepared air fryer basket in a single layer.
7. Air Fry for about 15 minutes and then another 1¼ hours at 320 degrees F.
8. Remove from air fryer and transfer the roast onto a platter.
9. With a piece of foil, cover the roast for about 10 minutes before slicing.
10. Cut the roast into desired size slices and serve.

## Nutrition Values (Per Serving)

- Calories: 418
- Carbohydrate: 0.9g
- Protein: 57.4g
- Fat: 14.9g
- Sugar: 0g
- Sodium: 165mg

# CHAPTER 5 | FISH AND SEAFOOD

## Simple Salmon

**(Yields:** 2 servings / **Prep Time:** 5 minutes / **Cooking Time:** 10 minutes)

### Ingredients

- 2 (6-ounces) salmon fillets
- Salt and ground black pepper, as required
- 1 tablespoon olive oil

### Instructions

1. Set the temperature of air fryer to 360 degrees F. Grease an air fryer basket.
2. Season each salmon fillet with salt and black pepper and then, coat with the oil.
3. Arrange salmon fillets into the prepared air fryer basket in a single layer.
4. Air fry for about 8-10 minutes.
5. Remove from air fryer and place the salmon fillets onto the serving plates.
6. Serve hot.

### Nutrition Values (Per Serving)

- Calories: 285
- Carbohydrate: 0g
- Protein: 33g
- Fat: 17.5g
- Sugar: 0g
- Sodium: 153mg

---

## Cajun Spiced Salmon

**(Yields:** 2 servings / **Prep Time:** 10 minutes / **Cooking Time:** 7 minutes)

### Ingredients

- 2 (7-ounces) (¾-inch thick) salmon fillets
- 1 tablespoon Cajun seasoning
- ½ teaspoon sugar
- 1 tablespoon fresh lemon juice

### Instructions

1. Set the temperature of air fryer to 356 degrees F. Grease an air fryer grill pan.
2. Sprinkle the salmon evenly with Cajun seasoning and sugar.
3. Arrange fish into the prepared air fryer grill pan, skin-side up.

4. Air fry for about 7 minutes.
5. Remove from air fryer and place the salmon fillets onto the serving plates.
6. Drizzle with the lemon juice and serve hot.

## Nutrition Values (Per Serving)

- Calories: 268
- Carbohydrate: 1.2g
- Protein: 38.6g
- Fat: 12.3g
- Sugar: 1.2g
- Sodium: 164mg

---

# Spicy Salmon

(**Yields:** 2 servings / **Prep Time:** 10 minutes / **Cooking Time:** 11 minutes)

## Ingredients

- 1 teaspoon smoked paprika
- 1 teaspoon cayenne pepper
- 1 teaspoon onion powder
- 1 teaspoon garlic powder
- Salt and ground black pepper, as required
- 2 (6-ounces) (1½-inch thick) salmon fillets
- 2 teaspoons olive oil

## Instructions

1. Add the spices in a bowl and mix well.
2. Drizzle the salmon fillets with oil and then, rub with the spice mixture.
3. Set the temperature of air fryer to 390 degrees F. Grease an air fryer basket.
4. Arrange salmon fillets into the prepared air fryer basket in a single layer.
5. Air fry for about 9-11 minutes.
6. Remove from air fryer and place the salmon fillets onto the serving plates.
7. Serve hot.

## Nutrition Values (Per Serving)

- Calories: 277
- Carbohydrate: 2.5g
- Protein: 33.5g
- Fat: 15.4g
- Sugar: 0.9g
- Sodium: 154mg

# Zesty Salmon

**(Yields:** 3 servings / **Prep Time:** 10 minutes / **Cooking Time:** 8 minutes)

## Ingredients

- 1½ pounds salmon
- ½ teaspoon red chili powder
- Salt and ground black pepper, as required
- 1 lemon, cut into slices
- 1 tablespoon fresh dill, chopped

## Instructions

1. Set the temperature of air fryer to 375 degrees F. Grease an air fryer basket.
2. Season the salmon evenly with chili powder, salt, and black pepper.
3. Arrange salmon into the prepared air fryer basket.
4. Place the lemon slices over the salmon.
5. Air fry for about 8 minutes.
6. Remove from air fryer and place the salmon fillets onto serving plates.
7. Garnish with fresh dill and serve.

## Nutrition Values (Per Serving)

- Calories: 206
- Carbohydrate: 1.3g
- Protein: 29.7g
- Fat: 9.5g
- Sugar: 0.2g
- Sodium: 124mg

---

# Maple Glazed Salmon

**(Yields:** 2 servings / **Prep Time:** 10 minutes / **Cooking Time:** 8 minutes)

## Ingredients

- 2 (6-ounces) salmon fillets
- Salt, as required
- 2 tablespoons maple syrup

## Instructions

1. Sprinkle the salmon fillets evenly with salt and then, coat with maple syrup.
2. Set the temperature of air fryer to 355 degrees F. Grease an air fryer basket.
3. Arrange salmon fillets into the prepared air fryer basket in a single layer.
4. Air Fry for about 8 minutes.

5. Remove from air fryer and place the salmon fillets onto serving plates.
6. Serve hot.

### Nutrition Values (Per Serving)
- Calories: 277
- Carbohydrate: 13.4g
- Protein: 33g
- Fat: 10.5g
- Sugar: 11.9g
- Sodium: 154mg

---

# Sweet & Sour Glazed Salmon

**(Yields:** 2 servings / **Prep Time:** 20 minutes / **Cooking Time:** 12 minutes)

## Ingredients
- 1/3 cup soy sauce
- 1/3 cup honey
- 3 teaspoons rice wine vinegar
- 1 teaspoon water
- 4 (3½-ounces) salmon fillets

## Instructions
1. In a small bowl, mix together the soy sauce, honey, vinegar, and water.
2. In another bowl, reserve about half of the mixture.
3. Add salmon fillets in the remaining mixture and coat well.
4. Cover the bowl and refrigerate to marinate for about 2 hours.
5. Set the temperature of air fryer to 355 degrees F. Grease an air fryer basket.
6. Arrange salmon fillets into the prepared air fryer basket in a single layer.
7. Air fry for about 12 minutes, flipping once halfway through and coating with the reserved marinade after every 3 minutes.
8. Remove from air fryer and place the salmon fillets onto serving plates.
9. Serve hot.

## Nutrition Values (Per Serving)
- Calories: 462
- Carbohydrate: 49.8g
- Protein: 41.3g
- Fat: 12.3g
- Sugar: 47.1g
- Sodium: 2000mg

# Salmon with Broccoli

**(Yields:** 2 servings / **Prep Time:** 15 minutes / **Cooking Time:** 12 minutes)

## Ingredients

- 1½ cups small broccoli florets
- 2 tablespoons vegetable oil, divided
- Salt and ground black pepper, as required
- 1 (½-inch) piece fresh ginger, grated
- 1 tablespoon soy sauce
- 1 teaspoon rice vinegar
- 1 teaspoon light brown sugar
- ¼ teaspoon cornstarch
- 2 (6-ounces) skin-on salmon fillets
- 1 scallion, thinly sliced

## Instructions

1. In a bowl, mix together the broccoli, 1 tablespoon of oil, salt, and black pepper.
2. In another bowl, mix well the ginger, soy sauce, vinegar, sugar, and cornstarch.
3. Coat the salmon fillets evenly with remaining oil and then with the ginger mixture.
4. Set the temperature of air fryer to 375 degrees F. Grease an air fryer basket.
5. Arrange broccoli florets into the prepared air fryer basket.
6. Place the salmon fillets on top of broccoli, flesh-side down.
7. Air fry for about 12 minutes.
8. Remove from air fryer and place the salmon fillets onto serving plates.
9. Serve hot alongside the broccoli.

## Nutrition Values (Per Serving)

- Calories: 385
- Carbohydrate: 7.8g
- Protein: 35.6g
- Fat: 24.4g
- Sugar: 3g
- Sodium: 628mg

# Salmon with Asparagus

**(Yields:** 2 servings / **Prep Time:** 15 minutes / **Cooking Time:** 11 minutes)

## Ingredients

- 2 (6-ounces) boneless salmon fillets
- 1½ tablespoons fresh lemon juice
- 1 tablespoon olive oil
- 2 tablespoons fresh parsley, roughly chopped

- 2 tablespoons fresh dill, roughly chopped
- 1 bunch asparagus
- Salt and ground black pepper, as required

## Instructions

1. In a small bowl, mix well the lemon juice, oil, herbs, salt, and black pepper.
2. In another large bowl, mix together the salmon and ¾ of oil mixture.
3. In a second large bowl, add the asparagus and remaining oil mixture. Mix them well.
4. Set the temperature of air fryer to 400 degrees F. Grease an air fryer basket.
5. Arrange asparagus into the prepared air fryer basket.
6. Air fry for about 2-3 minutes.
7. Now, place the salmon fillets on top of asparagus and air fry for about 8 minutes.
8. Remove from air fryer and place the salmon fillets onto serving plates.
9. Serve hot alongside the asparagus.

## Nutrition Values (Per Serving)

- Calories: 331
- Carbohydrate: 8.8g
- Protein: 37.6g
- Fat: 18g
- Sugar: 3.5g
- Sodium: 167mg

# Salmon with Green Beans

**(Yields:** 4 servings / **Prep Time:** 15 minutes / **Cooking Time:** 12 minutes)

## Ingredients

**For Green Beans**
- 5 cups green beans (I use frozen)
- 1 tablespoon avocado oil
- Salt, as required

**For Salmon**
- 2 garlic cloves, minced
- 2 tablespoons fresh dill, chopped
- 2 tablespoons fresh lemon juice
- 1 tablespoon olive oil
- Salt, as required
- 4 (6-ounces) salmon fillets

## Instructions

1. Set the temperature of air fryer to 375 degrees F. Grease an air fryer basket.
2. In a large bowl, mix well the green beans, oil, and salt.
3. Arrange green beans into the prepared air fryer basket.
4. Air fry for about 6 minutes.
5. Meanwhile, for salmon: in a bowl, mix together the garlic, dill, lemon juice, and olive oil.
6. Remove the basket from air fryer.
7. Flip the green beans and top with salmon fillets.
8. Place the garlic mixture evenly on top of each salmon fillet and then, sprinkle with the salt.
9. Air fry for about 6 minutes.
10. Remove from air fryer and place the salmon fillets onto serving plates.
11. Serve hot alongside the green beans.

## Nutrition Values (Per Serving)

- Calories: 310
- Carbohydrate: 11.5g
- Protein: 326g
- Fat: 14.8g
- Sugar: 2.1
- Sodium: 127mg

# Salmon with Shrimp & Pasta

(**Yields:** 4 servings / **Prep Time:** 20 minutes / **Cooking Time:** 18 minutes)

## Ingredients

- 14 ounces pasta (of your choice)
- 4 tablespoons pesto, divided
- 4 (4-ounces) salmon steaks
- 2 tablespoons olive oil
- ½ pound cherry tomatoes, chopped
- 8 large prawns, peeled and deveined
- 2 tablespoons fresh lemon juice
- 2 tablespoons fresh thyme, chopped

## Instructions

1. In a large pan of salted boiling water, add the pasta and cook for about 8-10 minutes or until desired doneness.
2. Meanwhile, in the bottom of a baking dish, spread 1 tablespoon of pesto.

3. Place salmon steaks and tomatoes over pesto in a single layer and drizzle evenly with the oil.
4. Now, add the prawns on top in a single layer.
5. Drizzle with lemon juice and sprinkle with thyme.
6. Set the temperature of air fryer to 390 degrees F.
7. Arrange the baking dish in air fryer and air fry for about 8 minutes.
8. Once done, remove the salmon mixture from air fryer.
9. Drain the pasta and transfer into a large bowl.
10. Add the remaining pesto and toss to coat well.
11. Add the pasta evenly onto each serving plate and top with salmon mixture.
12. Serve immediately.

## **Nutrition Values (Per Serving)**

- Calories: 592
- Carbohydrate: 58.7g
- Protein: 37.7g
- Fat: 23.2g
- Sugar: 2.7g
- Sodium: 203mg

---

# **Salmon Patties**

**(Yields:** 6 servings / **Prep Time:** 20 minutes / **Cooking Time:** 27 minutes)

## **Ingredients**

- 3 large russet potatoes, peeled and cubed
- 1 (6-ounces) salmon fillet
- 1 egg
- ¾ cup frozen vegetables (of your choice), parboiled and drained
- 2 tablespoons fresh parsley, chopped
- 1 teaspoon fresh dill, chopped
- Salt and ground black pepper, as required
- 1 cup breadcrumbs
- ¼ cup olive oil

## **Instructions**

1. In a pan of boiling water, cook the potatoes for about 10 minutes.
2. Drain the potatoes well.
3. Transfer the potatoes into a bowl and mash them using a potato masher.
4. Set aside to cool completely.
5. Set the temperature of air fryer to 355 degrees F. Grease an air fryer basket.
6. Arrange salmon fillet into the prepared air fryer basket.
7. Air fry for about 5 minutes.

8. Remove from air fryer and transfer the salmon fillet into a large bowl. With a fork, flake the salmon.
9. Add the mashed potatoes, egg, vegetables, herbs, salt, and black pepper into the bowl of salmon and mix until well combined.
10. Make 6 equal-sized patties from the mixture.
11. Coat patties evenly with breadcrumbs and then, drizzle with the oil.
12. Transfer the patties into air fryer basket
13. Once again, set the temperature of air fryer to 355 degrees F. Line an air fryer basket with a lightly greased piece of foil.
14. Arrange patties into the prepared air fryer basket in a single layer.
15. Air fry for about 10-12 minutes, flipping once halfway through.
16. Remove from air fryer and place the patties onto serving plates.
17. Serve warm.

## **Nutrition Values (Per Serving)**

- Calories: 334
- Carbohydrate: 45.2g
- Protein: 12.6g
- Fat: 12.1g
- Sugar: 40g
- Sodium: 202mg

---

# **Chinese Style Cod**

(**Yields:** 2 servings / **Prep Time:** 20 minutes / **Cooking Time:** 15 minutes)

## **Ingredients**

- 2 (7-ounces) cod fillets
- Salt and ground black pepper, as required
- ¼ teaspoon sesame oil
- 1 cup water
- 5 little squares rock sugar
- 5 tablespoons light soy sauce
- 1 teaspoon dark soy sauce
- 2 scallions (green part), sliced
- ¼ cup fresh cilantro, chopped
- 3 tablespoons olive oil
- 5 ginger slices

## **Instructions**

1. Season each cod fillet evenly with salt, and black pepper and drizzle with sesame oil.
2. Set aside at room temperature for about 15-20 minutes.
3. Set the temperature of air fryer to 355 degrees F. Grease an air fryer basket.
4. Arrange cod fillets into the prepared air fryer basket in a single layer.
5. Air fry for about 12 minutes.
6. Meanwhile, in a small pan, add the water and bring it to a boil.

7. Add the rock sugar and both soy sauces and cook until sugar is dissolved, stirring continuously.
8. Remove from the heat and set aside.
9. Remove cod fillets from air fryer and transfer them onto serving plates. Top each fillet with scallion and cilantro.
10. Heat the olive oil in a small frying pan over medium heat and sauté ginger slices for about 2-3 minutes.
11. Remove the frying pan from heat and discard the ginger slices.
12. Carefully, pour the hot oil evenly over cod fillets.
13. Top with the sauce mixture and serve.

## Nutrition Values (Per Serving)

- Calories: 433
- Carbohydrate: 7.6g
- Protein: 48.2g
- Fat: 23.4g
- Sugar: 4.2g
- Sodium: 2001mg

# Cod & Veggie Parcel

(**Yields:** 4 servings / **Prep Time:** 20 minutes / **Cooking Time:** 15 minutes)

## Ingredients

- 2 tablespoons butter, melted
- 1 tablespoon fresh lemon juice
- ½ teaspoon dried tarragon
- Salt and ground black pepper, as required
- ½ cup red bell peppers, seeded and thinly sliced
- ½ cup carrots, peeled and julienned
- ½ cup fennel bulbs, julienned
- 2 (5-ounces) frozen cod fillets, thawed
- 1 tablespoon olive oil

## Instructions

1. In a large bowl, mix well butter, lemon juice, tarragon, salt, and black pepper.
2. Add the bell pepper, carrot, and fennel bulb and generously coat with the mixture.
3. Arrange 2 large parchment squares onto a smooth surface.
4. Coat the cod fillets with oil and then, sprinkle evenly with salt and black pepper.
5. Arrange 1 cod fillet onto each parchment square and top each evenly with the vegetables.

6. Top with any remaining sauce from the bowl.
7. Fold the parchment paper and crimp the sides to secure fish and vegetables.
8. Set the temperature of air fryer to 350 degrees F.
9. Arrange fish parcels into the air fryer basket.
10. Air fry for about 15 minutes.
11. Remove from air fryer and place the parcels onto serving plates.
12. Carefully, open each parcel and serve warm.

## Nutrition Values (Per Serving)
- Calories: 344
- Carbohydrate: 6.8g
- Protein: 33.4g
- Fat: 19.9g
- Sugar: 3g
- Sodium: 225mg

# Crispy Cod Sticks

**(Yields:** 2 servings / **Prep Time:** 20 minutes / **Cooking Time:** 7 minutes)

## Ingredients
- 3 (4-ounces) skinless cod fillets, cut into rectangular pieces
- ¾ cup flour
- 4 eggs
- 2 garlic cloves, minced
- 1 green chili, finely chopped
- 2 teaspoons light soy sauce
- Salt and ground black pepper, as required

## Instructions
1. In a shallow bowl, add the flour.
2. In another bowl, mix well eggs, garlic, green chili, soy sauce, salt, and black pepper.
3. Coat each piece with flour and then, dip into the egg mixture.
4. Set the temperature of air fryer to 375 degrees F. Grease an air fryer basket.
5. Arrange cod pieces into the prepared air fryer basket in a single layer.
6. Air fry for about 7 minutes.
7. Remove from air fryer and place the cod sticks onto serving plates.
8. Serve warm.

## Nutrition Values (Per Serving)
- Calories: 483
- Carbohydrate: 38g
- Protein: 55.3g
- Fat: 10.7g
- Sugar: 1.1g
- Sodium: 634mg

# Cod Cakes

**(Yields:** 6 servings / **Prep Time:** 20 minutes / **Cooking Time:** 14 minutes)

## Ingredients

- 1 pound cod fillet
- 1 teaspoon fresh lime zest, finely grated
- 1 egg
- 1 teaspoon red chili paste
- Salt, as required
- 1 tablespoon fresh lime juice
- 1/3 cup coconut, grated and divided
- 1 scallion, finely chopped
- 2 tablespoons fresh parsley, chopped

## Instructions

1. For cod cakes: in a food processor, add the cod fillet, lime zest, egg, chili paste, salt, and lime juice and pulse until smooth.
2. Transfer the cod mixture into a bowl.
3. Add 2 tablespoons of coconut, scallion, and parsley. Mix until well combined.
4. Make 12 equal-sized round cakes from the mixture.
5. In a shallow bowl, place the remaining coconut.
6. Coat the cod cakes evenly with coconut.
7. Set the temperature of air fryer to 375 degrees F. Grease an air fryer basket.
8. Arrange cod cakes into the prepared air fryer basket in 2 batches in a single layer.
9. Air fry for about 7 minutes.
10. Remove from air fryer and place 2 cod cakes onto each serving plate.
11. Serve warm.

## Nutrition Values (Per Serving)

- Calories: 165
- Carbohydrate: 2.1g
- Protein: 27.7g
- Fat: 4.5g
- Sugar: 1g
- Sodium: 161mg

---

# Glazed Halibut

**(Yields:** 3 servings / **Prep Time:** 20 minutes / **Cooking Time:** 15 minutes)

## Ingredients

- 1 garlic clove, minced
- ¼ teaspoon fresh ginger, finely grated
- ½ cup cooking wine
- ½ cup low-sodium soy sauce
- ¼ cup fresh orange juice

- 2 tablespoons lime juice
- ¼ cup sugar
- ¼ teaspoon red pepper flakes, crushed
- 1 pound halibut steak

## Instructions

1. In a medium pan, add the garlic, ginger, wine, soy sauce, juices, sugar, and red pepper flakes and bring to a boil.
2. Cook for about 3-4 minutes, stirring continuously.
3. Remove the pan of marinade from heat and let it cool.
4. In a small bowl, add half of the marinade and reserve in a refrigerator.
5. In a resealable bag, add the remaining marinade and halibut steak.
6. Seal the bag and shake to coat well.
7. Refrigerate for about 30 minutes.
8. Set the temperature of air fryer to 390 degrees F. Grease an air fryer basket.
9. Place halibut steak into the prepared air fryer basket.
10. Air fry for about 9-11 minutes.
11. Remove from air fryer and place the halibut steak onto a platter.
12. Cut the steak into 3 equal-sized pieces and coat with the remaining glaze.
13. Serve immediately.

## Nutrition Values (Per Serving)

- Calories: 289
- Carbohydrate: 23.2g
- Protein: 34.8g
- Fat: 3.6g
- Sugar: 21.6g
- Sodium: 2400mg

# Crispy Halibut Strips

(**Yields:** 2 servings / **Prep Time:** 20 minutes / **Cooking Time:** 14 minutes)

## Ingredients

- 4 tablespoons taco seasoning mix*
- 2 eggs
- 1 tablespoon water
- ¾ cup plain panko breadcrumbs
- ¾ pound skinless halibut fillets, cut into 1-inch strips

## Instructions

1. In a shallow bowl, add the taco seasoning mix.
2. In a second bowl, beat eggs and water.

3. In a third bowl, place the breadcrumbs.
4. Coat fish with taco seasoning mix, then, dip into the egg mixture and finally, coat with the breadcrumb.
5. Set the temperature of air fryer to 350 degrees F. Line air fryer basket with a lightly greased parchment paper.
6. Arrange halibut strips into the prepared air fryer basket in a single layer.
7. Air fry for about 12-14 minutes, flipping once halfway through.
8. Remove from air fryer and transfer the halibut strips onto serving plates.
9. Serve warm.

## Nutrition Values (Per Serving)

- Calories: 443
- Carbohydrate: 15.5g
- Protein: 42.4g
- Fat: 11.2g
- Sugar: 0.4g
- Sodium: 961mg

(**Note: Taco seasoning mix\*** - In a small bowl, mix together chili powder, garlic powder, onion powder, red pepper flakes, oregano, paprika, cumin, salt and pepper. Store in an airtight container.)

---

# Pesto Haddock

(**Yields:** 2 servings / **Prep Time:** 15 minutes / **Cooking Time:** 8 minutes)

## Ingredients

- 2 (6-ounces) haddock fillets
- 1 tablespoon olive oil
- Salt and ground black pepper, as required
- 2 tablespoons pine nuts
- 3 tablespoons fresh basil, chopped
- 1 tablespoon Parmesan cheese, grated
- 1/3 cup extra-virgin olive oil

## Instructions

1. Set the temperature of air fryer to 355 degrees F. Grease an air fryer basket.
2. Coat the fish fillets evenly with oil and then, sprinkle with salt and black pepper.
3. Arrange fish fillets into the prepared air fryer basket in a single layer.

4. Air fry for about 8 minutes.
5. Meanwhile, for the pesto: add the remaining ingredients in a food processor and pulse until smooth.
6. Remove from air fryer and transfer the flounder fillets onto serving plates.
7. Top with the pesto and serve.

## Nutrition Values (Per Serving)

- Calories: 606
- Carbohydrate: 1.2g
- Protein: 43.5g
- Fat: 48.7g
- Sugar: 0.3g
- Sodium: 247g

---

# Breaded Flounder

(**Yields:** 3 servings / **Prep Time:** 15 minutes / **Cooking Time:** 12 minutes)

## Ingredients

- 1 egg
- 1 cup dry breadcrumbs
- ¼ cup vegetable oil
- 3 (6-ounces) flounder fillets
- 1 lemon, sliced

## Instructions

1. In a shallow bowl, beat the egg
2. In another bowl, add the breadcrumbs and oil. Mix until crumbly mixture is formed.
3. Dip flounder fillets into the beaten egg and then, coat with the breadcrumb mixture.
4. Set the temperature of air fryer to 356 degrees F. Grease an air fryer basket.
5. Arrange flounder fillets into the prepared air fryer basket in a single layer.
6. Air fry for about 12 minutes.
7. Remove from air fryer and transfer the flounder fillets onto serving plates.
8. Garnish with the lemon slices and serve hot.

## Nutrition Values (Per Serving)

- Calories: 524
- Carbohydrate: 26.5g
- Protein: 47.8g
- Fat: 24.4g
- Sugar: 2.5g
- Sodium: 463g

# 3-Ingredients Catfish

**(Yields:** 4 servings / **Prep Time:** 10 minutes / **Cooking Time:** 23 minutes)

## Ingredients

- 4 (6-ounces) catfish fillets
- ¼ cup seasoned fish fry*
- 1 tablespoon olive oil

## Instructions

1. Set the temperature of air fryer to 400 degrees F. Grease an air fryer basket.
2. In a bowl, add the catfish fillets and seasoned fish fry. Toss to coat well.
3. Then, drizzle each fillet evenly with oil.
4. Arrange catfish fillets into the prepared air fryer basket in a single layer.
5. Air fry for about 10 minutes.
6. Flip the side and spray with the cooking spray.
7. Air fry for another 10 minutes.
8. Flip one last time and air fry for about 2-3 more minutes.
9. Remove from air fryer and transfer the catfish fillets onto serving plates.
10. Serve hot.

## Nutrition Values (Per Serving)

- Calories: 294
- Carbohydrate: 2.6g
- Protein: 28.7g
- Fat: 18.3g
- Sugar: 0g
- Sodium: 170g

(**Note: Seasoned Fish Fry*** - LOUISIANA Fish Fry (Seasoned) is a flavorful blend of corn meal, corn flour, garlic, salt and other spices traditionally used as a total seasoning for your favorite fish, oysters, shrimp, meat or vegetables.)

---

# Cajun Coated Catfish

**(Yields:** 4 servings / **Prep Time:** 15 minutes / **Cooking Time:** 14 minutes)

## Ingredients

- 2 tablespoons cornmeal polenta
- 2 teaspoons Cajun seasoning
- ½ teaspoon paprika

- ½ teaspoon garlic powder
- Salt, as required
- 2 (6-ounces) catfish fillets
- 1 tablespoon olive oil

## Instructions

1. In a bowl, mix together the cornmeal, Cajun seasoning, paprika, garlic powder, and salt.
2. Add the catfish fillets and coat evenly with the mixture.
3. Now, coat each fillet with oil.
4. Set the temperature of air fryer to 400 degrees F. Grease an air fryer basket.
5. Arrange catfish fillets into the prepared air fryer basket in a single layer.
6. Air fry for about 13-14 minutes, flipping once halfway through.
7. Remove from air fryer and transfer the catfish fillets onto serving plates.
8. Serve hot.

## Nutrition Values (Per Serving)

- Calories: 321
- Carbohydrate: 6.7g
- Protein: 27.3g
- Fat: 20.3g
- Sugar: 0.3g
- Sodium: 221g

(**Note:** Do not keep the fish sit in the coating mixture for long or it will get soggy).

---

# Southern Style Catfish

(**Yields:** 5 servings / **Prep Time:** 15 minutes / **Cooking Time:** 15 minutes)

## Ingredients

- 5 (6-ounces) catfish fillets
- 1 cup milk
- 2 teaspoons fresh lemon juice
- ½ cup yellow mustard
- ½ cup cornmeal
- ¼ cup all-purpose flour
- 2 tablespoons dried parsley flakes
- ¼ teaspoon red chili powder
- ¼ teaspoon cayenne pepper
- ¼ teaspoon onion powder
- ¼ teaspoon garlic powder
- Salt and ground black pepper, as required
- Olive oil cooking spray

## Instructions

1. In a large bowl, place the catfish, milk, and lemon juice and refrigerate for about 15 minutes.

2. In a shallow bowl, add the mustard.
3. In another bowl, mix together the cornmeal, flour, parsley flakes, and spices.
4. Remove the catfish fillets from milk mixture and with paper towels, pat them dry.
5. Coat each fish fillet with mustard and then, roll evenly into cornmeal mixture.
6. Set the temperature of air fryer to 400 degrees F. Grease an air fryer basket.
7. Arrange catfish fillets into the prepared air fryer basket in a single layer and spray with the cooking spray.
8. Air fry for about 10 minutes.
9. Flip the side and spray with the cooking spray.
10. Air fry for about 3-5 minutes.
11. Remove from air fryer and transfer the catfish fillets onto serving plates.
12. Serve hot.

## Nutrition Values (Per Serving)

- Calories: 340
- Carbohydrate: 18.3g
- Protein: 30.9g
- Fat: 15.5g
- Sugar: 2.7g
- Sodium: 435g

## Sesame Seeds Coated Haddock

(**Yields:** 4 servings / **Prep Time:** 15 minutes / **Cooking Time:** 14 minutes)

## Ingredients

- 4 tablespoons plain flour
- 2 eggs
- ½ cup sesame seeds, toasted
- ½ cup breadcrumbs
- 1/8 teaspoon dried rosemary, crushed
- Salt and ground black pepper, as required
- 3 tablespoons olive oil
- 4 (6-ounces) frozen haddock fillets

## Instructions

1. In a shallow bowl, place the flour
2. In a second bowl, whisk the eggs
3. In a third bowl, add the sesame seeds, breadcrumbs, rosemary, salt, black pepper and oil and mix until a crumbly mixture forms.
4. Coat each fillet with flour, then dip into beaten egg and finally, coat with the breadcrumbs mixture.
5. Set the temperature of air fryer to 390 degrees F. Line an air fryer basket with a lightly greased piece of foil.

6. Arrange haddock fillets into the prepared air fryer basket in a single layer.
7. Air fry for about 14 minutes, flipping once halfway through.
8. Remove from air fryer and transfer the haddock fillets onto serving plates.
9. Serve hot.

## Nutrition Values (Per Serving)

- Calories: 497
- Carbohydrate: 20.1g
- Protein: 49.8g
- Fat: 24g
- Sugar: 1.1g
- Sodium: 319g

---

# Breaded Hake

**(Yields:** 2 servings / **Prep Time:** 15 minutes / **Cooking Time:** 12 minutes)

## Ingredients

- 1 egg
- 4 ounces breadcrumbs
- 2 tablespoons vegetable oil
- 4 (6-ounces) hake fillets
- 1 lemon, cut into wedges

## Instructions

1. In a shallow bowl, whisk the egg.
2. In another bowl, add the breadcrumbs, and oil and mix until a crumbly mixture forms.
3. Dip fish fillets into the egg and then, coat with the breadcrumbs mixture.
4. Set the temperature of air fryer to 350 degrees F. Grease an air fryer basket.
5. Arrange haddock fillets into the prepared air fryer basket in a single layer.
6. Air fry for about 12 minutes.
7. Remove from air fryer and transfer the hake fillets onto serving plates.
8. Garnish with lemon wedges and serve hot.

## Nutrition Values (Per Serving)

- Calories: 27
- Carbohydrate: 22.1g
- Protein: 29.2g
- Fat: 10.6g
- Sugar: 1.9g
- Sodium: 439g

# Ranch Tilapia

**(Yields:** 4 servings / **Prep Time:** 15 minutes / **Cooking Time:** 13 minutes)

## Ingredients

- ¾ cup cornflakes, crushed
- 1 (1-ounce) packet dry ranch-style dressing mix*
- 2½ tablespoons vegetable oil
- 2 eggs
- 4 (6-ounces) tilapia fillets

## Instructions

1. In a shallow bowl, beat the eggs.
2. In another bowl, add the cornflakes, ranch dressing, and oil and mix until a crumbly mixture forms.
3. Dip the fish fillets into egg and then, coat with the breadcrumbs mixture.
4. Set the temperature of air fryer to 356 degrees F. Grease an air fryer basket.
5. Arrange tilapia fillets into the prepared air fryer basket in a single layer.
6. Air fry for about 12-13 minutes.
7. Remove from air fryer and transfer the tilapia fillets onto serving plates.
8. Serve hot.

## Nutrition Values (Per Serving)

- Calories: 532
- Carbohydrate: 4.9g
- Protein: 34.8g
- Fat: 41.8g
- Sugar: 0.7g
- Sodium: 160g

**(Note: Ranch-style dressing mix\*** -

1/2 cup Dry Buttermilk Powder

1 Tablespoon Dried Parsley

2 teaspoons Dried Dill Weed

1 teaspoon Freeze Dried Chives

1 Tablespoon Garlic Powder

1 Tablespoon Onion Powder

1 teaspoon Sea Salt

1/2 teaspoon Ground Black Pepper

In a medium bowl, whisk all ingredients to combine. Transfer the mixture to an airtight container. Or, you can buy ready-made mix at your local store or on Amazon.)

# Sesame Seeds Coated Tuna

**(Yields:** 2 servings / **Prep Time:** 15 minutes / **Cooking Time:** 6 minutes)

## Ingredients

- ¼ cup white sesame seeds
- 1 tablespoon black sesame seeds
- Salt and ground black pepper, as required
- 1 egg white
- 2 (6-ounces) tuna steaks

## Instructions

1. In a shallow bowl, whisk the egg white.
2. In another bowl, mix together the sesame seeds, salt, and black pepper.
3. Dip the tuna steaks into egg white and then, coat with the sesame seeds mixture.
4. Set the temperature of air fryer to 400 degrees F. Grease an air fryer basket.
5. Arrange tuna steaks into the prepared air fryer basket in a single layer.
6. Air fry for about 3 minutes per side.
7. Remove from air fryer and transfer the tuna steaks onto serving plates.
8. Serve hot.

## Nutrition Values (Per Serving)

- Calories: 450
- Carbohydrate: 5.4g
- Protein: 56.7g
- Fat: 21.9g
- Sugar: 0.2g
- Sodium: 182g

---

# Tuna & Potato Cakes

**(Yields:** 4 servings / **Prep Time:** 20 minutes / **Cooking Time:** 12 minutes)

## Ingredients

- ½ tablespoon olive oil
- 1 onion, chopped
- 1 tablespoon fresh ginger, grated
- 1 green chili, seeded and finely chopped
- 2 (6-ounces) cans tuna, drained
- 1 medium boiled potato, mashed
- 2 tablespoons celery, finely chopped
- Salt, as required
- 1 cup breadcrumbs
- 1 egg

## Instructions

1. Heat the olive oil in a frying pan and sauté onions, ginger, and green chili for about 30 seconds.

2. Add the tuna and stir fry for about 2-3 minutes or until all the liquid is absorbed.
3. Remove from heat and transfer the tuna mixture onto a large bowl. Set aside to cool.
4. In the bowl of tuna mixture, mix well mashed potato, celery, and salt.
5. Make 4 equal-sized patties from the mixture.
6. In a shallow bowl, place the breadcrumbs.
7. In another bowl, beat the egg.
8. Coat each patty with breadcrumbs, then dip into egg and finally, again coat with the breadcrumbs.
9. Set the temperature of air fryer to 390 degrees F. Grease an air fryer basket.
10. Arrange tuna cakes into the prepared air fryer basket in a single layer.
11. Air fry for about 2-3 minutes.
12. Flip the side and air fry for about 4-5 minutes.
13. Remove from air fryer and transfer the tuna cakes onto serving plates.
14. Serve warm.

## Nutrition Values (Per Serving)

- Calories: 353
- Carbohydrate: 32.6g
- Protein: 29.1g
- Fat: 11.3g
- Sugar: 3.5g
- Sodium: 302mg

---

# Creamy Tuna Cakes

(**Yields:** 4 servings / **Prep Time:** 15 minutes / **Cooking Time:** 15 minutes)

## Ingredients

- 2 (6-ounces) cans tuna, drained
- 1½ tablespoons mayonnaise
- 1½ tablespoon almond flour
- 1 tablespoon fresh lemon juice
- 1 teaspoon dried dill
- 1 teaspoon garlic powder
- ½ teaspoon onion powder
- Pinch of salt and ground black pepper

## Instructions

1. In a large bowl, mix together the tuna, mayonnaise, flour, lemon juice, dill, and spices.
2. Make 4 equal-sized patties from the mixture.
3. Set the temperature of air fryer to 400 degrees F. Grease an air fryer basket.
4. Arrange tuna cakes into the prepared air fryer basket in a single layer.
5. Air fry for about 10 minutes.
6. Flip the side and air fry for another 4-5 minutes.

7. Remove from air fryer and transfer the tuna cakes onto serving plates.
8. Serve warm.

## Nutrition Values (Per Serving)

- Calories: 200
- Carbohydrate: 2.9g
- Protein: 23.4g
- Fat: 10.1g
- Sugar: 0.8g
- Sodium: 122mg

---

## Spicy Shrimp

(**Yields:** 2 servings / **Prep Time:** 13 minutes / **Cooking Time:** 5 minutes)

## Ingredients

- ¾ pound tiger shrimp, peeled and deveined
- 1½ tablespoons olive oil
- ½ teaspoon old bay seasoning
- ¼ teaspoon smoked paprika
- ¼ teaspoon cayenne pepper
- Salt, as required

## Instructions

1. Set the temperature of air fryer to 390 degrees F. Grease an air fryer basket.
2. In a large bowl, mix well shrimp, oil, and spices.
3. Arrange shrimp into the prepared air fryer basket in a single layer.
4. Air fry for about 5 minutes.
5. Remove from air fryer and transfer the shrimp onto serving plates.
6. Serve hot.

## Nutrition Values (Per Serving)

- Calories: 260
- Carbohydrate: 0.3g
- Protein: 135.6g
- Fat: 12.4g
- Sugar: 0.1g
- Sodium: 619mg

# Lemon Garlic Shrimp

**(Yields:** 2 servings / **Prep Time:** 15 minutes / **Cooking Time:** 8 minutes)

## Ingredients

- 1½ tablespoons fresh lemon juice
- 1 tablespoon olive oil
- 1 teaspoon lemon pepper
- ¼ teaspoon paprika
- ¼ teaspoon garlic powder
- ¾ pound medium shrimp, peeled and deveined

## Instructions

1. In a large bowl, mix well lemon juice, oil, and spices.
2. Add the shrimp and toss to combine.
3. Set the temperature of air fryer to 400 degrees F. Grease an air fryer basket.
4. Arrange shrimp into the prepared air fryer basket in a single layer.
5. Air fry for about 6-8 minutes.
6. Remove from air fryer and transfer the shrimp onto serving plates.
7. Serve hot.

## Nutrition Values (Per Serving)

- Calories: 260
- Carbohydrate: 0.3g
- Protein: 135.6g
- Fat: 12.4g
- Sugar: 0.1g
- Sodium: 619mg

---

# Cheesy Shrimp

**(Yields:** 4 servings / **Prep Time:** 20 minutes / **Cooking Time:** 20 minutes)

## Ingredients

- 2/3 cup Parmesan cheese, grated
- 4 garlic cloves, minced
- 2 tablespoons olive oil
- 1 teaspoon dried basil
- ½ teaspoon dried oregano
- 1 teaspoon onion powder
- ½ teaspoon red pepper flakes, crushed
- Ground black pepper, as required
- 2 pounds shrimp, peeled and deveined
- 1-2 tablespoons fresh lemon juice

## Instructions

1. In a large bowl, mix well Parmesan cheese, garlic, oil, herbs, and spices.
2. Add the shrimp and toss to combine.

3. Set the temperature of air fryer to 350 degrees F. Grease an air fryer basket.
4. Arrange shrimp into the prepared air fryer basket in 2 batches in a single layer.
5. Air fry for about 8-10 minutes.
6. Remove from air fryer and transfer the shrimp onto serving plates.
7. Drizzle with lemon juice and serve immediately.

## Nutrition Values (Per Serving)

- Calories: 386
- Carbohydrate: 5.3g
- Protein: 57.3g
- Fat: 14.2g
- Sugar: 0.4g
- Sodium: 670mg

---

# Creamy Breaded Shrimp

**(Yields:** 3 servings / **Prep Time:** 15 minutes / **Cooking Time:** 20 minutes)

## Ingredients

- ¼ cup all-purpose flour
- ½ cup mayonnaise
- ¼ cup sweet chili sauce
- 1 tablespoon Sriracha sauce
- 1 cup panko breadcrumbs
- 1 pound shrimp, peeled and deveined

## Instructions

1. In a shallow bowl, place the flour.
2. In a second bowl, mix together the mayonnaise, chili sauce, and Sriracha sauce.
3. In a third bowl, add the breadcrumbs.
4. Coat each shrimp with the flour, then dip into mayonnaise mixture and finally, coat with the breadcrumbs.
5. Set the temperature of air fryer to 400 degrees F. Grease an air fryer basket.
6. Arrange shrimp into the prepared air fryer basket in 2 batches in a single layer.
7. Air fry for about 10 minutes.
8. Remove from air fryer and transfer the shrimp onto serving plates.
9. Serve hot.

## Nutrition Values (Per Serving)

- Calories: 540
- Carbohydrate: 33.1g
- Protein: 36.8g
- Fat: 18.2g
- Sugar: 10.6g
- Sodium: 813mg

# Breaded Shrimp with Lemon

**(Yields:** 3 servings / **Prep Time:** 15 minutes / **Cooking Time:** 14 minutes)

## Ingredients

- ½ cup plain flour
- Salt and ground black pepper, as required
- 2 egg whites
- 1 cup breadcrumbs
- ¼ teaspoon lemon zest
- ¼ teaspoon cayenne pepper
- ¼ teaspoon red pepper flakes, crushed
- 1 pound large shrimp, peeled and deveined
- 2 tablespoons vegetable oil

## Instructions

1. In a shallow bowl, mix together the flour, salt, and black pepper.
2. In a second bowl, whisk the egg whites.
3. In a third bowl, mix well breadcrumbs, lime zest and spices.
4. Coat each shrimp with flour, then dip into egg whites and finally, coat with the breadcrumbs mixture.
5. Drizzle the shrimp evenly with oil.
6. Set the temperature of air fryer to 400 degrees F. Grease an air fryer basket.
7. Arrange shrimp into the prepared air fryer basket in 2 batches in a single layer.
8. Air fry for about 6-7 minutes.
9. Remove from air fryer and transfer the shrimp onto serving plates.
10. Serve hot.

## Nutrition Values (Per Serving)

- Calories: 432
- Carbohydrate: 44.8g
- Protein: 37.7g
- Fat: 11.3g
- Sugar: 2.5g
- Sodium: 526mg

---

# Coconut Crusted Shrimp

**(Yields:** 3 servings / **Prep Time:** 15 minutes / **Cooking Time:** 40 minutes)

## Ingredients

- 8 ounces coconut milk
- Salt and ground black pepper, as required
- ½ cup sweetened coconut, shredded

- ½ cup panko breadcrumbs
- 1 pound large shrimp, peeled and deveined

## Instructions

1. In a shallow bowl, add the coconut milk.
2. In another bowl, mix well coconut, breadcrumbs, salt, and black pepper.
3. Dip the shrimp into coconut milk and then, coat with the coconut mixture.
4. Set the temperature of air fryer to 350 degrees F. Grease an air fryer basket.
5. Arrange shrimp into the prepared air fryer basket in 2 batches in a single layer.
6. Air fry for about 17-20 minutes.
7. Remove from air fryer and transfer the shrimp onto serving plates.
8. Serve hot.

## Nutrition Values (Per Serving)

- Calories: 408
- Carbohydrate: 11.7g
- Protein: 31g
- Fat: 23.7g
- Sugar: 3.4g
- Sodium: 253mg

# Bacon Wrapped Shrimp

**(Yields:** 4 servings / **Prep Time:** 20 minutes / **Cooking Time:** 14 minutes**)**

## Ingredients

- 1 pound bacon
- 1½ pounds tiger shrimp, peeled and deveined

## Instructions

1. With a slice of bacon, wrap each shrimp.
2. Refrigerate for about 20 minutes.
3. Set the temperature of air fryer to 390 degrees F. Grease an air fryer basket.
4. Arrange shrimp into the prepared air fryer basket in 2 batches in a single layer.
5. Air fry for about 5-7 minutes.
6. Remove from air fryer and transfer the shrimp onto serving plates.
7. Serve hot.

## Nutrition Values (Per Serving)

- Calories: 782
- Carbohydrate: 1.6g
- Protein: 77.6g
- Fat: 49.2g
- Sugar: 0g
- Sodium: 3000mg

# Shrimp Scampi

**(Yields:** 4 servings / **Prep Time:** 20 minutes / **Cooking Time:** 7 minutes)

## Ingredients

- 4 tablespoons salted butter
- 1 tablespoon fresh lemon juice
- 1 tablespoon garlic, minced
- 2 teaspoons red pepper flakes, crushed
- 1 pound shrimp, peeled and deveined
- 2 tablespoons fresh basil, chopped
- 1 tablespoon fresh chives, chopped
- 2 tablespoons dry white wine

## Instructions

1. Arrange a 7-inch round baking pan in the air fryer basket. Set the temperature of air fryer to 325 degrees F for about 8 minutes.
2. Carefully remove the pan from air fryer basket.
3. In the heated pan, place butter, lemon juice, garlic, and red pepper flakes and return the pan to air fryer basket.
4. Air fry for about 2 minutes, stirring once halfway through.
5. Carefully remove the pan from air fryer basket and stir in shrimp, basil, chives and wine.
6. Return the pan to air fryer basket and air fry for about 5 minutes, stirring once halfway through.
7. Remove from air fryer and place the pan onto a wire rack for about 1 minute.
8. Stir the mixture and transfer onto serving plates.
9. Serve hot.

## Nutrition Values (Per Serving)

- Calories: 250
- Carbohydrate: 3.3g
- Protein: 26.3g
- Fat: 13.7g
- Sugar: 0.3g
- Sodium: 360mg

# Rice Flour Coated Shrimp

**(Yields:** 3 servings / **Prep Time:** 20 minutes / **Cooking Time:** 20 minutes)

## Ingredients

- 3 tablespoons rice flour
- 2 tablespoons olive oil
- 1 teaspoon powdered sugar
- Salt and ground black pepper, as required
- 1 pound shrimp, peeled and deveined

## Instructions

1. In a bowl, mix well flour, oil, sugar, salt, and black pepper.
2. Add the shrimp and toss to coat well.
3. Set the temperature of air fryer to 325 degrees F. Grease an air fryer basket.
4. Arrange shrimp into the prepared air fryer basket in 2 batches in a single layer.
5. Air fry for about 8-10 minutes, tossing once halfway through.
6. Remove from air fryer and transfer the shrimp onto serving plates.
7. Serve hot.

## Nutrition Values (Per Serving)

- Calories: 299
- Carbohydrate: 11.1g
- Protein: 35g
- Fat: 12g
- Sugar: 0.8g
- Sodium: 419mg

---

# Shrimp Kebabs

**(Yields:** 2 servings / **Prep Time:** 15 minutes / **Cooking Time:** 8 minutes)

## Ingredients

- ¾ pound shrimp, peeled and deveined
- 2 tablespoons fresh lemon juice
- 1 teaspoon garlic, minced
- ½ teaspoon paprika
- ½ teaspoon ground cumin
- Salt and ground black pepper, as required
- 1 tablespoon fresh cilantro, chopped

## Instructions

1. Set the temperature of air fryer to 350 degrees F. Grease an air fryer basket.
2. In a bowl, mix together the lemon juice, garlic, and spices.
3. Add the shrimp and mix well.
4. Thread the shrimp onto presoaked wooden skewers.

5. Arrange shrimp skewers into the prepared air fryer basket.
6. Air fry for about 5-8 minutes, flipping once halfway through.
7. Remove from air fryer and transfer the shrimp kebabs onto serving plates.
8. Garnish with fresh cilantro and serve immediately.

## Nutrition Values (Per Serving)

- Calories: 212
- Carbohydrate: 3.9g
- Protein: 39.1g
- Fat: 3.2g
- Sugar: 0.4g
- Sodium: 497mg

# Nacho Chips Crusted Prawns

**(Yields:** 2 servings / **Prep Time:** 15 minutes / **Cooking Time:** 8 minutes)

## Ingredients

- ¾ pound prawns, peeled and deveined
- 1 large egg
- 5 ounces Nacho flavored chips, finely crushed

## Instructions

1. In a shallow bowl, beat the egg.
2. In another bowl, place the nacho chips
3. Dip each prawn into the beaten egg and then, coat with the crushed nacho chips.
4. Set the temperature of air fryer to 350 degrees F. Grease an air fryer basket.
5. Arrange prawns into the prepared air fryer basket.
6. Air fry for about 8 minutes.
7. Remove from air fryer and transfer the prawns onto serving plates.
8. Serve hot.

## Nutrition Values (Per Serving)

- Calories: 602
- Carbohydrate: 46.5g
- Protein: 11.3g
- Fat: 23.9g
- Sugar: 2.9g
- Sodium: 886mg

# Prawn Burgers

**(Yields:** 2 servings / **Prep Time:** 20 minutes / **Cooking Time:** 6 minutes)

## Ingredients

- ½ cup prawns, peeled, deveined and finely chopped
- ½ cup breadcrumbs
- 2-3 tablespoons onion, finely chopped
- ½ teaspoon ginger, minced
- ½ teaspoon garlic, minced
- ½ teaspoon red chili powder
- ½ teaspoon ground cumin
- ¼ teaspoon ground turmeric
- Salt and ground black pepper, as required
- 3 cups fresh baby greens

## Instructions

1. In a large bowl, mix together the prawns, breadcrumbs, onion, ginger, garlic, and spices.
2. Make small-sized patties from the mixture.
3. Set the temperature of air fryer to 390 degrees F. Grease an air fryer basket.
4. Arrange patties into the prepared air fryer basket in a single layer.
5. Air fry for about 5-6 minutes.
6. Remove from air fryer and transfer the prawn burgers onto serving plates.
7. Serve warm alongside the baby greens.

## Nutrition Values (Per Serving)

- Calories: 240
- Carbohydrate: 37.4g
- Protein: 18g
- Fat: 2.7g
- Sugar: 4g
- Sodium: 371mg

---

# Buttered Scallops

**(Yields:** 2 servings / **Prep Time:** 15 minutes / **Cooking Time:** 4 minutes)

## Ingredients

- ¾ pound sea scallops, cleaned and patted very dry
- 1 tablespoon butter, melted
- ½ tablespoon fresh thyme, minced
- Salt and ground black pepper, as required

## Instructions

1. In a large bowl, add the scallops, butter, thyme, salt, and black pepper. Toss to coat well.
2. Set the temperature of air fryer to 390 degrees F. Grease an air fryer basket.
3. Arrange scallops into the prepared air fryer basket in a single layer.
4. Air fry for about 4 minutes.
5. Remove from air fryer and transfer the scallops onto serving plates.
6. Serve hot.

## Nutrition Values (Per Serving)

- Calories: 202
- Carbohydrate: 4.4g
- Protein: 28.7g
- Fat: 7.1g
- Sugar: 0g
- Sodium: 393mg

---

# Scallops with Capers Sauce

**(Yields:** 2 servings / **Prep Time:** 15 minutes / **Cooking Time:** 6 minutes)

## Ingredients

- 10 (1-ounce) sea scallops, cleaned and patted very dry
- Salt and ground black pepper, as required
- ¼ cup extra-virgin olive oil
- 2 tablespoons fresh parsley, finely chopped
- 2 teaspoons capers, finely chopped
- 1 teaspoon fresh lemon zest, finely grated
- ½ teaspoon garlic, finely chopped

## Instructions

1. Season each scallop evenly with salt and black pepper.
2. Set the temperature of air fryer to 400 degrees F. Grease an air fryer basket.
3. Arrange scallops into the prepared air fryer basket in a single layer.
4. Air fry for about 6 minutes.
5. Meanwhile, for the sauce: in a bowl, mix the remaining ingredients.
6. Remove from air fryer and transfer the scallops onto serving plates.
7. Top with the sauce and serve immediately.

## Nutrition Values (Per Serving)

- Calories: 344
- Carbohydrate: 4.2g
- Protein: 24g
- Fat: 26.3g
- Sugar: 0.1g
- Sodium: 393mg

---

# Crispy Scallops

**(Yields:** 4 servings / **Prep Time:** 15 minutes / **Cooking Time:** 6 minutes)

## Ingredients

- 18 sea scallops, cleaned and patted very dry
- 1/8 cup all-purpose flour
- ½ teaspoon paprika
- Salt and ground black pepper, as required
- 1 tablespoon 2% milk
- ½ egg
- ¼ cup cornflakes, crushed
- Olive oil cooking spray

## Instructions

1. In a shallow bowl, mix together the flour, paprika, salt, and black pepper.
2. In another bowl, add the milk and egg. Beat until well combined.
3. In a third bowl, place the cornflakes.
4. Coat each scallop with the flour mixture, then dip into the egg mixture and finally, coat with the cornflakes.
5. Spray the scallops evenly with cooking spray.
6. Set the temperature of air fryer to 400 degrees F. Grease an air fryer basket.
7. Arrange scallops into the prepared air fryer basket in a single layer.
8. Air fry for about 5-6 minutes, flipping once halfway through.
9. Remove from air fryer and transfer the scallops onto serving plates.
10. Serve hot.

## Nutrition Values (Per Serving)

- Calories: 150
- Carbohydrate: 8g
- Protein: 24g
- Fat: 1.7g
- Sugar: 0.4g
- Sodium: 278mg

# Scallops with Spinach

**(Yields:** 2 servings / **Prep Time:** 20 minutes / **Cooking Time:** 10 minutes)

## Ingredients

- 1 (12-ounces) package frozen spinach, thawed and drained
- 8 jumbo sea scallops
- Olive oil cooking spray
- Salt and ground black pepper, as required
- ¾ cup heavy whipping cream
- 1 tablespoon tomato paste
- 1 teaspoon garlic, minced
- 1 tablespoon fresh basil, chopped

## Instructions

1. In the bottom of a 7-inch heatproof pan, place the spinach.
2. Spray each scallop evenly with cooking spray and then, sprinkle with a little salt and black pepper.
3. Arrange scallops on top of the spinach in a single layer.
4. In a bowl, mix well cream, tomato paste, garlic, basil, salt, and black pepper.
5. Add cream mixture evenly over the spinach and scallops.
6. Set the temperature of air fryer to 350 degrees F.
7. Air fry for about 10 minutes.
8. Remove from air fryer and transfer the scallops mixture onto serving plates.
9. Serve hot.

## Nutrition Values (Per Serving)

- Calories: 203
- Carbohydrate: 12,3g
- Protein: 26.4g
- Fat: 18.3g
- Sugar: 1.7g
- Sodium: 101mg

# Bacon Wrapped Scallops

**(Yields:** 4 servings / **Prep Time:** 15 minutes / **Cooking Time:** 12 minutes)

## Ingredients

- 5 center-cut bacon slices, cut each in 4 pieces
- 20 sea scallops, cleaned and patted very dry
- 1 teaspoon lemon pepper seasoning
- ½ teaspoon paprika
- Olive oil cooking spray
- Salt and ground black pepper, as required

## Instructions

1. With a piece of bacon, wrap each scallop and secure each with a toothpick.
2. Sprinkle each scallop evenly with lemon pepper seasoning and paprika.
3. Set the temperature of air fryer to 400 degrees F. Grease an air fryer basket.
4. Arrange scallops into the prepared air fryer basket in 2 batches in a single layer.
5. Spray the scallops evenly with cooking spray and sprinkle with salt and black pepper.
6. Air fry for about 5-6 minutes, flipping once halfway through.
7. Remove from air fryer and transfer the scallops onto a paper towel-lined plate.
8. Serve hot.

## Nutrition Values (Per Serving)

- Calories: 330
- Carbohydrate: 4.5g
- Protein: 38.7g
- Fat: 16.3g
- Sugar: 0g
- Sodium: 1118mg

---

# Glazed Calamari

**(Yields:** 3 servings / **Prep Time:** 20 minutes / **Cooking Time:** 13 minutes)

## Ingredients

### For Calamari

- ½ pound calamari tubes
- 1 cup club soda
- 1 cup flour
- ½ tablespoon red pepper flakes, crushed
- Salt and ground black pepper, as required

### For Sauce

- ½ cup honey
- 2 tablespoons Sriracha sauce
- ¼ teaspoon red pepper flakes, crushed

## Instructions

1. Wash calamari and cut into ¼ inch rings.
2. Transfer the calamari into a bowl and cover with club soda.
3. Set aside for about 10 minutes.
4. In another bowl, mix well flour, red pepper flakes, salt, and black pepper.
5. Drain the club soda from calamari.
6. With the paper towels, pat dry the calamari rings.
7. Coat the calamari rings evenly with flour mixture.
8. Set the temperature of air fryer to 375 degrees F. Grease an air fryer basket.
9. Arrange calamari rings into the prepared air fryer basket.
10. Air fry for about 11 minutes, shaking occasionally.
11. Meanwhile, in a bowl, mix together the honey, Sriracha sauce, and red pepper flakes.
12. Remove from air fryer and coat calamari rings with the sauce.
13. Air fry for about 2 minutes.
14. Remove from air Fryer and transfer the calamari rings onto serving plates.
15. Serve hot.

## Nutrition Values (Per Serving)

- Calories: 307
- Carbohydrate: 62.1g
- Protein: 12g
- Fat: 1.4g
- Sugar: 35g
- Sodium: 131mg

---

# Buttered Crab Shells

**(Yields:** 4 servings / **Prep Time:** 20 minutes / **Cooking Time:** 20 minutes)

## Ingredients

- 4 soft crab shells, cleaned
- 1 cup buttermilk
- 3 eggs
- 2 cups panko breadcrumb
- 2 teaspoons seafood seasoning*
- 1½ teaspoons lemon zest, grated
- 2 tablespoons butter, melted

## Instructions

1. In a shallow bowl, place the buttermilk.
2. In a second bowl, whisk the eggs.
3. In a third bowl, mix together the breadcrumbs, seafood seasoning, and lemon zest.
4. Soak the crab shells into the buttermilk for about 10 minutes.

5. Now, dip the crab shells into beaten eggs and then, coat with the breadcrumbs mixture.
6. Set the temperature of air fryer to 375 degrees F. Grease an air fryer basket.
7. Arrange crab shells into the prepared air fryer basket in a single layer.
8. Air fry for about 8-10 minutes.
9. Remove from air Fryer and transfer the crab shells onto serving plates.
10. Drizzle crab shells with the melted butter and serve immediately.

## **Nutrition Values (Per Serving)**

- Calories: 521
- Carbohydrate: 11.5g
- Protein: 47.8g
- Fat: 16.8g
- Sugar: 3.3g
- Sodium: 1100mg

(**Note: Seafood Seasoning*** - Mix the salt, celery seed, dry mustard powder, red pepper, black pepper, bay leaves, paprika, cloves, allspice, ginger, cardamom, and cinnamon together in a bowl until thoroughly combined. Or, you can buy at your local store or on Amazon.)

# **Crab Cakes**

(**Yields:** 4 servings / **Prep Time:** 20 minutes / **Cooking Time:** 20 minutes)

## **Ingredients**

- 1 pound lump crab meat
- 1/3 cup panko breadcrumbs
- ¼ cup scallion, finely chopped
- 2 large eggs
- 2 tablespoons mayonnaise
- 1 teaspoon Dijon mustard
- 1 teaspoon Worcestershire sauce
- 1½ teaspoons Old Bay seasoning
- Ground black pepper, as required

## **Instructions**

1. In a large bowl, add all the ingredients and gently, stir to combine.
2. Cover the bowl and refrigerate for about 1 hour.
3. Make 8 equal-sized patties from the mixture.
4. Set the temperature of air fryer to 375 degrees F. Grease an air fryer basket.
5. Arrange crab cakes into the prepared air fryer basket in 2 batches in a single layer.
6. Air fry for about 5 minutes per side.
7. Remove from air fryer and transfer the crab cakes onto serving plates.
8. Serve warm.

## Nutrition Values (Per Serving)

- Calories: 183
- Carbohydrate: 5.9g
- Protein: 20.1g
- Fat: 14.8g
- Sugar: 1.1g
- Sodium: 996mg

# Wasabi Crab Cakes

**(Yields:** 6 servings / **Prep Time:** 20 minutes / **Cooking Time:** 24 minutes)

## Ingredients

- 3 scallions, finely chopped
- 1 medium sweet red pepper, finely chopped
- 1 celery rib*, finely chopped
- 1/3 cup plus ½ cup dry breadcrumbs, divided
- 2 large egg whites
- 3 tablespoons mayonnaise
- ¼ teaspoon prepared wasabi
- Salt, to taste
- 1½ cups lump crab meat, drained
- Olive oil cooking spray

## Instructions

1. In a bowl, add the scallions, red pepper, celery, 1/3 cup of breadcrumbs, egg whites, mayonnaise, wasabi, and salt. Mix until well combined.
2. Gently fold in the crab meat.
3. In a shallow bowl, place the remaining breadcrumbs.
4. Make ¾-inch thick patties from the mixture.
5. Set the temperature of air fryer to 375 degrees F. Grease an air fryer basket.
6. Arrange crab cakes into the prepared air fryer basket in 2 batches in a single layer.
7. Air fry for about 8-12 minutes, flipping once halfway through and spraying with the cooking spray.
8. Remove from air fryer and transfer the crab cakes onto serving plates.
9. Serve warm.

## Nutrition Values (Per Serving)

- Calories: 112
- Carbohydrate: 15.5g
- Protein: 4.9g
- Fat: 4g
- Sugar: 2.7g
- Sodium: 253mg

(**Note: Celery Rib*** - By most definitions, a whole head of celery is a stalk and a single "stick" from the stalk is a rib. Some dictionaries use the accurate but clunky term "leafstalk" for a single rib.)

# CHAPTER 6 | VEGETARIAN AND VEGAN

## Vegetarian Mains

### Brussel Sprout Salad

**(Yields:** 4 servings / **Prep Time:** 20 minutes / **Cooking Time:** 15 minutes)

## Ingredients

**For Salad**

- 1 pound fresh medium Brussels sprouts, trimmed and halved vertically
- 3 teaspoons olive oil
- Salt and ground black pepper, as required
- 2 apples, cored and chopped
- 1 red onion, sliced
- 4 cups lettuce, torn

**For Dressing**

- 2 tablespoons extra-virgin olive oil
- 2 tablespoons fresh lemon juice
- 1 tablespoon apple cider vinegar
- 1 tablespoon honey
- 1 teaspoon Dijon mustard
- Salt and ground black pepper, as required

## Instructions

1. Set the temperature of air fryer to 360 degrees F.
2. For Brussels sprout: in a bowl, add the Brussels sprout, oil, salt, and black pepper and toss to coat well.
3. Spread the Brussels sprouts onto a large baking sheet.
4. Arrange the baking sheet into air fryer basket and air fryer for about 15 minutes, flipping once halfway through.
5. Remove from air fryer and transfer the Brussel sprouts onto a plate.
6. Set aside to cool slightly.
7. In a serving bowl, mix together the Brussel sprouts, apples, onion, and lettuce.
8. For dressing: in a bowl, add all the ingredients and beat until well combined.
9. Add the dressing and gently, stir to combine.
10. Serve immediately.

## Nutrition Values (Per Serving)

- Calories: 235
- Carbohydrate: 34.5g
- Protein: 4.9g
- Fat: 11.3g
- Sugar: 20.3g
- Sodium: 88mg

# Eggplant Salad

(**Yields:** 2 servings / **Prep Time:** 15 minutes / **Cooking Time:** 15 minutes)

## Ingredients

### For Salad

- 1 eggplant, cut into ½-inch-thick slices crosswise
- 2 tablespoons canola oil
- Salt and ground black pepper, as required
- 1 avocado, peeled, pitted and chopped
- 1 teaspoon fresh lemon juice

### For Dressing

- 1 tablespoon extra-virgin olive oil
- 1 tablespoon red wine vinegar
- 1 tablespoon honey
- 1 tablespoon fresh oregano leaves, chopped
- 1 teaspoon fresh lemon zest, grated
- 1 teaspoon Dijon mustard
- Salt and ground black pepper, as required

## Instructions

1. Set the temperature of air fryer to 400 degrees F. Grease an air fryer basket.
2. For salad: in a bowl, add the eggplant, oil, salt, and black pepper and toss to coat well.
3. Arrange eggplants pieces into the prepared air fryer basket in a single layer.
4. Air fry for about 15 minutes, shaking after every 5 minutes.
5. Remove from air fryer and transfer the eggplant pieces onto a plate.
6. Set aside to cool slightly.
7. In a bowl, mix together the avocado and lemon juice.
8. In a serving bowl, mix together the eggplants pieces and avocado mixture.
9. For dressing: in a bowl, add all the ingredients and beat until well combined.
10. Add the dressing and gently, stir to combine.
11. Serve immediately.

## Nutrition Values (Per Serving)

- Calories: 489
- Carbohydrate: 32.7g
- Protein: 4.6g
- Fat: 41.4g
- Sugar: 16.2g
- Sodium: 118mg

# Potato Salad

**(Yields:** 6 servings / **Prep Time:** 10 minutes / **Cooking Time:** 40 minutes)

## Ingredients

- 4 Russet potatoes
- 1 tablespoon olive oil
- Salt, as required
- 3 hard-boiled eggs, peeled and chopped
- 1 cup celery, chopped
- ½ cup red onion, chopped
- 1 tablespoon prepared mustard
- ¼ teaspoon celery salt
- ¼ teaspoon garlic salt
- ¼ cup mayonnaise

## Instructions

1. Set the temperature of air fryer to 390 degrees F. Grease an air fryer basket.
2. With a fork, prick the potatoes.
3. Drizzle with oil and rub with the salt.
4. Arrange potatoes into the prepared air fryer basket.
5. Air fry for about 35-40 minutes.
6. Remove from air fryer and transfer the potatoes into a bowl.
7. Set aside to cool.
8. After cooling, chop the potatoes.
9. In a serving bowl, add the potatoes and remaining ingredients and gently, mix them well.
10. Refrigerate to chill before serving.
11. Serve.

## Nutrition Values (Per Serving)

- Calories: 196
- Carbohydrate: 26.5g
- Protein: 5.6g
- Fat: 8.1g
- Sugar: 3.1g
- Sodium: 18`0mg

# Cauliflower Salad

**(Yields:** 4 servings / **Prep Time:** 20 minutes / **Cooking Time:** 10 minutes)

## Ingredients

### For Salad

- ¼ cup golden raisins
- 1 cup boiling water
- ¼ cup olive oil
- 1 head cauliflower, cut into small florets
- 1 tablespoon curry powder
- Salt, to taste
- ¼ cup pecans, toasted and chopped
- 2 tablespoons fresh mint leaves, chopped

### For Dressing

- 1 cup mayonnaise
- 2 tablespoons sugar
- 1 tablespoon fresh lemon juice

## Instructions

1. For salad: in a bowl, add the cauliflower, curry powder, salt, and oil and toss to coat well.
2. Set the temperature of air fryer to 390 degrees F. Grease an air fryer basket.
3. Arrange cauliflower florets into the prepared air fryer basket in a single layer.
4. Air fry for about 8-10 minutes.
5. Meanwhile, in a bowl, add the raisins, and boiling water and set aside until using.
6. Remove from air fryer and transfer the cauliflower florets onto a plate.
7. Set aside to cool.
8. Drain the raisins well.
9. For dressing: in a bowl, add all the ingredients and mix until well combined.
10. In another bowl, mix together the cauliflower, raisins and pecans.
11. Add the dressing and gently, stir to combine.
12. Refrigerate to chill before serving.
13. Garnish with mint and serve

## Nutrition Values (Per Serving)

- Calories: 162
- Carbohydrate: 25.3g
- Protein: 11.3g
- Fat: 3.1g
- Sugar: 1.6g
- Sodium: 160mg

# Radish Salad

**(Yields:** 4 servings / **Prep Time:** 15 minutes / **Cooking Time:** 30 minutes)

## Ingredients

### For Radishes:

- 1½ pounds radishes, trimmed and halved
- Salt and ground black pepper, as required
- 2 tablespoons olive oil

### For Salad:

- ½ pound fresh mozzarella, sliced
- 6 cups fresh salad greens
- 1 teaspoon honey
- 1 teaspoon olive oil
- 1 tablespoon balsamic vinegar
- Salt and ground black pepper, as required

## Instructions

1. In a bowl, add the radishes, salt, black pepper, and oil and toss to coat well.
2. Set the temperature of air fryer to 350 degrees F. Grease an air fryer basket.
3. Arrange radishes into the prepared air fryer basket in a single layer.
4. Air fry for about 30 minutes, tossing 2-3 times.
5. Remove from air fryer and place the radishes into a bowl to cool.
6. For salad: in a large serving bowl, mix together the cooked radishes, mozzarella, and greens.
7. For dressing: in a small bowl, mix together the honey, oil, vinegar, salt, and black pepper.
8. Place the dressing over salad and toss to coat well.
9. Serve immediately.

## Nutrition Values (Per Serving)

- Calories: 468
- Carbohydrate: 33.1g
- Protein: 3.3g
- Fat: 38.5g
- Sugar: 17.1g
- Sodium: 482mg

# Zucchini Salad

**(Yields:** 4 servings / **Prep Time:** 15 minutes / **Cooking Time:** 30 minutes)

## Ingredients

- 1 pound zucchini, cut into rounds
- 2 tablespoons olive oil
- 1 teaspoon garlic powder
- Salt and ground black pepper, as required
- 5 cups fresh spinach, chopped
- ¼ cup feta cheese, crumbled
- 2 tablespoons fresh lemon juice

## Instructions

1. Set the temperature of air fryer to 400 degrees F. Grease an air fryer basket.
2. In a bowl, mix together the zucchini, oil, garlic powder, salt, and black pepper.
3. Arrange zucchini slices into the prepared air fryer basket in a single layer.
4. Air fry for about 30 minutes, tossing 3 times.
5. Remove from air fryer and transfer the zucchini slices onto a plate.
6. Set aside to cool.
7. In another bowl, add the cooked zucchini slices, spinach, feta cheese, lemon juice, a little bit of salt, and black pepper and toss to coat well.
8. Serve immediately.

## Nutrition Values (Per Serving)

- Calories: 116
- Carbohydrate: 6.2g
- Protein: 4g
- Fat: 9.4g
- Sugar: 2.8g
- Sodium: 186mg

# Mixed Veggie Salad

**(Yields:** 8 servings / **Prep Time:** 25 minutes / **Cooking Time:** 1 hour 35 minutes)

## Ingredients

- 2 tablespoons olive oil, divided
- 3 medium zucchinis, sliced into ½-inch thick rounds
- 3 small eggplants, sliced into ½-inch thick rounds
- 4 medium tomatoes, cut in eighths
- 1 cup cherry tomatoes, quartered
- 2 red bell peppers, seeded and chopped
- 4 fresh basil leaves, chopped
- ½ cup Italian dressing
- Salt, as required
- ½ cup Parmesan cheese, grated

## Instructions

1. Set the temperature of air fryer to 355 degrees F. Grease an air fryer basket.
2. In a bowl, mix together the zucchini and one tablespoon of oil.
3. Place zucchini slices into the prepared air fryer basket.
4. Air fry for about 25 minutes.
5. Remove from air fryer and place the zucchini slices into a bowl. Set aside.
6. In another bowl, mix well eggplant and one tablespoon of oil.
7. Place eggplant slices into the greased air fryer basket.
8. Air fry for about 30-40 minutes.
9. Remove from air fryer and place the eggplant slices into a bowl with zucchini. Set aside.
10. Now, set the temperature of air fryer to 320 degrees F.
11. Place tomatoes into the greased air fryer basket.
12. Air fry for about 30 minutes.
13. Remove from air fryer and place the tomatoes into a bowl with veggies.
14. In the bowl of cooked vegetables, add the bell pepper, basil, salt, dressing, and salt and gently, stir to combine.
15. Cover the bowl of salad and refrigerate for 2 hours before serving.
16. Garnish with Parmesan cheese and serve.

## Nutrition Values (Per Serving)

- Calories: 179
- Carbohydrate: 21.6g
- Protein: 6g
- Fat: 9.6g
- Sugar: 12.4g
- Sodium: 83mg

# Honey Glazed Carrots

**(Yields:** 4 servings / **Prep Time:** 15 minutes / **Cooking Time:** 12 minutes)

## Ingredients

- 3 cups carrots, peeled and cut into large chunks
- 1 tablespoon olive oil
- 1 tablespoon honey
- 1 tablespoon fresh thyme, finely chopped
- Salt and ground black pepper, as required

## Instructions

1. Set the temperature of air fryer to 390 degrees F. Grease an air fryer basket.
2. In a bowl, mix well carrot, oil, honey, thyme, salt, and black pepper.
3. Arrange carrot chunks into the prepared air fryer basket in a single layer.
4. Air fry for about 12 minutes.
5. Remove from air fryer and transfer the carrot chunks onto serving plates.
6. Serve hot.

## Nutrition Values (Per Serving)

- Calories: 82
- Carbohydrate: 12.9g
- Protein: 0.8g
- Fat: 3.6g
- Sugar: 8.4g
- Sodium: 96mg

# Caramelized Carrots

**(Yields:** 3 servings / **Prep Time:** 10 minutes / **Cooking Time:** 15 minutes)

## Ingredients

- ½ cup butter, melted
- ½ cup brown sugar
- 1 small bag baby carrots

## Instructions

1. Set the temperature of air fryer to 400 degrees F. Grease an air fryer basket.
2. In a bowl, mix together the butter and brown sugar.
3. Add the carrots and coat well.
4. Arrange carrots into the prepared air fryer basket in a single layer.
5. Air fry for about 15 minutes.

6. Remove from air fryer and transfer the carrots onto serving plates.
7. Serve hot.

## Nutrition Values (Per Serving)

- Calories: 416
- Carbohydrate: 36.2g
- Protein: 1.3g
- Fat: 30.9g
- Sugar: 30.7g
- Sodium: 343mg

---

# Cheesy Brussel Sprouts

**(Yields:** 3 servings / **Prep Time:** 15 minutes / **Cooking Time:** 10 minutes)

## Ingredients

- 1 pound Brussels sprouts, trimmed and halved
- 1 tablespoon balsamic vinegar
- 1 tablespoon extra-virgin olive oil
- Salt and ground black pepper, as required
- ¼ cup whole wheat breadcrumbs
- ¼ cup Parmesan cheese, shredded

## Instructions

1. Set the temperature of air fryer to 400 degrees F. Grease an air fryer basket.
2. In a bowl, mix well Brussel sprouts, vinegar, oil, salt, and black pepper.
3. Arrange Brussel sprouts into the prepared air fryer basket in a single layer.
4. Air fry for about 5 minutes.
5. Remove from air fryer and flip the Brussel sprouts.
6. Sprinkle the Brussel sprouts evenly with breadcrumbs, followed by the cheese.
7. Air fryer for about 5 more minutes.
8. Remove from air fryer and transfer the Brussels sprouts onto serving plates.
9. Serve hot.

## Nutrition Values (Per Serving)

- Calories: 240
- Carbohydrate: 19.4g
- Protein: 16.3g
- Fat: 12.6g
- Sugar: 3.4g
- Sodium: 548mg

# Sweet & Sour Brussel Sprouts

**(Yields:** 2 servings / **Prep Time:** 10 minutes / **Cooking Time:** 10 minutes)

## Ingredients

- 2 cups Brussels sprouts, trimmed and halved lengthwise
- 1 tablespoon balsamic vinegar
- 1 tablespoon maple syrup
- Salt, as required

## Instructions

1. Set the temperature of air fryer to 400 degrees F. Grease an air fryer basket.
2. In a bowl, add all the ingredients and toss to coat well.
3. Arrange Brussels sprouts into the prepared air fryer basket in a single layer.
4. Air fry for about 8-10 minutes, shaking once halfway through.
5. Remove from air fryer and transfer the Brussels sprouts onto serving plates.
6. Serve hot.

## Nutrition Values (Per Serving)

- Calories: 66
- Carbohydrate: 14.8g
- Protein: 3g
- Fat: 0.3g
- Sugar: 7.9g
- Sodium: 101mg

===

# Spiced Eggplant

**(Yields:** 3 servings / **Prep Time:** 15 minutes / **Cooking Time:** 27 minutes)

## Ingredients

- 2 medium eggplants, cubed
- 2 tablespoons butter, melted
- 1 tablespoon Maggi seasoning sauce
- 1 teaspoon sumac*
- 1 teaspoon garlic powder
- 1 teaspoon onion powder
- Salt and ground black pepper, as required
- 1 tablespoon fresh lemon juice
- 2 tablespoons Parmesan cheese, shredded

## Instructions

1. Set the temperature of air fryer to 320 degrees F. Grease an air fryer basket.
2. In a bowl, mix together the eggplant cubes, butter, seasoning sauce and spices.
3. Arrange eggplant cubes into the prepared air fryer basket in a single layer.
4. Air fry for about 15 minutes.
5. Remove from air fryer and toss the eggplant cubes.

6. Now, set the temperature of air fryer to 350 degrees F and air fry for about 10-12 minutes, tossing once halfway through.
7. Remove from air fryer and transfer the eggplant cubes into a bowl.
8. Add the lemon juice, and Parmesan and toss to coat well.
9. Serve immediately.

## Nutrition Values (Per Serving)

- Calories: 173
- Carbohydrate: 23g
- Protein: 4.6g
- Fat: 8.9g
- Sugar: 11.6g
- Sodium: 276mg

(**Note: Sumac\*** - The sumac bush, native to the Middle East, produces deep red berries, which are dried and ground into coarse powder. Lemon zest is the most easily available ingredient that can be used as a sumac substitute.)

# Veggies Stuffed Eggplants

(**Yields:** 5 servings / **Prep Time:** 20 minutes / **Cooking Time:** 14 minutes)

## Ingredients

- 10 small eggplants, halved lengthwise
- 1 tablespoon fresh lime juice
- 1 tablespoon vegetable oil
- 1 onion, chopped
- ½ teaspoon garlic, chopped
- 1 tomato, chopped
- Salt and ground black pepper, as required
- ¼ cup cottage cheese, chopped
- ½ green bell pepper, seeded and chopped
- 2 tablespoons tomato paste
- 2 tablespoons fresh cilantro, chopped

## Instructions

1. Carefully, cut a slice from one side of each eggplant lengthwise.
2. Now, with a small spoon, scoop out the flesh from each eggplant leaving a thick shell.
3. Transfer the eggplant flesh into a bowl.
4. Drizzle the eggplants evenly with lime juice.
5. Set the temperature of air fryer to 320 degrees F. Grease an air fryer basket.
6. Arrange hollowed eggplants into the prepared air fryer basket in a single layer.
7. Air fry for about 3-4 minutes.
8. Meanwhile, heat the oil in a skillet over medium heat and sauté the onion and garlic for about 2 minutes.

9. Add the eggplant flesh, tomato, salt, and black pepper and sauté for about 2 minutes.
10. Stir in the cheese, bell pepper, tomato paste, and cilantro and cook for about 1 minute.
11. Remove the pan of veggie mixture from heat.
12. Stuff the hollowed eggplant shells with veggie mixture and close each with its cut part.
13. Set the temperature of air fryer to 356 degrees F. Grease the air fryer basket.
14. Arrange eggplant shells into the prepared air fryer basket in a single layer.
15. Air fry for about 4-5 minutes.
16. Remove from air fryer and transfer the eggplants onto serving plates.
17. Serve hot.

## Nutrition Values (Per Serving)

- Calories: 83
- Carbohydrate: 11.9g
- Protein: 3.4g
- Fat: 3.2g
- Sugar: 6.1g
- Sodium: 87mg

---

# Buttered Broccoli

**(Yields:** 4 servings / **Prep Time:** 10 minutes / **Cooking Time:** 7 minutes)

## Ingredients

- 4 cups fresh broccoli florets
- 2 tablespoons butter, melted
- Salt and ground black pepper, as required
- ¼ cup water

## Instructions

1. Set the temperature of air fryer to 400 degrees F. Grease an air fryer basket.
2. In a bowl, mix well broccoli, butter, salt, and black pepper.
3. In the bottom of air fryer pan, place the water.
4. Arrange broccoli florets into the prepared air fryer basket in a single layer.
5. Air fry for about 7 minutes.
6. Remove from air fryer and transfer the broccoli onto serving plates.
7. Serve hot.

## Nutrition Values (Per Serving)

- Calories: 82
- Carbohydrate: 6g
- Protein: 2.6g
- Fat: 6.1g
- Sugar: 1.6g
- Sodium: 110mg

# Garlic Broccoli

**(Yields:** 3 servings / **Prep Time:** 15 minutes / **Cooking Time:** 20 minutes)

## Ingredients

- 1 tablespoon butter
- 2 teaspoons vegetable bouillon granules
- 1 tablespoon fresh lemon juice
- 3 garlic cloves, sliced
- 1 large head broccoli, cut into bite-sized pieces
- ½ teaspoon fresh lemon zest, finely grated
- ½ teaspoon red pepper flakes, crushed

## Instructions

1. Set the temperature of air fryer to 355 degrees F.
2. In an air fryer pan, add the butter, bouillon granules, and lemon juice and air fry for about 1-1½ minutes.
3. Stir in the garlic and air fry for about 30 seconds.
4. Stir in the broccoli and air fry for about 13 minutes.
5. Stir in the lemon zest, and red pepper flakes and air fry for about 5 minutes.
6. Remove from air fryer and transfer the broccoli onto serving plates.
7. Serve hot.

## Nutrition Values (Per Serving)

- Calories: 80
- Carbohydrate: 8.9g
- Protein: 3.5g
- Fat: 4.3g
- Sugar: 2.1g
- Sodium: 85mg

# Parmesan Broccoli

**(Yields:** 2 servings / **Prep Time:** 10 minutes / **Cooking Time:** 40 minutes)

## Ingredients

- 10 ounces frozen broccoli
- 3 tablespoons balsamic vinegar
- 1 tablespoon olive oil
- 1/8 teaspoon cayenne pepper
- Salt and ground black pepper, as required
- 2 tablespoons Parmesan cheese, grated

## Instructions

1. In a bowl, add the broccoli, vinegar, oil, cayenne, salt, and black pepper and toss to coat well.
2. Set the temperature of air fryer to 400 degrees F. Grease an air fryer basket.
3. Arrange broccoli into the prepared air fryer basket.
4. Air fry for about 20 minutes, tossing several times while frying.
5. Remove from air fryer and transfer the broccoli onto serving plates.
6. Immediately, sprinkle with cheese and serve hot.

## Nutrition Values (Per Serving)

- Calories: 173
- Carbohydrate: 10.7g
- Protein: 10g
- Fat: 11.5g
- Sugar: 2.5g
- Sodium: 505mg

# Broccoli with Olives

(**Yields:** 4 servings / **Prep Time:** 15 minutes / **Cooking Time:** 19 minutes)

## Ingredients

- 2 pounds broccoli, stemmed and cut into 1 inch florets
- 2 tablespoons olive oil
- Salt and ground black pepper, as required
- 1/3 cup Kalamata olives, halved and pitted
- 2 teaspoons fresh lemon zest, grated
- ¼ cup Parmesan cheese, grated

## Instructions

1. In a pan of boiling water, add the broccoli and cook for about 3-4 minutes.
2. Drain the broccoli well.
3. Set the temperature of air fryer to 400 degrees F. Grease an air fryer basket.
4. In a bowl, mix together broccoli, oil, salt, and black pepper.
5. Arrange broccoli into the prepared air fryer basket.
6. Air fry for about 15 minutes, tossing once halfway through.
7. Remove from air fryer and immediately stir in the olives, lemon zest and cheese.
8. Serve immediately.

## Nutrition Values (Per Serving)

- Calories: 169
- Carbohydrate: 16g
- Protein: 8.5g
- Fat: 10.2g
- Sugar: 3.9g
- Sodium: 254mg

# Pesto Tomatoes

**(Yields:** 4 servings / **Prep Time:** 15 minutes / **Cooking Time:** 16 minutes)

## Ingredients

### For Pesto:
- ½ cup plus 1 tablespoon olive oil, divided
- 3 tablespoons pine nuts
- Salt, to taste
- ½ cup fresh basil, chopped
- ½ cup fresh parsley, chopped
- 1 garlic clove, chopped
- ½ cup Parmesan cheese, grated

### For Tomatoes:
- 2 heirloom tomatoes, cut into ½ inch thick slices
- 8 ounces feta cheese, cut into ½ inch thick slices.
- ½ cup red onions, thinly sliced
- 1 tablespoon olive oil
- Salt, to taste

## Instructions

1. Set the temperature of air fryer to 390 degrees F. Grease an air fryer basket.
2. In a bowl, mix together one tablespoon of oil, pine nuts and pinch of salt.
3. Arrange pine nuts into the prepared air fryer basket.
4. Air fry for about 1-2 minutes.
5. Remove from air fryer and transfer the pine nuts onto a paper towel-lined plate.
6. In a food processor, add the toasted pine nuts, fresh herbs, garlic, Parmesan, and salt and pulse until just combined.
7. While motor is running, slowly add the remaining oil and pulse until smooth.
8. Transfer into a bowl, covered and refrigerate until serving.
9. Spread about one tablespoon of pesto onto each tomato slice.
10. Top each tomato slice with one feta and onion slice and drizzle with oil.
11. Arrange tomato slices into the prepared air fryer basket in a single layer.
12. Air fry for about 12-14 minutes.
13. Remove from air fryer and transfer the tomato slices onto serving plates.
14. Sprinkle with a little salt and serve with the remaining pesto.

## Nutrition Values (Per Serving)

- Calories: 633
- Carbohydrate: 9.7g
- Protein: 22g
- Fat: 59.6g
- Sugar: 4.9g
- Sodium: 1200mg

# Cheese Stuffed Tomatoes

**(Yields:** 2 servings / **Prep Time:** 15 minutes / **Cooking Time:** 15 minutes)

## Ingredients

- 2 large tomatoes
- ½ cup broccoli, finely chopped
- ½ cup cheddar cheese, shredded
- 1 tablespoon unsalted butter, melted
- ½ teaspoon dried thyme, crushed

## Instructions

1. Slice the top of each tomato and scoop out pulp and seeds.
2. In a bowl, mix together the chopped broccoli and cheese.
3. Stuff each tomato evenly with broccoli mixture.
4. Set the temperature of air fryer to 355 degrees F. Grease an air fryer basket.
5. Arrange tomatoes into the prepared air fryer basket.
6. Drizzle evenly with butter.
7. Air fry for about 12-15 minutes.
8. Remove from air fryer and transfer the tomatoes onto a serving platter.
9. Set aside to cool slightly.
10. Garnish with thyme and serve.

## Nutrition Values (Per Serving)

- Calories: 206
- Carbohydrate: 9.1g
- Protein: 9.4g
- Fat: 15.6g
- Sugar: 5.3g
- Sodium: 233mg

---

# Jacket Potatoes

**(Yields:** 2 servings / **Prep Time:** 15 minutes / **Cooking Time:** 15 minutes)

## Ingredients

- 2 potatoes
- 1 tablespoon mozzarella cheese, shredded
- 3 tablespoons sour cream
- 1 tablespoon butter, softened
- 1 teaspoon chives, minced
- Salt and ground black pepper, as required

### Instructions

1. Set the temperature of air fryer to 355 degrees F. Grease an air fryer basket.
2. With a fork, prick the potatoes.
3. Arrange potatoes into the prepared air fryer basket.
4. Air fry for about 15 minutes.
5. In a bowl, add the remaining ingredients and mix until well combined.
6. Remove from air fryer and transfer the potatoes onto a platter.
7. Open potatoes from the center and stuff them with cheese mixture.
8. Serve immediately

### Nutrition Values (Per Serving)

- Calories: 277
- Carbohydrate: 34.8g
- Protein: 8.2g
- Fat: 12.2g
- Sugar: 2.5g
- Sodium: 226mg

---

## Stuffed Potatoes

**(Yields:** 4 servings / **Prep Time:** 15 minutes / **Cooking Time:** 31 minutes)

### Ingredients

- 4 potatoes, peeled
- 2-3 tablespoons canola oil
- 1 tablespoon butter
- ½ of brown onion, chopped
- 2 tablespoons chives, chopped
- ½ cup Parmesan cheese, grated

### Instructions

1. Set the temperature of air fryer to 390 degrees F.
2. Coat the potatoes with oil.
3. Arrange potatoes into the air fryer basket.
4. Air fry for about 20 minutes, coating twice with the remaining oil.
5. Meanwhile, in a frying pan, melt the butter over medium heat and sauté the onion for about 4-5 minutes.
6. Remove from heat and transfer the onion into a bowl.
7. Remove the potatoes from air fryer and transfer onto a platter.
8. Carefully, cut each potato in half.
9. With a small scooper, scoop out the flesh from each half.

10. In the bowl of onion, add the potato flesh, chives, and half of cheese and stir to combine.
11. Stuff the potato halves evenly with potato mixture.
12. Sprinkle with the remaining cheese.
13. Arrange potato halves into the air fryer basket.
14. Air fry for another 6 minutes.
15. Remove from air fryer and transfer the potatoes onto a platter.
16. Serve immediately.

## Nutrition Values (Per Serving)

- Calories: 258
- Carbohydrate: 34.8g
- Protein: 5.8g
- Fat: 11.3g
- Sugar: 3.1g
- Sodium: 77mg

---

# Hasselback Potatoes

**(Yields:** 4 servings / **Prep Time:** 20 minutes / **Cooking Time:** 30 minutes)

## Ingredients

- 4 potatoes
- 2 tablespoons olive oil
- 2 tablespoons Parmesan cheese, shredded
- 1 tablespoon fresh chives, chopped

## Instructions

1. With a sharp knife, cut slits along each potato the short way about ¼-inch apart, making sure slices should stay connected at the bottom.
2. Set the temperature of air fryer to 355 degrees F. Grease an air fryer basket.
3. Gently brush each potato evenly with oil.
4. Arrange potatoes into the prepared air fryer basket.
5. Air fry for about 30 minutes, coating with the oil once halfway through.
6. Remove from air fryer and transfer the potatoes onto a platter.
7. Garnish with the cheeses, and chives.
8. Serve immediately.

## Nutrition Values (Per Serving)

- Calories: 218
- Carbohydrate: 33.6g
- Protein: 4.6g
- Fat: 7.9g
- Sugar: 2.5g
- Sodium: 55mg

# Wine Infused Mushrooms

**(Yields:** 6 servings / **Prep Time:** 15 minutes / **Cooking Time:** 32 minutes)

## Ingredients

- 1 tablespoon butter
- 2 teaspoons Herbs de Provence
- ½ teaspoon garlic powder
- 2 pounds fresh mushrooms, quartered
- 2 tablespoons white vermouth*

## Instructions

1. Set the temperature of air fryer to 320 degrees F.
2. In an air fryer pan, mix together the butter, Herbs de Provence, and garlic powder and air fry for about 2 minutes.
3. Stir in the mushrooms and air fry for about 25 minutes.
4. Stir in the vermouth and air fry for 5 more minutes.
5. Remove from air fryer and transfer the mushrooms onto serving plates.
6. Serve hot.

## Nutrition Values (Per Serving)

- Calories: 54
- Carbohydrate: 5.3g
- Protein: 4.8g
- Fat: 2.4g
- Sugar: 2.7g
- Sodium: 23mg

(**Note: White vermouth*** - Vermouth is an aromatized, fortified white wine flavored with various botanicals and sometimes colored. The modern versions of the beverage were first produced in the mid to late 18th century in Turin, Italy.)

# Cheese Stuffed Mushrooms

**(Yields:** 4 servings / **Prep Time:** 15 minutes / **Cooking Time:** 8 minutes)

## Ingredients

- 4 fresh large mushrooms, stemmed and gills removed
- 4 ounces cream cheese, softened
- ¼ cup Parmesan cheese, shredded
- 2 tablespoons white cheddar cheese, shredded
- 2 tablespoons sharp cheddar cheese, shredded

- 1 teaspoon Worcestershire sauce
- 2 garlic cloves, chopped
- Salt and ground black pepper, as required

## Instructions

1. In a bowl, mix well cream cheese, Parmesan, cheddar cheeses, Worcestershire sauce, garlic, salt, and black pepper.
2. Set the temperature of air fryer to 370 degrees F. Grease an air fryer basket.
3. Stuff each mushroom with the cheese mixture.
4. Arrange stuffed mushrooms into the prepared air fryer basket.
5. Air fry for about 8 minutes.
6. Remove from air fryer and transfer the mushrooms onto a serving platter.
7. Set aside to cool slightly.
8. Serve warm.

## Nutrition Values (Per Serving)

- Calories: 156
- Carbohydrate: 2.6g
- Protein: 6.5g
- Fat: 13.6g
- Sugar: 0.7g
- Sodium: 267mg

---

# Cheesy Mushroom Pizza

**(Yields:** 2 servings / **Prep Time:** 15 minutes / **Cooking Time:** 6 minutes)

## Ingredients

- 2 Portobello mushroom caps, stemmed
- 2 tablespoons olive oil
- 1/8 teaspoon dried Italian seasonings
- Salt, to taste
- 2 tablespoons canned tomatoes, chopped
- 2 tablespoons mozzarella cheese, shredded
- 2 Kalamata olives, pitted and sliced
- 2 tablespoons Parmesan cheese, grated freshly
- 1 teaspoon red pepper flakes, crushed

## Instructions

1. Set the temperature of air fryer to 320 degrees F. Grease an air fryer basket.
2. With a spoon, scoop out the center of each mushroom cap.
3. Coat each mushroom cap with oil from both sides.

4. Sprinkle the inside of caps with Italian seasoning and salt.
5. Place the canned tomato evenly over both caps, followed by the olives and mozzarella cheese.
6. Arrange mushroom caps into the prepared air fryer basket.
7. Air fry for about 5-6 minutes.
8. Remove from air fryer and immediately sprinkle with the Parmesan cheese and red pepper flakes.
9. Serve.

## **Nutrition Values (Per Serving)**

- Calories: 251
- Carbohydrate: 5.7g
- Protein: 13.4g
- Fat: 21g
- Sugar: 0.7g
- Sodium: 330mg

# **Cheesy Spinach**

(**Yields:** 3 servings / **Prep Time:** 15 minutes / **Cooking Time:** 15 minutes)

## **Ingredients**

- 1 (10-ounces) package frozen spinach, thawed
- ½ cup onion, chopped
- 2 teaspoons garlic, minced
- 4 ounces cream cheese, chopped
- ½ teaspoon ground nutmeg
- Salt and ground black pepper, as required
- ¼ cup Parmesan cheese, shredded

## **Instructions**

1. In a bowl, mix well spinach, onion, garlic, cream cheese, nutmeg, salt, and black pepper.
2. Set the temperature of air fryer to 350 degrees F. Grease an air fryer pan.
3. Place spinach mixture into the prepared air fryer pan.
4. Air fry for about 10 minutes.
5. Remove from air fryer and stir the mixture well.
6. Sprinkle the spinach mixture evenly with Parmesan cheese.
7. Now, set the temperature of air fryer to 400 degrees F and air fry for 5 more minutes.
8. Remove from air fryer and transfer the spinach mixture onto serving plates.
9. Serve hot.

### Nutrition Values (Per Serving)

- Calories: 194
- Carbohydrate: 7.3g
- Protein: 8.4g
- Fat: 15.5g
- Sugar: 1.4g
- Sodium: 351mg

---

# Parmesan Asparagus

**(Yields:** 3 servings / **Prep Time:** 15 minutes / **Cooking Time:** 10 minutes)

## Ingredients

- 1 pound fresh asparagus, trimmed
- 1 tablespoon Parmesan cheese, grated
- 1 tablespoon butter, melted
- 1 teaspoon garlic powder
- Salt and ground black pepper, as required

## Instructions

1. In a bowl, mix together the asparagus, cheese, butter, garlic powder, salt, and black pepper.
2. Set the temperature of air fryer to 400 degrees F. Grease an air fryer basket.
3. Arrange asparagus into the prepared air fryer basket.
4. Air fry for about 10 minutes.
5. Remove from air fryer and transfer the asparagus onto serving plates.
6. Serve hot.

## Nutrition Values (Per Serving)

- Calories: 73
- Carbohydrate: 6.6g
- Protein: 4.2g
- Fat: 2.7g
- Sugar: 3.1g
- Sodium: 95mg

# Lemony Green Beans

**(Yields:** 3 servings / **Prep Time:** 15 minutes / **Cooking Time:** 12 minutes)

## Ingredients

- 1 pound green beans, trimmed and halved
- 1 teaspoon butter, melted
- 1 tablespoon fresh lemon juice
- ¼ teaspoon garlic powder
- Salt and ground black pepper, as required

## Instructions

1. In a large bowl, add all the ingredients and toss to coat well.
2. Set the temperature of air fryer to 400 degrees F. Grease an air fryer basket.
3. Arrange green beans into the prepared air fryer basket.
4. Air fry for about 10-12 minutes.
5. Remove from air fryer and transfer the green beans onto serving plates.
6. Serve hot.

## Nutrition Values (Per Serving)

- Calories: 60
- Carbohydrate: 11.1g
- Protein: 2.8g
- Fat: 1.5g
- Sugar: 2.3g
- Sodium: 70mg

# Veggie Stuffed Bell Peppers

**(Yields:** 6 servings / **Prep Time:** 20 minutes / **Cooking Time:** 25 minutes)

## Ingredients

- 6 large bell peppers
- 1 bread roll, finely chopped
- 1 carrot, peeled and finely chopped
- 1 onion, finely chopped
- 1 potato, peeled and finely chopped
- ½ cup fresh peas, shelled
- 2 garlic cloves, minced
- 2 teaspoons fresh parsley, chopped
- Salt and ground black pepper, as required
- 1/3 cup cheddar cheese, grated

## Instructions

1. Remove the tops of each bell pepper and discard the seeds.
2. Finely chop the bell pepper tops.
3. In a bowl, mix well chopped bell pepper tops, loaf, vegetables, garlic, parsley, salt and black pepper.
4. Stuff each bell pepper with the vegetable mixture.
5. Set the temperature of air fryer to 350 degrees F. Grease an air fryer basket.
6. Arrange peppers into the prepared air fryer basket.
7. Air fry for about 20 minutes.
8. Remove the air fryer basket and top each bell pepper with cheese.
9. Air fry for 5 more minutes.
10. Remove from air fryer and transfer the bell peppers onto a serving platter.
11. Set aside to cool slightly.
12. Serve warm.

## Nutrition Values (Per Serving)

- Calories: 123
- Carbohydrate: 21.7g
- Protein: 4.8g
- Fat: 2.7g
- Sugar: 8.7g
- Sodium: 105mg

# Rice & Beans Stuffed Bell Peppers

(**Yields:** 5 servings / **Prep Time:** 15 minutes / **Cooking Time:** 15 minutes)

## Ingredients

- ½ small bell pepper, seeded and chopped
- 1 (15-ounces) can diced tomatoes with juice
- 1 (15-ounces) can red kidney beans, rinsed and drained
- 1 cup cooked rice
- 1½ teaspoons Italian seasoning
- 5 large bell peppers, tops removed and seeded
- ½ cup mozzarella cheese, shredded
- 1 tablespoon Parmesan cheese, grated

## Instructions

1. In a bowl, mix well chopped bell pepper, tomatoes with juice, beans, rice, and Italian seasoning.
2. Stuff each bell pepper evenly with the rice mixture.
3. Set the temperature of air fryer to 360 degrees F. Grease an air fryer basket.
4. Arrange bell peppers into the air fryer basket in a single layer.

5. Air fry for about 12 minutes.
6. Meanwhile, in a bowl, mix together the mozzarella and Parmesan cheese.
7. Remove the air fryer basket and top each bell pepper with cheese mixture.
8. Air fry for 3 more minutes.
9. Remove from air fryer and transfer the bell peppers onto a serving platter.
10. Set aside to cool slightly.
11. Serve warm.

## Nutrition Values (Per Serving)

- Calories: 288
- Carbohydrate: 55g
- Protein: 11.3g
- Fat: 3.1g
- Sugar: 9.7g
- Sodium: 286mg

# Stuffed Pumpkin

(**Yields:** 5 servings / **Prep Time:** 20 minutes / **Cooking Time:** 30 minutes)

## Ingredients

- 1 sweet potato, peeled and chopped
- 1 parsnip, peeled and chopped
- 1 carrot, peeled and chopped
- ½ cup fresh peas, shelled
- 1 onion, chopped
- 2 garlic cloves, minced
- 1 egg, beaten
- 2 teaspoons mixed dried herbs
- Salt and ground black pepper, as required
- ½ of butternut pumpkin, seeded

## Instructions

1. In a large bowl, mix well vegetables, garlic, egg, herbs, salt, and black pepper.
2. Stuff the pumpkin half with vegetable mixture.
3. Set the temperature of air fryer to 355 degrees F. Grease an air fryer basket.
4. Arrange pumpkin half into the prepared air fryer basket.
5. Air fry for about 30 minutes.
6. Remove from air fryer and transfer the pumpkin onto a serving platter.
7. Set aside to cool slightly.
8. Serve warm.

## Nutrition Values (Per Serving)

- Calories: 157
- Carbohydrate: 35.9g
- Protein: 4.6g
- Fat: 1.1g
- Sugar: 4.6g
- Sodium: 64mg

# Glazed Veggies

**(Yields:** 4 servings / **Prep Time:** 20 minutes / **Cooking Time:** 20 minutes)

## Ingredients

- 2 ounces cherry tomatoes
- 1 large parsnip, peeled and chopped
- 1 large carrot, peeled and chopped
- 1 large zucchini, chopped
- 1 green bell pepper, seeded and chopped
- 6 tablespoons olive oil, divided
- 3 tablespoons honey
- 1 teaspoon Dijon mustard
- 1 teaspoon mixed dried herbs
- 1 teaspoon garlic paste
- Salt and ground black pepper, as required

## Instructions

1. Set the temperature of air fryer to 350 degrees F. Grease an air fryer pan.
2. Arrange vegetables into the prepared air fryer pan and drizzle with 3 tablespoons of oil.
3. Air fry for about 15 minutes.
4. Meanwhile, in a baking dish, mix well remaining oil, honey, mustard, herbs, garlic, salt, and black pepper.
5. Remove the vegetables from air fryer.
6. Transfer the vegetables into baking dish with honey mixture and mix until well combined.
7. Now, set the temperature of air fryer to 392 degrees F.
8. Arrange the baking dish into air fryer and air fry for about 5 minutes.
9. Remove from air fryer and transfer the vegetable mixture into a serving bowl.
10. Serve immediately.

## Nutrition Values (Per Serving)

- Calories: 288
- Carbohydrate: 26.7g
- Protein: 2.1g
- Fat: 21.4g
- Sugar: 18.7g
- Sodium: 79mg

# Tofu with Capers Sauce

**(Yields:** 4 servings / **Prep Time:** 20 minutes / **Cooking Time:** 20 minutes)

## Ingredients

**For Marinade:**

- ¼ cup fresh lemon juice
- 2 tablespoons fresh parsley
- 1 garlic clove, peeled
- Salt and ground black pepper, as required

**For Tofu:**

- 1 (14-ounces) block extra-firm tofu, pressed and cut into 8 rectangular cutlets
- ½ cup mayonnaise
- 1 cup panko breadcrumbs

**For Sauce:**

- 1 cup vegetable broth
- ¼ cup lemon juice
- 1 garlic clove, peeled
- 2 tablespoons fresh parsley
- 2 teaspoons cornstarch
- Salt and ground black pepper, as required
- 2 tablespoons capers

## Instructions

1. For marinade: in a food processor, add all the ingredients and pulse until smooth.
2. In a bowl, mix together the marinade and tofu.
3. Set aside for about 15-30 minutes.
4. In two shallow bowls, place the mayonnaise and panko breadcrumbs respectively.
5. Coat the tofu pieces with mayonnaise and then, roll into the panko.
6. Set the temperature of air fryer to 375 degrees F. Grease an air fryer basket.
7. Arrange tofu pieces into the prepared air fryer basket in a single layer.
8. Air fry for about 20 minutes, shaking once halfway through.
9. Meanwhile, for the sauce: add broth, lemon juice, garlic, parsley, cornstarch, salt and black pepper in a food processor and pulse until smooth.
10. Transfer the sauce into a small pan and stir in the capers.
11. Place the sauce over medium heat and bring to a boil.
12. Reduce the heat to low and simmer for about 5-7 minutes, stirring continuously.
13. Remove the tofu from air fryer and transfer onto serving plates.
14. Top with the sauce and serve.

## Nutrition Values (Per Serving)

- Calories: 307
- Carbohydrate: 15.6g
- Protein: 10.8g
- Fat: 16.5g
- Sugar: 3.4g
- Sodium: 586mg

---

# Tofu with Orange Sauce

**(Yields:** 4 servings / **Prep Time:** 20 minutes / **Cooking Time:** 20 minutes)

## Ingredients

**For Tofu:**

- 1 pound extra-firm tofu, pressed and cubed
- 1 tablespoon cornstarch
- 1 tablespoon tamari*

**For Sauce:**

- ½ cup water
- 1/3 cup fresh orange juice
- 1 tablespoon honey
- 1 teaspoon orange zest, grated
- 1 teaspoon garlic, minced
- 1 teaspoon fresh ginger, minced
- 2 teaspoons cornstarch
- ¼ teaspoon red pepper flakes, crushed

**For Garnishing:**

- 2 scallions (green part), chopped

## Instructions

1. In a bowl, add the tofu, cornstarch, and tamari and toss to coat well.
2. Set the tofu aside to marinate for at least 15 minutes.
3. Set the temperature of air fryer to 390 degrees F. Grease an air fryer basket.
4. Arrange tofu pieces into the prepared air fryer basket in 2 batches in a single layer.
5. Air fry for about 10 minutes, shaking once halfway through.
6. Meanwhile, for the sauce: in a small pan, add all the ingredients over medium-high heat and bring to a boil, stirring continuously.
7. Remove from air fryer and transfer the tofu into a serving bowl.
8. Top with the sauce and gently stir to combine.
9. Garnish with scallions and serve.

### Nutrition Values (Per Serving)

- Calories: 148
- Carbohydrate: 13g
- Protein: 12.1g
- Fat: 6.7g
- Sugar: 6.9g
- Sodium: 263mg

(**Note: Tamari*** - Tamari is soy sauce without the normally added wheat.)

---

## Buttered Dinner Rolls

(**Yields:** 12 servings / **Prep Time:** 15 minutes / **Cooking Time:** 30 minutes)

### Ingredients

- 1 cup milk
- 1 tablespoon coconut oil
- 1 tablespoon olive oil
- 3 cups plain flour
- 7½ tablespoons unsalted butter
- 1 teaspoon yeast
- Salt and ground black pepper, as required

### Instructions

1. In a pan, add the milk, coconut oil, and olive oil and cook until lukewarm.
2. Remove from the heat and stir well.
3. In a large bowl, add the flour, butter, yeast, salt, black pepper, and milk mixture and mix until a dough forms.
4. With your hands, knead for about 4-5 minutes
5. With a damp cloth, cover the dough and set aside in a warm place for about 5 minutes.
6. Again, with your hands, knead the dough for about 4-5 minutes
7. With a damp cloth, cover the dough and set aside in a warm place for about 30 minutes.
8. Place the dough onto a lightly floured surface.
9. Divide the dough into 12 equal pieces and form each into a ball.
10. Set the temperature of air fryer to 360 degrees F. Grease an air fryer basket.
11. Arrange rolls into the prepared air fryer basket in 2 batches in a single layer.
12. Air fry for about 15 minutes.
13. Remove from the air fryer and serve warm.

### Nutrition Values (Per Serving)

- Calories: 208
- Carbohydrate: 25g
- Protein: 4.1g
- Fat: 10.3g
- Sugar: 1g
- Sodium: 73mg

# Cheesy Dinner Rolls

**(Yields:** 2 servings / **Prep Time:** 10 minutes / **Cooking Time:** 5 minutes)

## Ingredients

- 2 dinner rolls
- ½ cup Parmesan cheese, grated
- 2 tablespoons unsalted butter, melted
- ½ teaspoon garlic bread seasoning mix

## Instructions

1. Cut the dinner rolls into cross style, but not the all way through.
2. Stuff the slits evenly with cheese.
3. Coat the tops of each roll with butter and then, sprinkle with the seasoning mix.
4. Set the temperature of air fryer to 355 degrees F. Grease an air fryer basket.
5. Arrange dinner rolls into the prepared air fryer basket.
6. Air fry for about 5 minutes or until cheese melts completely.
7. Remove from the air fryer and serve hot.

## Nutrition Values (Per Serving)

- Calories: 608
- Carbohydrate: 48.8g
- Protein: 33.5g
- Fat: 33.1g
- Sugar: 4.8g
- Sodium: 2000mg

# Croissant Rolls

**(Yields:** 8 servings / **Prep Time:** 10 minutes / **Cooking Time:** 6 minutes)

## Ingredients

- 1 (8-ounces) can croissant rolls
- 4 tablespoons butter, melted

## Instructions

1. Set the temperature of air fryer to 320 degrees F. Grease an air fryer basket.
2. Arrange croissant rolls into the prepared air fryer basket.
3. Air fry for about 4 minutes.
4. Flip the side and air fry for 1-2 more minutes.
5. Remove from the air fryer and transfer onto a platter.
6. Drizzle with the melted butter and serve hot.

### Nutrition Values (Per Serving)
- Calories: 152
- Carbohydrate: 11.1g
- Protein: 2.1g
- Fat: 10.8g
- Sugar: 3g
- Sodium: 223mg

## Sweet & Spicy Parsnips

**(Yields:** 6 servings / **Prep Time:** 15 minutes / **Cooking Time:** 44 minutes)

### Ingredients
- 2 pounds parsnip, peeled and cut into 1-inch chunks
- 1 tablespoon butter, melted
- 2 tablespoons honey
- 1 tablespoon dried parsley flakes, crushed
- ¼ teaspoon red pepper flakes, crushed
- Salt and ground black pepper, as required

### Instructions
1. Set the temperature of air fryer to 355 degrees F. Grease an air fryer basket.
2. In a large bowl, mix together the parsnips and butter.
3. Arrange parsnip chunks into the prepared air fryer basket in a single layer.
4. Air fry for about 40 minutes.
5. Meanwhile, in another large bowl, mix well remaining ingredients.
6. After 40 minutes, transfer parsnips into the bowl of honey mixture and toss to coat well.
7. Again, arrange the parsnip chunks into air fryer basket in a single layer.
8. Air fry for 3-4 more minutes.
9. Remove from air fryer and transfer the parsnip chunks onto serving plates.
10. Serve hot.

### Nutrition Values (Per Serving)
- Calories: 155
- Carbohydrate: 33.1g
- Protein: 1.9g
- Fat: 2.4g
- Sugar: 13g
- Sodium: 57mg

# Vegan

## Herbed Carrots

**(Yields:** 8 servings / **Prep Time:** 15 minutes / **Cooking Time:** 14 minutes)

### Ingredients

- 6 large carrots, peeled and sliced lengthwise
- 2 tablespoons olive oil
- ½ tablespoon fresh oregano, chopped
- ½ tablespoon fresh parsley, chopped
- Salt and ground black pepper, as required

### Instructions

1. Set the temperature of air fryer to 360 degrees F. Grease an air fryer basket.
2. In a bowl, mix together the carrot slices, and oil.
3. Arrange carrot slices into the prepared air fryer basket in a single layer.
4. Air fry for about 12 minutes.
5. Remove from air fryer and sprinkle the carrots evenly with herbs, salt and black pepper.
6. Air fry for 2 more minutes.
7. Remove from air fryer and transfer the carrot slices onto serving plates.
8. Serve hot.

### Nutrition Values (Per Serving)

- Calories: 53
- Carbohydrate: 5.5g
- Protein: 0.5g
- Fat: 3.5g
- Sugar: 2.7g
- Sodium: 57mg

---

## Curried Eggplant

**(Yields:** 2 servings / **Prep Time:** 15 minutes / **Cooking Time:** 10 minutes)

### Ingredients

- 1 large eggplant, cut into ½-inch thick slices
- 1 garlic clove, minced
- ½ fresh red chili, chopped
- 1 tablespoon vegetable oil

- ¼ teaspoon curry powder
- Salt, as required

## Instructions

1. Set the temperature of air fryer to 300 degrees F. Grease an air fryer basket.
2. In a bowl, add all the ingredients and toss to coat well.
3. Arrange eggplant slices into the prepared air fryer basket in a single layer.
4. Air fry for about 10 minutes, shaking once halfway through.
5. Remove from air fryer and transfer the eggplant slices onto serving plates.
6. Serve hot.

## Nutrition Values (Per Serving)

- Calories: 121
- Carbohydrate: 14.2g
- Protein: 2.4g
- Fat: 7.3g
- Sugar: 7g
- Sodium: 83mg

# Herbed Eggplant

**(Yields:** 2 servings / **Prep Time:** 15 minutes / **Cooking Time:** 15 minutes)

## Ingredients

- ½ teaspoon dried marjoram, crushed
- ½ teaspoon dried oregano, crushed
- ½ teaspoon dried thyme, crushed
- ½ teaspoon garlic powder
- Salt and ground black pepper, as required
- 1 large eggplant, cubed
- Olive oil cooking spray

## Instructions

1. Set the temperature of air fryer to 390 degrees F. Grease an air fryer basket.
2. In a small bowl, mix well herbs, garlic powder, salt, and black pepper.
3. Spray the eggplant cubes evenly with cooking spray and then, rub with the herbs mixture.
4. Arrange eggplant cubes into the prepared air fryer basket in a single layer.
5. Air fry for about 6 minutes.
6. Flip and spray the eggplant cubes with cooking spray.
7. Air fry for another 6 minutes.
8. Flip and again, spray the eggplant cubes with cooking spray.

9. Air fry for 2-3 more minutes.
10. Remove from air fryer and transfer the eggplant cubes onto serving plates.
11. Serve hot.

## **Nutrition Values (Per Serving)**
- Calories: 62
- Carbohydrate: 14.5g
- Protein: 2.4g
- Fat: 0.5g
- Sugar: 7.1g
- Sodium: 83mg

---

# **Spices Stuffed Eggplants**

(**Yields:** 4 servings / **Prep Time:** 15 minutes / **Cooking Time:** 12 minutes)

## **Ingredients**
- 4 teaspoons olive oil, divided
- ¾ tablespoon dry mango powder
- ¾ tablespoon ground coriander
- ½ teaspoon ground cumin
- ½ teaspoon ground turmeric
- ½ teaspoon garlic powder
- Salt, to taste
- 8 baby eggplants

## **Instructions**
1. In a small bowl, mix together one teaspoon of oil, and spices.
2. From the bottom of each eggplant, make 2 slits, leaving the stems intact.
3. With a small spoon, fill each slit of eggplants with spice mixture.
4. Now, brush the outer side of each eggplant with remaining oil.
5. Set the temperature of air fryer to 369 degrees F. Grease an air fryer basket.
6. Arrange eggplants into the prepared air fryer basket in a single layer.
7. Air fry for about 8-12 minutes.
8. Remove from air fryer and transfer the eggplants onto serving plates.
9. Serve hot.

## **Nutrition Values (Per Serving)**
- Calories: 317
- Carbohydrate: 65g
- Protein: 10.9g
- Fat: 6.7g
- Sugar: 33g
- Sodium: 61mg

# Salsa Stuffed Eggplants

**(Yields:** 2 servings / **Prep Time:** 15 minutes / **Cooking Time:** 25 minutes)

## Ingredients

- 1 large eggplant
- 2 teaspoons olive oil, divided
- 2 teaspoons fresh lemon juice, divided
- 8 cherry tomatoes, quartered
- 2 tablespoons tomato salsa
- ½ tablespoon fresh parsley
- Salt and ground black pepper, as required

## Instructions

1. Set the temperature of air fryer to 390 degrees F. Grease an air fryer basket.
2. Place eggplant into the prepared air fryer basket.
3. Air fry for about 15 minutes.
4. Remove from air fryer and cut the eggplant in half lengthwise.
5. Drizzle the eggplant halves evenly with one teaspoon of oil.
6. Now, set the temperature of air fryer to 355 degrees F. Grease the air fryer basket.
7. Arrange eggplant into the prepared air fryer basket, cut-side up.
8. Air fry for another 10 minutes.
9. Remove eggplant from the air fryer and set aside for about 5 minutes.
10. Carefully, scoop out the flesh, leaving about ¼-inch away from edges.
11. Drizzle the eggplant halves with one teaspoon of lemon juice.
12. Transfer the eggplant flesh into a bowl.
13. Add the tomatoes, salsa, parsley, salt, black pepper, remaining oil, and lemon juice and mix well.
14. Stuff the eggplant haves with salsa mixture and serve.

## Nutrition Values (Per Serving)

- Calories: 192
- Carbohydrate: 33.8g
- Protein: 6.9g
- Fat: 6.1g
- Sugar: 20.4g
- Sodium: 204mg

# Sesame Seeds Bok Choy

**(Yields:** 4 servings / **Prep Time:** 10 minutes / **Cooking Time:** 6 minutes)

## Ingredients

- 4 bunches baby bok choy, bottoms removed and leaves separated
- Olive oil cooking spray
- 1 teaspoon garlic powder
- 1 teaspoon sesame seeds

## Instructions

1. Set the temperature of air fryer to 325 degrees F.
2. Arrange bok choy leaves into the air fryer basket in a single layer.
3. Spray with the cooking spray and sprinkle with garlic powder.
4. Air fry for about 5-6 minutes, shaking after every 2 minutes.
5. Remove from air fryer and transfer the bok choy onto serving plates.
6. Garnish with sesame seeds and serve hot.

## Nutrition Values (Per Serving)

- Calories: 26
- Carbohydrate: 4g
- Protein: 2.5g
- Fat: 0.7g
- Sugar: 1.9g
- Sodium: 98mg

---

# Basil Tomatoes

**(Yields:** 2 servings / **Prep Time:** 10 minutes / **Cooking Time:** 10 minutes)

## Ingredients

- 2 tomatoes, halved
- Olive oil cooking spray
- Salt and ground black pepper, as required
- 1 tablespoon fresh basil, chopped

## Instructions

1. Set the temperature of air fryer to 320 degrees F. Grease an air fryer basket.
2. Spray the tomato halves evenly with cooking spray and sprinkle with salt, black pepper and basil.
3. Arrange tomato halves into the prepared air fryer basket, cut sides up.
4. Air fry for about 10 minutes or until desired doneness.

5. Remove from air fryer and transfer the tomatoes onto serving plates.
6. Serve warm.

## Nutrition Values (Per Serving)

- Calories: 22
- Carbohydrate: 4.8g
- Protein: 1.1g
- Fat: 4.8g
- Sugar: 3.2g
- Sodium: 84mg

---

# Stuffed Tomatoes

(**Yields:** 4 servings / **Prep Time:** 15 minutes / **Cooking Time:** 22 minutes)

## Ingredients

- 4 tomatoes
- 1 teaspoon olive oil
- 1 carrot, peeled and finely chopped
- 1 onion, chopped
- 1 cup frozen peas, thawed
- 1 garlic clove, minced
- 2 cups cold cooked rice
- 1 tablespoon soy sauce

## Instructions

1. Cut the top of each tomato and scoop out pulp and seeds.
2. In a skillet, heat oil over low heat and sauté the carrot, onion, garlic, and peas for about 2 minutes.
3. Stir in the soy sauce and rice and remove from heat.
4. Set the temperature of air fryer to 355 degrees F. Grease an air fryer basket.
5. Stuff each tomato with the rice mixture.
6. Arrange tomatoes into the prepared air fryer basket.
7. Air fry for about 20 minutes.
8. Remove from air fryer and transfer the tomatoes onto a serving platter.
9. Set aside to cool slightly.
10. Serve warm.

## Nutrition Values (Per Serving)

- Calories: 421
- Carbohydrate: 89.1g
- Protein: 10.5g
- Fat: 2.2g
- Sugar: 7.2g
- Sodium: 277mg

# Sweet & Spicy Cauliflower

**(Yields:** 4 servings / **Prep Time:** 15 minutes / **Cooking Time:** 30 minutes)

## Ingredients

- 1 head cauliflower, cut into florets
- ¾ cup onion, thinly sliced
- 5 garlic cloves, finely sliced
- 1½ tablespoons soy sauce
- 1 tablespoon hot sauce
- 1 tablespoon rice vinegar
- 1 teaspoon coconut sugar
- Pinch of red pepper flakes
- Ground black pepper, as required
- 2 scallions, chopped

## Instructions

1. Set the temperature of air fryer to 350 degrees F. Grease an air fryer pan.
2. Arrange cauliflower florets into the prepared air fryer pan in a single layer.
3. Air fry for about 10 minutes.
4. Remove from air fryer and stir in the onions.
5. Air fry for another 10 minutes.
6. Remove from air fryer and stir in the garlic.
7. Air fry for 5 more minutes.
8. Meanwhile, in a bowl, mix well soy sauce, hot sauce, vinegar, coconut sugar, red pepper flakes, and black pepper.
9. Remove from the air fryer and stir in the sauce mixture.
10. Air fry for about 5 minutes.
11. Remove from air fryer and transfer the cauliflower mixture onto serving plates.
12. Garnish with scallions and serve.

## Nutrition Values (Per Serving)

- Calories: 72
- Carbohydrate: 13.8g
- Protein: 3.6g
- Fat: 0.2g
- Sugar: 3.1g
- Sodium: 1300mg

# Spiced Butternut Squash

**(Yields:** 4 servings / **Prep Time:** 15 minutes / **Cooking Time:** 20 minutes)

## Ingredients

- 1 medium butternut squash, peeled, seeded and cut into chunk
- 2 teaspoons cumin seeds
- 1/8 teaspoon garlic powder
- 1/8 teaspoon chili flakes, crushed
- Salt and ground black pepper, as required
- 1 tablespoon olive oil
- 2 tablespoons pine nuts
- 2 tablespoons fresh cilantro, chopped

## Instructions

1. Set the temperature of air fryer to 375 degrees F. Grease an air fryer basket.
2. In a bowl, mix together the squash, spices, and oil.
3. Arrange butternut squash chunks into the prepared fryer basket.
4. Air fry for about 20 minutes, flipping occasionally.
5. Remove from air fryer and transfer the squash chunks onto serving plates.
6. Garnish with pine nuts and cilantro.
7. Serve.

## Nutrition Values (Per Serving)

- Calories: 165
- Carbohydrate: 27.6g
- Protein: 3.1g
- Fat: 6.9g
- Sugar: 5.2g
- Sodium: 50mg

---

# Herbed Potatoes

**(Yields:** 4 servings / **Prep Time:** 10 minutes / **Cooking Time:** 16 minutes)

## Ingredients

- 6 small potatoes, chopped
- 3 tablespoons olive oil
- 2 teaspoons mixed dried herbs
- Salt and ground black pepper, as required
- 2 tablespoons fresh parsley, chopped

### Instructions

1. Set the temperature of air fryer to 356 degrees F. Grease an air fryer basket.
2. In a large bowl, add the potatoes, oil, herbs, salt and black pepper and toss to coat well.
3. Arrange the chopped potatoes into the prepared air fryer basket in a single layer.
4. Air fry for about 16 minutes, tossing once halfway through.
5. Remove from air fryer and transfer the potatoes onto serving plates.
6. Garnish with parsley and serve.

### Nutrition Values (Per Serving)

- Calories: 268
- Carbohydrate: 40.4g
- Protein: 4.4g
- Fat: 10.8g
- Sugar: 3g
- Sodium: 55mg

---

# Spicy Potatoes

(**Yields:** 6 servings / **Prep Time:** 10 minutes / **Cooking Time:** 20 minutes)

### Ingredients

- 1¾ pounds waxy potatoes, peeled and cubed
- 1 tablespoon olive oil
- ½ teaspoon ground cumin
- ½ teaspoon ground coriander
- ½ teaspoon paprika
- Salt and freshly ground black pepper, as required

### Instructions

1. In a large bowl of water, add the potatoes and set aside for about 30 minutes.
2. Drain the potatoes completely and dry with paper towels.
3. In a bowl, add the potatoes, oil, and spices and toss to coat well.
4. Set the temperature of air fryer to 355 degrees F. Grease an air fryer basket.
5. Arrange potato pieces into the prepared air fryer basket in a single layer.
6. Air fry for about 20 minutes.
7. Remove from air fryer and transfer the potato pieces onto serving plates.
8. Serve hot.

### Nutrition Values (Per Serving)

- Calories: 113
- Carbohydrate: 21g
- Protein: 2.3g
- Fat: 2.5g
- Sugar: 1.5g
- Sodium: 35mg

# Mushrooms with Peas

**(Yields:** 4 servings / **Prep Time:** 15 minutes / **Cooking Time:** 15 minutes)

## Ingredients

- ½ cup soy sauce
- 4 tablespoons maple syrup
- 4 tablespoons rice vinegar
- 4 garlic cloves, finely chopped
- 2 teaspoons Chinese five spice powder
- ½ teaspoon ground ginger
- 16 ounces cremini mushrooms, halved
- ½ cup frozen peas

## Instructions

1. In a bowl, mix well soy sauce, maple syrup, vinegar, garlic, five spice powder, and ground ginger.
2. Set the temperature of air fryer to 350 degrees F. Grease an air fryer pan.
3. Arrange mushroom into the prepared air fryer pan in a single layer.
4. Air fry for about 10 minutes.
5. Remove from air fryer and stir the mushrooms.
6. Add the peas and vinegar mixture and stir to combine.
7. Air fry for about 5 more minutes.
8. Remove from air fryer and transfer the mushroom mixture onto serving plates.
9. Serve hot.

## Nutrition Values (Per Serving)

- Calories: 132
- Carbohydrate: 25g
- Protein: 6.1g
- Fat: 0.3g
- Sugar: 15.4g
- Sodium: 6.1mg

---

# Breadcrumbs Stuffed Mushrooms

**(Yields:** 4 servings / **Prep Time:** 15 minutes / **Cooking Time:** 10 minutes)

## Ingredients

- 1½ spelt bread slices
- 1½ tablespoons olive oil
- 1 garlic clove, crushed
- 1 tablespoon flat-leaf parsley, finely chopped
- Salt and ground black pepper, as required
- 16 small button mushrooms, stemmed and gills removed

## Instructions

1. In a food processor, add the bread slices and pulse until fine crumbs form.
2. Transfer the crumbs into a bowl.
3. Add the garlic, parsley, salt, and black pepper and stir to combine.
4. Stir in the olive oil.
5. Set the temperature of air fryer to 390 degrees F. Grease an air fryer basket.
6. Stuff each mushroom cap with the breadcrumbs mixture.
7. Arrange mushroom caps into the prepared air fryer basket.
8. Air fry for about 9-10 minutes.
9. Remove from air fryer and transfer the mushrooms onto a serving platter.
10. Set aside to cool slightly.
11. Serve warm.

## Nutrition Values (Per Serving)

- Calories: 64
- Carbohydrate: 3.3g
- Protein: 1.6g
- Fat: 5.5g
- Sugar: 0.5g
- Sodium: 65mg

---

# Hummus Mushroom Pizza

(**Yields:** 4 servings / **Prep Time:** 20 minutes / **Cooking Time:** 6 minutes)

## Ingredients

- 4 Portobello mushroom caps, stemmed and gills removed
- 1 tablespoon balsamic vinegar
- Salt and ground black pepper, as required
- 4 tablespoons pasta sauce
- 1 garlic clove, minced
- 3 ounces zucchini, shredded
- 2 tablespoons sweet red pepper, seeded and chopped
- 4 Kalamata olives, sliced
- 1 teaspoon dried basil
- ½ cup hummus

## Instructions

1. Coat both sides of each mushroom cap with vinegar.
2. Now, sprinkle the inside of each mushroom cap with salt and black pepper.
3. Place one tablespoon of pasta sauce inside each mushroom and sprinkle with garlic.

4. Set the temperature of air fryer to 330 degrees F. Grease an air fryer basket.
5. Arrange mushroom caps into the prepared air fryer basket.
6. Air fry for about 3 minutes.
7. Remove from the air fryer and top each mushroom cap with zucchini, peppers and olives.
8. Then, sprinkle with basil, salt, and black pepper.
9. Place back mushroom caps into the air fryer basket.
10. Air fry for about 3 more minutes.
11. Remove from air fryer and transfer the mushrooms onto a serving platter.
12. Top each mushroom pizza with hummus and serve.

## **Nutrition Values (Per Serving)**

- Calories: 115
- Carbohydrate: 15.4g
- Protein: 6.7g
- Fat: 4.1g
- Sugar: 4.8g
- Sodium: 264mg

(**Note: Kalamata olive*** - The Kalamata olive is a large black or brown olive with a smooth, meaty texture named after the city of Kalamata in the southern Peloponnese, Greece.)

---

# **Sautéed Spinach**

(**Yields:** 2 servings / **Prep Time:** 15 minutes / **Cooking Time:** 9 minutes)

## **Ingredients**

- 2 tablespoons olive oil
- 1 small onion, chopped
- 1 garlic clove, minced
- 6 ounces fresh spinach
- Salt and ground black pepper, as required

## **Instructions**

1. Set the temperature of air fryer to 340 degrees F.
2. In an air fryer pan, heat the oil for about 2 minutes.
3. Add the onion, and garlic and air fry for about 3 minutes.
4. Add the spinach, salt, and black pepper and air fry for about 4 more minutes.
5. Remove from air fryer and transfer the spinach mixture onto serving plates.
6. Serve hot.

### Nutrition Values (Per Serving)

- Calories: 156
- Carbohydrate: 6.9g
- Protein: 2.9g
- Fat: 14.4g
- Sugar: 1.9g
- Sodium: 146mg

## Almond Asparagus

**(Yields:** 3 servings / **Prep Time:** 15 minutes / **Cooking Time:** 6 minutes)

### Ingredients

- 1 pound asparagus
- 2 tablespoons olive oil
- 2 tablespoons balsamic vinegar
- Salt and ground black pepper, as required
- 1/3 cup almonds, sliced

### Instructions

1. In a bowl, mix together the asparagus, oil, vinegar, salt, and black pepper.
2. Set the temperature of air fryer to 400 degrees F. Grease an air fryer basket.
3. Arrange asparagus into the prepared air fryer basket in a single layer and top with the almond slices.
4. Air fry for about 5-6 minutes.
5. Remove from air fryer and transfer the asparagus onto serving plates.
6. Serve hot.

### Nutrition Values (Per Serving)

- Calories: 173
- Carbohydrate: 8.2g
- Protein: 5.6g
- Fat: 14.8g
- Sugar: 3.3g
- Sodium: 54mg

## Sautéed Green Beans

**(Yields:** 2 servings / **Prep Time:** 10 minutes / **Cooking Time:** 10 minutes)

### Ingredients

- 8 ounces fresh green beans, trimmed and cut in half
- 1 tablespoon soy sauce
- 1 teaspoon sesame oil

### Instructions

1. In a bowl, mix well green beans, soy sauce, and sesame oil.
2. Set the temperature of air fryer to 390 degrees F. Lightly, grease an air fryer basket.
3. Arrange green beans into the prepared air fryer basket.
4. Air fry for about 10 minutes, tossing once halfway through.
5. Remove from air fryer and transfer the green beans onto serving plates.
6. Serve hot.

### Nutrition Values (Per Serving)

- Calories: 59
- Carbohydrate: 8.7g
- Protein: 2.6g
- Fat: 2.4g
- Sugar: 1.7g
- Sodium: 458mg

## Green Beans & Mushroom Casserole

**(Yields:** 6 servings / **Prep Time:** 15 minutes / **Cooking Time:** 12 minutes)

### Ingredients

- 24 ounces fresh green beans, trimmed
- 2 cups fresh button mushrooms, sliced
- 3 tablespoons olive oil
- 2 tablespoons fresh lemon juice
- 1 teaspoon ground sage
- 1 teaspoon garlic powder
- 1 teaspoon onion powder
- Salt and ground black pepper, as required
- 1/3 cup French fried onions*

### Instructions

1. In a bowl, add the green beans, mushrooms, oil, lemon juice, sage, and spices and toss to coat well.
2. Set the temperature of air fryer to 400 degrees F. Lightly, grease an air fryer basket.
3. Arrange mushroom mixture into the prepared air fryer basket.
4. Air fry for about 10-12 minutes, shaking several times while frying.
5. Remove from air fryer and transfer the mushroom mixture into a serving dish.
6. Top with fried onions and serve.

### Nutrition Values (Per Serving)

- Calories: 65
- Carbohydrate: 11g
- Protein: 3g
- Fat: 1.6g
- Sugar: 2.4g
- Sodium: 52mg

(**Note: French fried onions*** - French fried onions is usually found in the condiments section or aisle of the grocery store or supermarket.)

---

# Okra with Green Beans

(**Yields:** 2 servings / **Prep Time:** 10 minutes / **Cooking Time:** 20 minutes)

## Ingredients

- ½ (10-ounces) bag frozen cut okra*
- ½ (10-ounces) bag frozen cut green beans
- ¼ cup nutritional yeast
- 3 tablespoons balsamic vinegar
- Salt and ground black pepper, as required

## Instructions

1. In a bowl, add the okra, green beans, nutritional yeast, vinegar, salt, and black pepper and toss to coat well.
2. Set the temperature of air fryer to 400 degrees F. Grease an air fryer basket.
3. Arrange okra mixture into the prepared air fryer basket.
4. Air fry for about 20 minutes, tossing several times while frying.
5. Remove from air fryer and transfer the okra mixture onto serving plates.
6. Serve hot.

## Nutrition Values (Per Serving)

- Calories: 126
- Carbohydrate: 19.7g
- Protein: 11.9g
- Fat: 1.3g
- Sugar: 2.1g
- Sodium: 100mg

(**Note: Okra*** - Okra or okro, known in many English-speaking countries as ladies' fingers or ochro, is a flowering plant in the mallow family. It is valued for its edible green seed pods.)

# Stuffed Okra

**(Yields:** 2 servings / **Prep Time:** 15 minutes / **Cooking Time:** 12 minutes)

## Ingredients

- 8 ounces large okra
- ¼ cup chickpea flour
- ¼ of onion, chopped
- 2 tablespoons coconut, grated freshly
- 1 teaspoon garam masala powder
- ½ teaspoon ground turmeric
- ½ teaspoon red chili powder
- ½ teaspoon ground cumin
- Salt, to taste

## Instructions

1. With a knife, make a slit in each okra vertically without cutting in 2 halves.
2. In a bowl, mix together the flour, onion, grated coconut, and spices.
3. Stuff each okra with the mixture.
4. Set the temperature of air fryer to 390 degrees F. Grease an air fryer basket.
5. Arrange stuffed okra into the prepared air fryer basket.
6. Air fry for about 12 minutes.
7. Remove from air fryer and transfer the okra onto serving plates.
8. Serve hot.

## Nutrition Values (Per Serving)

- Calories: 166
- Carbohydrate: 26.6g
- Protein: 7.6g
- Fat: 3.7g
- Sugar: 5.3g
- Sodium: 103mg

---

# Oatmeal Stuffed Bell Peppers

**(Yields:** 2 servings / **Prep Time:** 15 minutes / **Cooking Time:** 16 minutes)

## Ingredients

- 2 large red bell peppers, halved lengthwise and seeded
- 2 cups cooked oatmeal
- 4 tablespoons canned red kidney beans, rinsed and drained
- 4 tablespoons coconut yogurt
- ¼ teaspoon ground cumin
- ¼ teaspoon smoked paprika
- Salt and ground black pepper, as required

## Instructions

1. Set the temperature of air fryer to 355 degrees F. Grease an air fryer basket.
2. Arrange bell peppers into the prepared air fryer basket, cut-side down.
3. Air fry for about 8 minutes.
4. Remove from the air fryer and set aside to cool.
5. Meanwhile, in a bowl, mix well oatmeal, beans, coconut yogurt, and spices.
6. Stuff each bell pepper half with the oatmeal mixture.
7. Now, set the air fryer to 355 degrees F.
8. Arrange bell peppers into the air fryer basket and air fry for about 8 minutes.
9. Remove from air fryer and transfer the bell peppers onto a serving platter.
10. Set aside to cool slightly.
11. Serve warm.

## Nutrition Values (Per Serving)

- Calories: 453
- Carbohydrate: 81g
- Protein: 19.1g
- Fat: 7.4g
- Sugar: 8.4g
- Sodium: 96mg

---

# Broccoli with Cauliflower

**(Yields:** 4 servings / **Prep Time:** 15 minutes / **Cooking Time:** 20 minutes)

## Ingredients

- 1½ cups broccoli, cut into 1-inch pieces
- 1½ cups cauliflower, cut into 1-inch pieces
- 1 tablespoon olive oil
- Salt, as required

## Instructions

1. In a bowl, add the vegetables, oil, and salt and toss to coat well.
2. Set the temperature of air fryer to 375 degrees F. Grease an air fryer basket.
3. Arrange veggie mixture into the prepared air fryer basket.
4. Air fry for about 15-20 minutes, tossing once halfway through.
5. Remove from air fryer and transfer the veggie mixture onto serving plates.
6. Serve hot.

## Nutrition Values (Per Serving)

- Calories: 51
- Carbohydrate: 4.3g
- Protein: 1.7g
- Fat: 3.7g
- Sugar: 1.5g
- Sodium: 61mg

# Herbed Veggies Combo

(**Yields:** 4 servings / **Prep Time:** 15 minutes / **Cooking Time:** 35 minutes)

## Ingredients

- 6 teaspoons olive oil, divided
- ½ pound carrots, peeled and sliced
- 1 pound yellow squash, sliced
- 1 pound zucchini, sliced
- Salt and ground white pepper, as required
- ½ tablespoon fresh basil, chopped
- ½ tablespoon tarragon leaves, chopped

## Instructions

1. Set the temperature of air fryer to 400 degrees F.
2. In a bowl, mix together two teaspoons of oil and carrot slices.
3. Place carrot slices into the air fryer basket
4. Air fry for about 5 minutes.
5. Meanwhile, in a large bowl, add the remaining oil, yellow squash, zucchini, salt, and white pepper and toss to coat well.
6. Transfer the zucchini mixture into air fryer basket with carrots.
7. Air fry for about 30 minutes, tossing 2-3 times.
8. Remove from air fryer and transfer the vegetable mixture into a serving bowl.
9. Add the herbs and mix until well combined.
10. Serve.

## Nutrition Values (Per Serving)

- Calories: 120
- Carbohydrate: 13.3g
- Protein: 3.3g
- Fat: 7.4g
- Sugar: 6.7g
- Sodium: 101mg

# Ratatouille

**(Yields:** 4 servings / **Prep Time:** 15 minutes / **Cooking Time:** 15 minutes)

## Ingredients

- 1 green bell pepper, seeded and chopped
- 1 yellow bell pepper, seeded and chopped
- 1 eggplant, chopped
- 1 zucchini, chopped
- 3 tomatoes, chopped
- 2 small onions, chopped
- 2 garlic cloves, minced
- 2 tablespoons Herbs de Provence
- 1 tablespoon olive oil
- 1 tablespoon balsamic vinegar
- Salt and ground black pepper, as required

## Instructions

1. Set the temperature of air fryer to 355 degrees F. Grease a baking dish.
2. In a large bowl, add the vegetables, garlic, Herbs de Provence, oil, vinegar, salt, and black pepper and toss to coat well.
3. Transfer vegetable mixture into the prepared baking dish.
4. Arrange the baking dish into air fryer and air fry for about 15 minutes.
5. Remove from air fryer and transfer the vegetable mixture into a serving bowl.
6. Serve immediately.

## Nutrition Values (Per Serving)

- Calories: 119
- Carbohydrate: 20.3g
- Protein: 3.6g
- Fat: 4.2g
- Sugar: 11.2g
- Sodium: 56mg

---

# Spicy Tofu

**(Yields:** 3 servings / **Prep Time:** 10 minutes / **Cooking Time:** 13 minutes)

## Ingredients

- 1 (14-ounces) block extra-firm tofu, pressed and cut into ¾-inch cubes
- 1½ tablespoons avocado oil
- 3 teaspoons cornstarch
- 1½ teaspoons paprika
- 1 teaspoon onion powder
- 1 teaspoon garlic powder
- Salt and ground black pepper, as required

### Instructions

1. In a bowl, mix well tofu, oil, cornstarch, and spices.
2. Set the temperature of air fryer to 390 degrees F. Grease an air fryer basket.
3. Arrange tofu pieces into the prepared air fryer basket in a single layer.
4. Air fry for about 13 minutes, shaking twice halfway through.
5. Remove from air fryer and transfer the tofu onto serving plates.
6. Serve hot.

### Nutrition Values (Per Serving)

- Calories: 121
- Carbohydrate: 7g
- Protein: 11.3g
- Fat: 6.6g
- Sugar: 1.4g
- Sodium: 68mg

---

# Rice Flour Crusted Tofu

**(Yields:** 3 servings / **Prep Time:** 15 minutes / **Cooking Time:** 28 minutes**)**

### Ingredients

- 1 (14-ounces) block firm tofu, pressed and cubed into ½-inch size
- 2 tablespoons cornstarch
- ¼ cup rice flour
- Salt and ground black pepper, as required
- 2 tablespoons olive oil

### Instructions

1. In a bowl, mix together cornstarch, rice flour, salt, and black pepper.
2. Coat the tofu evenly with flour mixture.
3. Drizzle the tofu with oil.
4. Set the temperature of air fryer to 360 degrees F. Grease an air fryer basket.
5. Arrange tofu cubes into the prepared air fryer basket in a single layer.
6. Air fry for about 14 minutes per side.
7. Remove from air fryer and transfer the tofu onto serving plates.
8. Serve warm.

### Nutrition Values (Per Serving)

- Calories: 241
- Carbohydrate: 17.7g
- Protein: 11.6g
- Fat: 15g
- Sugar: 0.8g
- Sodium: 67mg

# Crispy Marinated Tofu

**(Yields:** 3 servings / **Prep Time:** 15 minutes / **Cooking Time:** 20 minutes)

## Ingredients

- 1 (14-ounces) block firm tofu, pressed and cut into 1-inch cubes
- 2 tablespoons low sodium soy sauce
- 2 teaspoons sesame oil, toasted
- 1 teaspoon seasoned rice vinegar
- 1 tablespoon cornstarch

## Instructions

1. In a bowl, mix well tofu, soy sauce, sesame oil, and vinegar.
2. Set aside to marinate for about 25-30 minutes.
3. Coat the tofu cubes evenly with cornstarch.
4. Set the temperature of air fryer to 370 degrees F. Grease an air fryer basket.
5. Arrange tofu pieces into the prepared air fryer basket in a single layer.
6. Air fry for about 20 minutes, shaking once halfway through.
7. Remove from air fryer and transfer the tofu onto serving plates.
8. Serve warm.

## Nutrition Values (Per Serving)

- Calories: 136
- Carbohydrate: 5.8g
- Protein: 11.5g
- Fat: 8.6g
- Sugar: 1.1g
- Sodium: 423mg

---

# Tofu in Sweet & Spicy Sauce

**(Yields:** 3 servings / **Prep Time:** 20 minutes / **Cooking Time:** 23 minutes)

## Ingredients

**For Tofu:**

- 1 (14-ounces) block firm tofu, pressed and cubed
- ½ cup arrowroot flour
- ½ teaspoon sesame oil

**For Sauce:**

- 4 tablespoons low-sodium soy sauce
- 1½ tablespoons rice vinegar

- 1½ tablespoons chili sauce
- 1 tablespoon agave nectar
- 2 large garlic cloves, minced
- 1 teaspoon fresh ginger, peeled and grated
- 2 scallions (green part), chopped

## Instructions

1. In a bowl, mix together the tofu, arrowroot flour, and sesame oil.
2. Set the temperature of air fryer to 360 degrees F. Generously, grease an air fryer basket.
3. Arrange tofu pieces into the prepared air fryer basket in a single layer.
4. Air fry for about 20 minutes, shaking once halfway through.
5. Meanwhile, for the sauce: in a bowl, add all the ingredients except scallions and beat until well combined.
6. Remove from air fryer and transfer the tofu into a skillet with sauce over medium heat and cook for about 3 minutes, stirring occasionally.
7. Garnish with scallions and serve hot.

## Nutrition Values (Per Serving)

- Calories: 153
- Carbohydrate: 13.5g
- Protein: 13.4g
- Fat: 6.4g
- Sugar: 13.4g
- Sodium: 1300mg

---

# Tofu with Peanut Butter Sauce

(**Yields:** 3 servings / **Prep Time:** 20 minutes / **Cooking Time:** 15 minutes)

## Ingredients

### For Tofu:

- 2 tablespoons fresh lime juice
- 2 tablespoons soy sauce
- 1 tablespoon maple syrup
- 1 teaspoon Sriracha sauce
- 2 teaspoons fresh ginger, peeled
- 2 garlic cloves, peeled
- 1 (14-ounces) block tofu, pressed and cut into strips

### For Sauce:

- 1 (2-inches) piece fresh ginger, peeled
- 2 garlic cloves, peeled
- ½ cup creamy peanut butter
- 1 tablespoon soy sauce
- 1 tablespoon fresh lime juice
- 1-2 teaspoons Sriracha sauce
- 6 tablespoons of water

## Instructions

1. For tofu: in a food processor, put all the ingredients except tofu and pulse until smooth.
2. In a bowl, mix together the marinade and tofu.
3. Set aside to marinate for about 20-30 minutes.
4. Meanwhile, soak 6 bamboo skewers into water for about 30 minutes.
5. With a cutter, cut each skewer in half.
6. Thread one tofu strip onto each little bamboo stick.
7. Set the temperature of air fryer to 370 degrees F. Grease an air fryer basket.
8. Arrange tofu skewers into the prepared air fryer basket in a single layer.
9. Air fry for about 15 minutes.
10. For the sauce: add all the ingredients in a food processor and pulse until smooth.
11. Remove from air fryer and transfer the tofu onto serving plates.
12. Top with the sauce and serve.

## Nutrition Values (Per Serving)

- Calories: 385
- Carbohydrate: 9.3g
- Protein: 23g
- Fat: 27.3g
- Sugar: 9.1g
- Sodium: 1141mg

# Tofu with Cauliflower

(**Yields:** 2 servings / **Prep Time:** 15 minutes / **Cooking Time:** 15 minutes)

## Ingredients

- ½ (14-ounces) block firm tofu, pressed and cubed
- ½ small head cauliflower, cut into florets
- 1 tablespoon canola oil
- 1 tablespoon nutritional yeast*
- ¼ teaspoon dried parsley
- 1 teaspoon ground turmeric
- ¼ teaspoon paprika
- Salt and ground black pepper, as required

## Instructions

1. In a bowl, mix well tofu, cauliflower and the remaining ingredients.
2. Set the temperature of air fryer to 390 degrees F. Grease an air fryer basket.
3. Arrange tofu mixture into the prepared air fryer basket in a single layer.

4. Air fry for about 12-15 minutes, shaking once halfway through.
5. Remove from air fryer and transfer the tofu onto serving plates.
6. Serve hot.

## Nutrition Values (Per Serving)
- Calories: 170
- Carbohydrate: 8.3g
- Protein: 11.9g
- Fat: 11.6g
- Sugar: 2.3g
- Sodium: 113mg

(**Note: Nutritional Yeast\*** - Nutritional yeast is a deactivated yeast, often a strain of Saccharomyces cerevisiae, which is sold commercially as a food product.)

---

# Tofu with Veggies

(**Yields:** 3 servings / **Prep Time:** 25 minutes / **Cooking Time:** 22 minutes)

## Ingredients
- ½ (14-ounces) block firm tofu, pressed and crumbled
- 1 cup carrot, peeled and chopped
- ½ cup onion, chopped
- 4 tablespoons low-sodium soy sauce, divided
- 1 teaspoon ground turmeric
- 3 cups cauliflower rice*
- ½ cup broccoli, finely chopped
- ½ cup frozen peas
- 1 tablespoon fresh ginger, minced
- 2 garlic cloves, minced
- 1 tablespoon rice vinegar
- 1½ teaspoons sesame oil, toasted

## Instructions
1. In a bowl, mix well tofu, carrot, onion, 2 tablespoons of soy sauce, and turmeric.
2. Set the temperature of air fryer to 370 degrees F. Grease an air fryer pan.
3. Arrange tofu mixture into the prepared air fryer pan.

4. Air fry for about 10 minutes.
5. Meanwhile, in a large bowl, mix together the cauliflower rice, broccoli, peas, ginger, garlic, vinegar, sesame oil, and remaining soy sauce.
6. Remove the pan of tofu from air fryer and gently, stir in the vegetable mixture.
7. Air fry for about 10-12 minutes, shaking once halfway through.
8. Remove from air fryer and transfer the tofu mixture onto serving plates.
9. Serve hot.

## Nutrition Values (Per Serving)

- Calories: 162
- Carbohydrate: 20.4g
- Protein: 11.4g
- Fat: 5.5g
- Sugar: 8.3g
- Sodium: 1263mg

(**Note: Cauliflower rice\*** - Whole Foods also has its own 365 brand of riced cauliflower, and some Costco store carry the Farm Day Organic line of cauliflower "crumbles." So no need to buy a spare deep freezer for veggie hoarding: Just keep an eye open in any freezer aisle.)

---

# Spiced Soy Curls

(**Yields:** 2 servings / **Prep Time:** 15 minutes / **Cooking Time:** 10 minutes)

## Ingredients

- 3 cups boiling water
- 4 ounces soy curls
- ¼ cup nutritional yeast
- ¼ cup fine ground cornmeal
- 2 teaspoons Cajun seasoning
- 1 teaspoon poultry seasoning
- Salt and ground white pepper, as required

## Instructions

1. In a heatproof bowl, add the boiling water and soak the soy curls for about 10 minutes.
2. Through a strainer, drain the soy curls and then with a large spoon, press to release the extra water.
3. In a bowl, mix well nutritional yeast, cornmeal, seasonings, salt, and white pepper.

4. Add the soy curls and generously coat with the mixture.
5. Set the temperature of air fryer to 380 degrees F. Grease an air fryer basket.
6. Arrange soy curls into the prepared air fryer basket in a single layer.
7. Air fry for about 10 minutes, shaking once halfway through.
8. Remove from air fryer and transfer the soy curls onto serving plates.
9. Serve warm.

## **Nutrition Values (Per Serving)**

- Calories: 317
- Carbohydrate: 30.8g
- Protein: 29.4g
- Fat: 10.2g
- Sugar: 2g
- Sodium: 145mg

# **Veggie Rice**

(**Yields:** 2 servings / **Prep Time:** 20 minutes / **Cooking Time:** 18 minutes)

## **Ingredients**

- 2 cups cooked white rice
- 1 tablespoon vegetable oil
- 2 teaspoons sesame oil, toasted and divided
- 1 tablespoon water
- Salt and ground white pepper, as required
- 1 large egg, lightly beaten
- ½ cup frozen peas, thawed
- ½ cup frozen carrots, thawed
- 1 teaspoon soy sauce
- 1 teaspoon Sriracha sauce
- ½ teaspoon sesame seeds, toasted

## **Instructions**

1. In a large bowl, mix well rice, vegetable oil, one teaspoon of sesame oil, water, salt, and white pepper.
2. Set the temperature of air fryer to 380 degrees F. Lightly, grease an air fryer pan.
3. Transfer rice mixture into the prepared air fryer pan.
4. Air fryer for about 12 minutes, stirring once halfway through.
5. Remove the pan from air fryer and place the beaten egg over rice.
6. Air fry for another 4 minutes.
7. Again, remove the pan from air fryer and stir in the peas and carrots.
8. Air fry for 2 more minutes.

9. Meanwhile, in a bowl, mix together soy sauce, Sriracha sauce, sesame seeds and the remaining sesame oil.
10. Remove from air fryer and transfer the rice mixture into a serving bowl.
11. Drizzle with the sauce and serve.

## **Nutrition Values (Per Serving)**

- Calories: 369
- Carbohydrate: 48.9g
- Protein: 9.5g
- Fat: 14.7g
- Sugar: 3.6g
- Sodium: 328mg

# **Beans & Veggie Burgers**

(**Yields:** 4 servings / **Prep Time:** 20 minutes / **Cooking Time:** 22 minutes)

## **Ingredients**

- 1 cup cooked black beans
- 2 cups boiled potatoes, peeled and mashed
- 1 cup fresh spinach, chopped
- 1 cup fresh mushrooms, chopped
- 2 teaspoons Chile lime seasoning
- Olive oil cooking spray
- 6 cups fresh baby greens

## **Instructions**

1. In a large bowl, add the beans, potatoes, spinach, mushrooms, and seasoning and with your hands, mix until well combined.
2. Make 4 equal-sized patties from the mixture.
3. Set the temperature of air fryer to 370 degrees F. Grease an air fryer basket.
4. Arrange patties into the prepared air fryer basket in a single layer and spray with the cooking spray.
5. Air fry for about 12 minutes, shaking once halfway through.
6. Flip the patties and air fry for another 6-7 minutes.
7. Now, set the temperature of air fryer to 90 degrees F and air fry for 3 more minutes.
8. Remove from air fryer and transfer the burgers onto serving plates.
9. Serve warm alongside the baby greens.

## **Nutrition Values (Per Serving)**

- Calories: 249
- Carbohydrate: 48.8g
- Protein: 13.7g
- Fat: 1.1g
- Sugar: 2.9g
- Sodium: 47mg

# CHAPTER 7 | DESSERTS

## Chocolate Yogurt Muffins

**(Yields:** 9 servings / **Prep Time:** 15 minutes / **Cooking Time:** 10 minutes)

### Ingredients

- 1½ cups all-purpose flour
- ¼ cup sugar
- 2 teaspoons baking powder
- ½ teaspoon salt
- 1 cup yogurt
- 1/3 cup vegetable oil
- 1 egg
- 2 teaspoons vanilla extract
- ¼ cup mini chocolate chips
- ¼ cup pecans, chopped

### Instructions

1. In a bowl, mix well flour, sugar, baking powder, and salt.
2. In another bowl, add the yogurt, oil, egg, and vanilla extract and whisk until well combined.
3. Add the flour mixture and mix until just combined.
4. Fold in the chocolate chips and pecans.
5. Set the temperature of air fryer to 355 degrees F. Grease 9 muffin molds.
6. Place mixture evenly into the prepared muffin molds.
7. Arrange the muffin molds into an air fryer basket.
8. Air fry for 10 minutes or until a toothpick inserted in the center comes out clean.
9. Remove the muffin molds from air fryer and place onto a wire rack to cool for about 10 minutes.
10. Finally, invert the muffins onto wire rack to completely cool before serving.

### Nutrition Values (Per Serving)

- Calories: 246
- Carbohydrate: 27.3g
- Protein: 5g
- Fat: 12.9g
- Sugar: 10.2g
- Sodium: 159mg

---

## Brownies Muffins

**(Yields:** 12 servings / **Prep Time:** 10 minutes / **Cooking Time:** 10 minutes)

### Ingredients

- 1 package Betty Crocker fudge brownie mix
- ¼ cup walnuts, chopped

- 1 egg
- 1/3 cup vegetable oil
- 2 teaspoons water

## Instructions

1. In a bowl, mix well all the ingredients.
2. Set the temperature of air fryer to 300 degrees F. Grease 12 muffin molds.
3. Place mixture evenly into the prepared muffin molds.
4. Arrange the molds into an Air Fryer basket.
5. Air fry for 10 minutes or until a toothpick inserted in the center comes out clean.
6. Remove the muffin molds from air fryer and place onto a wire rack to cool for about 10 minutes.
7. Finally, invert the muffins onto wire rack to completely cool before serving.

## Nutrition Values (Per Serving)

- Calories: 241
- Carbohydrate: 36.9g
- Protein: 2.8g
- Fat: 9.6g
- Sugar: 25g
- Sodium: 155mg

---

## Double Chocolate Muffins

**(Yields:** 12 servings / **Prep Time:** 20 minutes / **Cooking Time:** 30 minutes)

### Ingredients

- 1 1/3 cups self-rising flour
- 2/3 cup plus 3 tablespoons caster sugar
- 2½ tablespoons cocoa powder
- 3½ ounces butter
- 5 tablespoons milk
- 2 medium eggs
- ½ teaspoon vanilla extract
- Water, as required
- 2½ ounces milk chocolate, finely chopped

### Instructions

1. In a bowl, mix well flour, sugar, and cocoa powder.
2. With a pastry cutter, cut in the butter until a breadcrumb like mixture forms.
3. In another bowl, mix together the milk, and eggs.
4. Add the egg mixture into flour mixture and mix until well combined.

5. Add the vanilla extract and a little water and mix until well combined.
6. Fold in the chopped chocolate.
7. Set the temperature of air fryer to 355 degrees F. Grease 12 muffin molds.
8. Transfer mixture evenly into the prepared muffin molds.
9. Arrange the molds into an air fryer basket in 2 batches.
10. Air fry for about 9 minutes.
11. Now, set the temperature of air fryer to 320 degrees F.
12. Air fry for another 6 minutes or until a toothpick inserted in the center comes out clean.
13. Remove the muffin molds from air fryer and place onto a wire rack to cool for about 10 minutes.
14. Now, invert the muffins onto wire rack to cool completely before serving.

## **Nutrition Values (Per Serving)**

- Calories: 207
- Carbohydrate: 28.1g
- Protein: 3.3g
- Fat: 9.6g
- Sugar: 16.5g
- Sodium: 66mg

# Fruity Oreo Muffins

**(Yields:** 6 servings / **Prep Time:** 15 minutes / **Cooking Time:** 10 minutes)

## Ingredients

- 1 cup milk
- 1 pack Oreo biscuits, crushed
- 1 teaspoon cocoa powder
- ¼ teaspoon baking soda
- ½ teaspoon baking powder
- 1 banana, peeled and chopped
- 1 apple, peeled, cored and chopped
- 1 teaspoon honey
- 1 teaspoon fresh lemon juice
- A pinch of ground cinnamon

## Instructions

1. In a bowl, add the milk, biscuits, cocoa powder, baking soda, and baking powder. Mix until a smooth mixture forms.
2. Set the temperature of air fryer to 320 degrees F. Grease 6 muffin cups.
3. Place mixture evenly into the prepared muffin cups.

4. Arrange the muffin cups into an air fryer basket.
5. Air fry for 10 minutes or until a toothpick inserted in the center comes out clean.
6. Remove from air fryer and place the muffin cups onto a wire rack to cool slightly.
7. Meanwhile, in another bowl, mix together the banana, apple, honey, lemon juice, and cinnamon.
8. Carefully, scoop some portion of muffins from the center to make a cup.
9. Fill each cup with fruit mixture.
10. Refrigerate to chill before serving.

## Nutrition Values (Per Serving)

- Calories: 182
- Carbohydrate: 31.4g
- Protein: 3.1g
- Fat: 5.9g
- Sugar: 19.5g
- Sodium: 196mg

# Strawberry Cupcakes

**(Yields:** 10 servings / **Prep Time:** 20 minutes / **Cooking Time:** 8 minutes)

## Ingredients

### For Cupcakes:
- ½ cup caster sugar
- 7 tablespoons butter
- 2 eggs
- ½ teaspoon vanilla essence
- 7/8 cup self-rising flour

### For Frosting:
- 1 cup icing sugar
- 3½ tablespoons butter
- 1 tablespoon whipped cream
- ¼ cup fresh strawberries, pureed
- ½ teaspoon pink food color

## Instructions

1. In a bowl, add butter, and sugar and whisk until fluffy and light.
2. Then, add the eggs, one at a time and whisk until well combined.
3. Stir in the vanilla extract.
4. Gradually, add the flour whisking continuously until well combined.
5. Place the mixture into silicon cups.
6. Set the temperature of air fryer to 340 degrees F.
7. Arrange the silicon cups into an air fryer basket.
8. Air fry for about 8 minutes or until a toothpick inserted in the center comes out clean.
9. Remove the silicon cups from air fryer and place onto a wire rack to cool for about 10 minutes.
10. Now, invert the cupcakes onto wire rack to completely cool before frosting.

11. For frosting: in another bowl, add the icing sugar, and butter and whisk until fluffy and light.
12. Add the whipped cream, strawberry puree, and color. Mix until well combined.
13. Fill the pastry bag with icing and decorate the cupcakes.

## **Nutrition Values (Per Serving)**

- Calories: 250
- Carbohydrate: 30.7g
- Protein: 2.4g
- Fat: 13.6g
- Sugar: 22.1g
- Sodium: 99mg

# Raspberry Cupcakes

**(Yields:** 10 servings / **Prep Time:** 15 minutes / **Cooking Time:** 15 minutes)

## **Ingredients**

- 4½ ounces self-rising flour
- ½ teaspoon baking powder
- A pinch of salt
- ½ ounce cream cheese, softened
- 4¾ ounces butter, softened
- 4¼ ounces caster sugar
- 2 eggs
- 2 teaspoons fresh lemon juice
- ½ cup fresh raspberries

## **Instructions**

1. In a bowl, mix well flour, baking powder, and salt.
2. In another bowl, mix together the cream cheese, and butter.
3. Add the sugar and whisk until fluffy and light.
4. Now, place the eggs, one at a time and whisk until just combined.
5. Add the flour mixture and stir until well combined.
6. Stir in the lemon juice.
7. Place the mixture evenly into silicon cups and top each with 2 raspberries.
8. Set the temperature of air fryer to 365 degrees F.
9. Arrange the silicon cups into an air fryer basket.
10. Air fry for about 15 minutes or until a toothpick inserted in the center comes out clean.
11. Remove the silicon cups from air fryer and place onto a wire rack to cool for about 10 minutes.
12. Now, invert the cupcakes onto wire rack to completely cool before serving.

## Nutrition Values (Per Serving)

- Calories: 209
- Carbohydrate: 22.8g
- Protein: 2.7g
- Fat: 12.5g
- Sugar: 12.5g
- Sodium: 110mg

---

# Red Velvet Cupcakes

**(Yields:** 12 servings / **Prep Time:** 20 minutes / **Cooking Time:** 12 minutes**)**

## Ingredients

### For Cupcakes:

- 2 cups refined flour
- ¾ cup icing sugar
- 2 teaspoons beet powder
- 1 teaspoon cocoa powder
- ¾ cup peanut butter
- 3 eggs

### For Frosting:

- 1 cup butter
- 1 (8-ounces) package cream cheese, softened
- 2 teaspoons vanilla extract
- ¼ teaspoon salt
- 4½ cups powdered sugar

### For Garnishing:

- ½ cup fresh raspberries

## Instructions

1. For cupcakes: in a bowl, put all the ingredients and with an electric whisker, whisk until well combined.
2. Place the mixture into silicon cups.
3. Set the temperature of air fryer to 340 degrees F.
4. Arrange the silicon cups into an air fryer basket.
5. Air fry for about 10-12 minutes or until a toothpick inserted in the center comes out clean.
6. Remove the silicon cups from air fryer and place onto a wire rack to cool for about 10 minutes.
7. Now, invert the cupcakes onto wire rack to completely cool before frosting.
8. For frosting: in a large bowl, mix well butter, cream cheese, vanilla extract, and salt.
9. Add the powdered sugar, one cup at a time, whisking well after each addition.
10. Spread frosting evenly over each cupcake.
11. Garnish with raspberries and serve.

## Nutrition Values (Per Serving)

- Calories: 599
- Carbohydrate: 73.2g
- Protein: 9.3g
- Fat: 31.5g
- Sugar: 53.4g
- Sodium: 308mg

---

# Semolina Cake

**(Yields:** 6 servings / **Prep Time:** 15 minutes / **Cooking Time:** 15 minutes)

## Ingredients

- 2½ cups semolina*
- ½ cup vegetable oil
- 1 cup milk
- 1 cup plain Greek yogurt
- 1 cup sugar
- ½ teaspoon baking soda
- 1½ teaspoons baking powder
- A pinch of salt
- ¼ cup raisins
- ¼ cup walnuts, chopped

## Instructions

1. In a bowl, mix well semolina, oil, milk, yogurt, and sugar.
2. Cover and set aside for about 15 minutes.
3. Add the baking soda, baking powder, and salt in the bowl of semolina mixture and mix until well combined.
4. Fold in the raisins and walnuts.
5. Set the temperature of air fryer to 390 degrees F. Grease a cake pan.
6. Place cake mixture evenly into the prepared cake pan.
7. Arrange the cake pan into an air fryer basket.
8. Now, set the temperature of air fryer to 320 degrees F.
9. Air fry for about 15 minutes or until a toothpick inserted in the center comes out clean.
10. Remove the cake pan from air fryer and place onto a wire rack to cool for about 10 minutes.
11. Now, invert the cake onto wire rack to completely cool before slicing.
12. Cut the cake into desired size slices and serve.

## Nutrition Values (Per Serving)
- Calories: 637
- Carbohydrate: 94.8g
- Protein: 13.9g
- Fat: 23.8g
- Sugar: 41.7g
- Sodium: 181mg

(**Note: Semolina*** - Semolina is the coarse, purified wheat middlings of durum wheat mainly used in making traditional pasta. The word semolina can also refer to sweet dessert made from semolina and milk.)

---

# Butter Cake

(**Yields:** 6 servings / **Prep Time:** 15 minutes / **Cooking Time:** 15 minutes)

## Ingredients
- 3 ounces butter, softened
- ½ cup caster sugar
- 1 egg
- 1 1/3 cups plain flour, sifted
- A pinch of salt
- ½ cup milk
- 1 tablespoon icing sugar

## Instructions
1. In a bowl, add the butter, and sugar and whisk until light and creamy.
2. Add in the egg and whisk until smooth and fluffy.
3. Now, add the flour, and salt and mix well alternately with the milk.
4. Set the temperature of air fryer to 350 degrees F. Grease a small Bundt cake pan.
5. Place mixture evenly into the prepared cake pan.
6. Arrange the cake pan in an air fryer basket.
7. Air fry for about 15 minutes or until a toothpick inserted into the center comes out clean.
8. Remove the cake pan from air fryer and place onto a wire rack to cool for about 10 minutes.
9. Now, invert the cake onto wire rack to completely cool before slicing.
10. Dust the cake with icing sugar and cut into desired size slices.
11. Serve.

## Nutrition Values (Per Serving)

- Calories: 291
- Carbohydrate: 40.3g
- Protein: 4.6g
- Fat: 12.9g
- Sugar: 19g
- Sodium: 129mg

===

# Apple Cake

**(Yields:** 6 servings / **Prep Time:** 15 minutes / **Cooking Time:** 45 minutes)

## Ingredients

- 1 cup all-purpose flour
- 1/3 cup brown sugar
- 1 teaspoon ground nutmeg
- 1 teaspoon ground cinnamon
- ½ teaspoon baking soda
- Salt, to taste
- 1 egg
- 5 tablespoons plus 1 teaspoon vegetable oil
- ¾ teaspoon vanilla extract
- 2 cups apples, peeled, cored and chopped

## Instructions

1. In a bowl, mix well flour, sugar, spices, baking soda, and salt.
2. In another bowl, add the egg, and oil and whisk until smooth.
3. Add the vanilla extract and whisk well.
4. Slowly, add the flour mixture, whisking continuously until well combined.
5. Fold in the chopped apples.
6. Set the temperature of air fryer to 355 degrees F. Lightly, grease a cake pan.
7. Place mixture evenly into the prepared cake pan.
8. With a piece of foil, cover the pan and poke some holes using a fork.
9. Arrange the cake pan into an air fryer basket.
10. Now, set the temperature of air fryer to 320 degrees F.
11. Air fry for about 40 minutes.
12. Remove the foil and air fry for another 5 minutes or until a toothpick inserted in the center comes out clean.
13. Remove the cake pan from air fryer and place onto a wire rack to cool for about 10 minutes.
14. Now, invert the cake onto wire rack to completely cool before slicing.
15. Cut the cake into desired size slices and serve.

### **Nutrition Values (Per Serving)**

- Calories: 260
- Carbohydrate: 34.7g
- Protein: 3.3g
- Fat: 12.5g
- Sugar: 15.9g
- Sodium: 145mg

---

# **Banana Cake**

(**Yields:** 6 servings / **Prep Time:** 15 minutes / **Cooking Time:** 40 minutes)

## **Ingredients**

- 1½ cups cake flour
- 1 teaspoon baking soda
- ½ teaspoon ground cinnamon
- Salt, to taste
- ½ cup vegetable oil
- 2 eggs
- ½ cup sugar
- ½ teaspoon vanilla extract
- 3 medium bananas, peeled and mashed
- ¼ cup walnuts, chopped
- ¼ cup raisins, chopped

## **Instructions**

1. In a large bowl, mix well flour, baking soda, cinnamon, and salt.
2. In another bowl, beat well eggs and oil.
3. Add the sugar, vanilla extract, and bananas. Whisk until well combined.
4. Add the flour mixture and stir until just combined.
5. Set the temperature of air fryer to 320 degrees F. Grease a cake pan.
6. Place mixture evenly into the prepared cake pan and top with walnuts and raisins.
7. With a piece of foil, cover the pan.
8. Arrange the cake pan into an air fryer basket.
9. Now, set the temperature of air fryer to 300 degrees F.
10. Air fry for about 30 minutes.
11. Remove the piece of foil and set the temperature to 285 degrees F.
12. Air fry for another 5-10 minutes or until a toothpick inserted in the center comes out clean.
13. Remove the cake pan from air fryer and place onto a wire rack to cool for about 10 minutes.
14. Now, invert the cake onto wire rack to completely cool before slicing.
15. Cut the cake into desired size slices and serve.

## **Nutrition Values (Per Serving)**
- Calories: 462
- Carbohydrate: 59.6g
- Protein: 7.2g
- Fat: 23.2g
- Sugar: 27.8g
- Sodium: 260mg

---

# **Chocolate Cake**

(**Yields:** 4 servings / **Prep Time:** 15 minutes / **Cooking Time:** 40 minutes)

## **Ingredients**

**For Cake:**
- 1/3 cup plain flour
- ¼ teaspoon baking powder
- 1½ tablespoons unsweetened cocoa powder
- 2 egg yolks
- ½ ounce caster sugar
- 2 tablespoons vegetable oil
- 3¾ tablespoons milk
- 1 teaspoon vanilla extract

**For Meringue:**
- 2 egg whites
- 1 ounce caster sugar
- 1/8 teaspoon cream of tartar

## **Instructions**

1. For cake: in a bowl, sift together the flour, baking powder, and cocoa powder.
2. In another bowl, add the remaining ingredients and whisk until well combined.
3. Add the flour mixture and whisk until well combined.
4. For meringue: in a clean glass bowl, add all the ingredients and with an electric whisker, whisk on high speed until stiff peaks form.
5. Place 1/3 of the meringue into flour mixture and with a hand whisker, whisk well.
6. Fold in the remaining meringue.
7. Set the temperature of air fryer to 355 degrees F.
8. Place the mixture into an ungreased chiffon pan.
9. With a piece of foil, cover the pan tightly and poke some holes using a fork.
10. Arrange the cake pan into an air fryer basket.
11. Now, set the temperature of air fryer to 320 degrees F.
12. Air fry for about 30-35 minutes.
13. Remove the piece of foil and set the temperature to 285 degrees F.
14. Air fry for another 5 minutes or until a toothpick inserted in the center comes out clean.

15. Remove the cake pan from air fryer and place onto a wire rack to cool for about 10 minutes.
16. Now, invert the cake onto wire rack to completely cool before slicing.
17. Cut the cake into desired size slices and serve.

## Nutrition Values (Per Serving)

- Calories: 189
- Carbohydrate: 21.2g
- Protein: 5.1g
- Fat: 9.8g
- Sugar: 11.6g
- Sodium: 28mg

# Chocolate Cream Cake

**(Yields:** 6 servings / **Prep Time:** 15 minutes / **Cooking Time:** 25 minutes)

## Ingredients

- 1 cup flour
- 1/3 cup cocoa powder
- 1 teaspoon baking powder
- ½ teaspoon baking soda
- 1/8 teaspoon salt
- 3 eggs
- 2/3 cup sugar
- ½ cup sour cream
- ½ cup butter, softened
- 2 teaspoons vanilla extract

## Instructions

1. In a large bowl, mix well flour, cocoa powder, baking powder, baking soda, and salt.
2. Add the remaining ingredients and with an electric whisker, whisk on low speed until well combined.
3. Set the temperature of air fryer to 320 degrees F. Lightly, grease a cake pan.
4. Place mixture evenly into the prepared cake pan.
5. Arrange the cake pan into an air fryer basket.
6. Air fry for about 25 minutes or until a toothpick inserted in the center comes out clean.
7. Remove the cake pan from air fryer and place onto a wire rack to cool for about 10 minutes.
8. Now, invert the cake onto wire rack to completely cool before slicing.
9. Cut the cake into desired size slices and serve.

## Nutrition Values (Per Serving)

- Calories: 383
- Carbohydrate: 42.3g
- Protein: 6.6g
- Fat: 22.4g
- Sugar: 22.8g
- Sodium: 307mg

# Chocolate Mug Cake

**(Yields:** 1 servings / **Prep Time:** 15 minutes / **Cooking Time:** 13 minutes)

## Ingredients

- ¼ cup self-rising flour
- 5 tablespoons caster sugar
- 1 tablespoon cocoa powder
- 3 tablespoons coconut oil
- 3 tablespoons whole milk

## Instructions

1. In a shallow mug, add all the ingredients and mix until well combined.
2. Set the temperature of air fryer to 392 degrees F.
3. Arrange the mug into an air fryer basket.
4. Air fry for about 13 minutes.
5. Remove from the air fryer and serve warm.

## Nutrition Values (Per Serving)

- Calories: 729
- Carbohydrate: 88.8g
- Protein: 5.7g
- Fat: 43.3g
- Sugar: 62.2g
- Sodium: 20mg

===

# Lava Cake

**(Yields:** 4 servings / **Prep Time:** 15 minutes / **Cooking Time:** 12½ minutes)

## Ingredients

- 2/3 cup chocolate chips
- ½ cup unsalted butter, softened
- 2 large eggs
- 2 large egg yolks
- 1 cup confectioners' sugar
- 1 teaspoon peppermint extract
- 1/3 cup all-purpose flour plus more for dusting
- 2 tablespoons powdered sugar
- 1/3 cup fresh raspberries

## Instructions

1. In a microwave-safe bowl, put the chocolate chips and butter. Microwave on high heat for about 30 seconds.
2. Remove the bowl from microwave and stir the mixture well.
3. Add the eggs, egg yolks and confectioners' sugar and whisk until well combined.
4. Add the flour and gently, stir to combine.

5. Set the temperature of air fryer to 375 degrees F. Grease 4 ramekins and dust each with a little flour.
6. Place mixture evenly into the prepared ramekins.
7. Arrange the ramekins into an air fryer basket.
8. Air fry for about 10-12 minutes.
9. Remove from air fryer and place the ramekins onto a wire rack for about 5 minutes.
10. Carefully run a knife around sides of each ramekin several times to loosen the cake.
11. Finally, invert each cake onto a dessert plate and dust with powdered sugar.
12. Garnish with raspberries and serve immediately.

## Nutrition Values (Per Serving)

- Calories: 598
- Carbohydrate: 60.4g
- Protein: 8.1g
- Fat: 36.2g
- Sugar: 19.2g
- Sodium: 225mg

---

# Layered Cake

(**Yields:** 8 servings / **Prep Time:** 20 minutes / **Cooking Time:** 25 minutes)

## Ingredients

**For Cake:**

- 3½ ounces plain flour
- 1 teaspoon ground cinnamon
- Pinch of salt
- 7 tablespoons sugar
- 3½ ounces butter, softened
- 2 medium eggs

**For Filling:**

- 1¾ ounces butter, softened
- 1 tablespoon whipped cream
- 2/3 cup icing sugar
- 2 tablespoons strawberry jam

## Instructions

1. In a large bowl, mix well flour, cinnamon, and salt.
2. In another bowl, add the sugar, and butter and whisk until creamy.
3. Add in the eggs and whisk until well combined.
4. Slowly, add the flour mixture whisking continuously until well combined
5. Set the temperature of air fryer to 355 degrees F. Grease a cake pan.
6. Place mixture evenly into the prepared cake pan.
7. Air fry for about 15 minutes and then, another 10 minutes at 335 degrees F.

8. Remove the cake pan from air fryer and place onto a wire rack to cool for about 10 minutes.
9. Now, invert the cake onto wire rack to completely cool before filling.
10. After cooling, cut the cake into 2 equal-sized portions.
11. For filling: in a bowl, add the butter and whisk until creamy.
12. Add the cream, and icing sugar and whisk until a thick creamy mixture forms.
13. Place one cake portion onto a serving platter, cut side up.
14. Spread the jam evenly over cake and top with butter mixture.
15. Arrange another cake over filling, cut side down.
16. Cut the cake into desired size slices and serve.

## **Nutrition Values (Per Serving)**

- Calories: 595
- Carbohydrate: 69.9g
- Protein: 5.8g
- Fat: 33.8g
- Sugar: 40.9g
- Sodium: 286mg

## Clafoutis

**(Yields:** 4 servings / **Prep Time:** 15 minutes / **Cooking Time:** 25 minutes)

## **Ingredients**

- 1½ cups fresh cherries, pitted
- 3 tablespoons vodka
- ¼ cup flour
- 2 tablespoons sugar
- Pinch of salt
- ½ cup sour cream
- 1 egg
- 1 tablespoon butter
- ¼ cup powdered sugar

## **Instructions**

1. In a bowl, mix together the cherries and vodka.
2. In another bowl, mix well flour, sugar, and salt.
3. Add the sour cream, and egg and mix until a smooth dough forms.
4. Set the temperature of air fryer to 355 degrees F. Grease a cake pan.
5. Place flour mixture evenly into the prepared cake pan.
6. Spread cherry mixture over the dough.
7. Place butter on top in the form of dots.
8. Arrange the cake pan in an air fryer basket.
9. Air fry for about 25 minutes or until a toothpick inserted in the center comes out clean.
10. Remove the cake pan from air fryer and place onto a wire rack to cool for about 10 minutes.

11. Now, invert the Clafoutis onto a platter and sprinkle with powdered sugar.
12. Cut the Clafoutis into desired size slices and serve warm.

## **Nutrition Values (Per Serving)**

- Calories: 226
- Carbohydrate: 25.5g
- Protein: 3.5g
- Fat: 10.2g
- Sugar: 0.8g
- Sodium: 191g

---

# **Simple Cheesecake**

(**Yields:** 14 servings / **Prep Time:** 15 minutes / **Cooking Time:** 19 minutes)

## **Ingredients**

- 1 cup honey graham cracker crumbs
- 2 tablespoons unsalted butter, softened
- 1 pound cream cheese, softened
- ½ cup sugar
- 2 large eggs
- ½ teaspoon vanilla extract

## **Instructions**

1. Line a round baking dish with parchment paper.
2. For crust: in a bowl, add the graham cracker crumbs, and butter.
3. Place the crust into baking dish and press to smooth.
4. Set the temperature of air fryer to 350 degrees F.
5. Arrange the baking dish into an air fryer basket.
6. Air fry for about 4 minutes.
7. Remove the crust from air fryer and set aside to cool slightly.
8. Meanwhile, in a bowl, add the cream cheese, and sugar and whisk until smooth.
9. Now, place the eggs, one at a time and whisk until mixture becomes creamy.
10. Add the vanilla extract and mix well.
11. Place the cream cheese mixture evenly over the crust.
12. Arrange baking dish into the air fryer basket.
13. Air fry for about 15 minutes.
14. Remove from the air fryer and set aside for about 1-2 hours to cool.
15. Refrigerate to chill for about 3 hours before serving.

## Nutrition Values (Per Serving)

- Calories: 201
- Carbohydrate: 14.9g
- Protein: 4g
- Fat: 14.5g
- Sugar: 9.4g
- Sodium: 182mg

---

# Strawberry Cheesecake

**(Yields:** 15 servings / **Prep Time:** 20 minutes / **Cooking Time:** 1 hour 37 minutes)

## Ingredients

### For Crust:

- 7 tablespoons almond flour
- 2 tablespoons natural peanut butter
- 1 tablespoon honey

### For Topping:

- 2 tablespoons fat-free plain Greek yogurt
- 1 tablespoon Splenda
- 2 tablespoons vanilla whey protein powder

### For Filling:

- 2 eggs
- 10½ ounces plain Greek yogurt
- 10½ ounces cream cheese
- 2 scoops vanilla whey protein powder
- 2 tablespoons strawberry preserves
- 2 tablespoons Splenda
- ¼ teaspoon vanilla extract
- 1 cup fresh strawberries, hulled and sliced

## Instructions

1. Line a greased round baking pan with a parchment paper.
2. For crust: in a bowl, add all the ingredients and mix until a dough ball forms.
3. Place the dough ball in the center of prepared baking pan.
4. With your fingers, press downwards until the dough spreads evenly in the bottom of pan.
5. Set the temperature of air fryer to 248 degrees F.
6. Arrange the baking pan into an air fryer basket.
7. Air fry for about 7 minutes.
8. Remove the crust from air fryer and set aside to cool slightly.
9. Meanwhile, for filling: in a large bowl, put all the ingredients except strawberries and whisk until smooth.

10. Fold in the strawberries.
11. Place strawberry mixture evenly over the crust.
12. With the back of spatula, smooth the top surface of strawberry mixture.
13. Again, set the temperature of air fryer to 248 degrees F.
14. Arrange baking pan into the air fryer basket.
15. Air fry for about 30 minutes and then, another 1 hour at 195 degrees F.
16. Remove from the air fryer and set aside for about 1-2 hours to cool.
17. For the topping: in a bowl, put all the ingredients and mix well.
18. After cooling, top the cheesecake with topping mixture.
19. Refrigerate for about 4-8 hours before serving.

## Nutrition Values (Per Serving)

- Calories: 167
- Carbohydrate: 8.9g
- Protein: 8.9g
- Fat: 10.8g
- Sugar: 6.4g
- Sodium: 88mg

# Lemon Cheesecake

(**Yields:** 8 servings / **Prep Time:** 15 minutes / **Cooking Time:** 25 minutes)

## Ingredients

- 17.6 ounces ricotta cheese
- 3 eggs
- ¾ cup sugar
- 3 tablespoons corn starch
- 1 tablespoon fresh lemon juice
- 2 teaspoons vanilla extract
- 1 teaspoon fresh lemon zest, finely grated

## Instructions

1. In a large bowl, put all ingredients and mix until well combined.
2. Place the mixture into a baking dish.
3. Set the temperature of air fryer to 320 degrees F.
4. Arrange the baking dish into an air fryer basket.
5. Air fry for about 25 minutes.
6. Remove from the air fryer and set aside for about 1-2 hours to cool.
7. Refrigerate to chill for about 2-3 hours before serving.

### Nutrition Values (Per Serving)

- Calories: 197
- Carbohydrate: 25.7g
- Protein: 9.2g
- Fat: 6.6g
- Sugar: 19.3g
- Sodium: 102mg

# White Chocolate Cheesecake

**(Yields:** 6 servings / **Prep Time:** 20 minutes / **Cooking Time:** 34 minutes)

## Ingredients

- 3 eggs, whites and yolks separated
- 1 cup white chocolate, chopped
- ½ cup cream cheese, softened
- 2 tablespoons cocoa powder
- 2 tablespoons powdered sugar
- ¼ cup apricot jam

## Instructions

1. In a bowl, add the egg whites and refrigerate to chill before using.
2. In a microwave-safe bowl, add the chocolate and microwave on high heat for about 2 minutes, stirring after every 30 seconds.
3. In the bowl of chocolate, add the cream cheese and microwave for about 1-2 minutes or until cream cheese melts completely.
4. Remove from microwave and stir in cocoa powder and egg yolks.
5. Remove the egg whites from refrigerator and whisk until firm peaks form.
6. Add 1/3 of the mixed egg whites into cheese mixture and gently, stir to combine.
7. Fold in the remaining egg whites.
8. Set the temperature of air fryer to 285 degrees F.
9. Place the mixture into a 6-inch cake pan.
10. Arrange the cake pan into an air fryer basket.
11. Air fry for about 30 minutes.
12. Remove from the air fryer and set aside to cool completely.
13. Refrigerate to chill before serving.
14. Just before serving, dust with the powdered sugar.
15. Finally, spread the jam evenly on top and serve.

### Nutrition Values (Per Serving)

- Calories: 298
- Carbohydrate: 29.7g
- Protein: 6.3g
- Fat: 18.3g
- Sugar: 24.5g
- Sodium: 119mg

# Apple Crumble

**(Yields:** 4 servings / **Prep Time:** 10 minutes / **Cooking Time:** 25 minutes)

## Ingredients

- 1 (14-ounces) can apple pie filling
- ¼ cup butter, softened
- 9 tablespoons self-rising flour
- 7 tablespoons caster sugar
- Pinch of salt

## Instructions

1. Set the temperature of air fryer to 320 degrees F. Lightly, grease a baking dish.
2. Place apple pie filling evenly into the prepared baking dish.
3. In a medium bowl, add the remaining ingredients and mix until a crumbly mixture forms.
4. Spread the mixture evenly over apple pie filling.
5. Arrange the baking dish in an air fryer basket.
6. Air fry for about 25 minutes.
7. Remove the baking dish from air fryer and place onto a wire rack to cool for about 10 minutes.
8. Serve warm.

## Nutrition Values (Per Serving)

- Calories: 340
- Carbohydrate: 60.3g
- Protein: 2g
- Fat: 11.8g
- Sugar: 34.8g
- Sodium: 167mg

---

# Fruity Crumble

**(Yields:** 4 servings / **Prep Time:** 15 minutes / **Cooking Time:** 20 minutes)

## Ingredients

- ½ pound fresh apricots, pitted and cubed
- 1 cup fresh blackberries
- 1/3 cup sugar, divided
- 1 tablespoon fresh lemon juice
- 7/8 cup flour
- Pinch of salt
- 1 tablespoon cold water
- ¼ cup chilled butter, cubed

## Instructions

1. Set the temperature of air fryer to 390 degrees F. Grease a baking pan.
2. In a large bowl, mix well apricots, blackberries, 2 tablespoons of sugar, and lemon juice.
3. Spread apricot mixture into the prepared baking pan.
4. In another bowl, add the flour, remaining sugar, salt, water, and butter. Mix until a crumbly mixture forms.
5. Spread the flour mixture evenly over apricot mixture.
6. Place the pan in an air fryer basket.
7. Air fry for about 20 minutes.
8. Remove the baking pan from air fryer and place onto a wire rack to cool for about 10 minutes.
9. Serve warm.

## Nutrition Values (Per Serving)

- Calories: 307
- Carbohydrate: 47.3g
- Protein: 4.2g
- Fat: 12.4g
- Sugar: 23.7g
- Sodium: 123mg

# Mini Apple Pies

(**Yields:** 6 servings / **Prep Time:** 20 minutes / **Cooking Time:** 30 minutes)

## Ingredients

**For Crust:**

- 1½ cups flour
- 1 teaspoon sugar
- Salt, to taste
- ½ cup unsalted butter
- ¼ cup chilled water

**For Topping:**

- 1 egg, beaten
- 3 tablespoons sugar
- 1 teaspoon ground cinnamon

**For Filling:**

- 4 Granny Smith apples, peeled and finely chopped
- 1 teaspoon fresh lemon zest, finely grated
- 2½ tablespoons sugar
- 2 tablespoons flour
- 1 teaspoon ground cinnamon
- ¼ teaspoon ground nutmeg
- Salt, to taste
- ¼ cup Nutella
- 2 tablespoons fresh lemon juice
- 2 tablespoons butter

## Instructions

1. In a bowl, mix well flour, sugar, butter, and salt.
2. With a pastry cutter, cut in the butter.
3. Add the chilled water and mix until a dough forms.
4. With a plastic wrapper, cover the bowl and refrigerate for about 30 minutes.
5. Meanwhile, for filling: in a large bowl, mix well all the ingredients. Set aside.
6. Now, place the dough onto a lightly floured surface and roll into ½-inch thickness.
7. With a ramekin, cut 12 circles from the dough.
8. Place 6 circles in the bottom of 6 ramekins and press slightly.
9. Add the filling mixture evenly into the ramekins and top with the remaining circles.
10. Pinch the edges to seal the pies.
11. Carefully, cut 3 slits in each pie and coat evenly with the beaten egg.
12. For topping: in a small bowl, mix together the cinnamon and sugar.
13. Sprinkle each pie with the cinnamon sugar.
14. Set the temperature of air fryer to 350 degrees F.
15. Arrange the ramekins into an air fryer basket.
16. Air fry for about 30 minutes.
17. Remove the ramekins from air fryer and place onto a wire rack to cool for about 10-15 minutes before serving.
18. Serve warm.

## Nutrition Values (Per Serving)

- Calories: 442
- Carbohydrate: 58.2g
- Protein: 5.2g
- Fat: 22.6g
- Sugar: 29.2g
- Sodium: 203mg

# Apple Pie

(**Yields:** 6 servings / **Prep Time:** 15 minutes / **Cooking Time:** 30 minutes)

## Ingredients

- 1 frozen pie crust, thawed
- 1 large apple, peeled, cored and chopped
- 3 tablespoons sugar, divided
- 1 tablespoon ground cinnamon
- 2 teaspoons fresh lemon juice
- ½ teaspoon vanilla extract
- 1 tablespoon butter, chopped
- 1 egg, beaten

## Instructions

1. Grease a pie pan.
2. With a smaller baking tin, cut 1 crust from thawed pie crust about 1/8-inch larger than pie pan.
3. Now, cut the second crust from the pie crust a little smaller than first one.
4. Arrange the large crust in the bottom of prepared pie pan.
5. In a bowl, mix together the apple, 2 tablespoons of sugar, cinnamon, lemon juice, and vanilla extract.
6. Place apple mixture evenly over the bottom crust.
7. Add the chopped butter over apple mixture.
8. Arrange the second crust on top and pinch the edges to seal.
9. Carefully, cut 3-4 slits in the top crust.
10. Spread the beaten egg evenly over top crust and sprinkle with the remaining sugar.
11. Set the temperature of air fryer to 320 degrees F.
12. Arrange the pie pan into an air fryer basket.
13. Air fry for about 30 minutes.
14. Remove from air fryer and place the pie pan onto a wire rack to cool for about 10-15 minutes before serving.
15. Serve warm.

## Nutrition Values (Per Serving)

- Calories: 190
- Carbohydrate: 25.3g
- Protein: 11.3g
- Fat: 3.1g
- Sugar: 1.6g
- Sodium: 160mg

## Sweet Potato Pie

**(Yields:** 6 servings / **Prep Time:** 25 minutes / **Cooking Time:** 60 minutes)

## Ingredients

- 6 ounces sweet potato
- 1 teaspoon olive oil
- 1 (9-inches) prepared frozen pie dough, thawed
- ¼ cup heavy cream
- 2 large eggs
- 2 tablespoons maple syrup
- 1 tablespoon butter, melted
- 1 tablespoon light brown sugar
- ½ teaspoon ground cinnamon
- 1/8 teaspoon ground nutmeg
- Salt, to taste
- ¾ teaspoon vanilla extract

## Instructions

1. Set the temperature of air fryer to 400 degrees F.
2. Coat the sweet potato evenly with oil.
3. Arrange the sweet potato into an air fryer basket.
4. Air fry for about 30 minutes.
5. Remove from air fryer and set aside to cool completely.
6. Peel the sweet potato and mash it completely.
7. Place the pie dough onto a floured surface and cut into 8-inch pie shell.
8. Arrange the dough shell into a greased pie pan.
9. In a large bowl, add the mashed sweet potato, and remaining ingredients and mix until well combined.
10. Place sweet potato mixture evenly over the pie shell.
11. Set the temperature of air fryer to 320 degrees F.
12. Arrange the pie pan into an air fryer basket.
13. Air fry for about 30 minutes.
14. Remove from air fryer and place the pie pan onto a wire rack to cool for about 10-15 minutes before serving.
15. Serve warm.

## Nutrition Values (Per Serving)

- Calories: 233
- Carbohydrate: 27.8g
- Protein: 3.8g
- Fat: 12.2g
- Sugar: 16.6g
- Sodium: 212mg

---

# Pecan Pie

(**Yields:** 5 servings / **Prep Time:** 15 minutes / **Cooking Time:** 35 minutes)

## Ingredients

- ¾ cup brown sugar
- ¼ cup caster sugar
- 1/3 cup butter, melted
- 2 large eggs
- 1¾ tablespoons flour
- 1 tablespoon milk
- 1 teaspoon vanilla extract
- 1 cup pecan halves
- 1 frozen pie crust, thawed

## Instructions

1. In a large bowl, mix well sugars, and butter.
2. Add the eggs and whisk until foamy.
3. Add the flour, milk, and vanilla extract and whisk until well combined.
4. Fold in the pecan halves.

5. Set the temperature of air fryer to 300 degrees F. Grease a pie pan.
6. Arrange the crust in the bottom of prepared pie pan.
7. Transfer pecan mixture evenly over the crust.
8. Arrange the pan in an air fryer basket.
9. Air fry for about 22 minutes and then, another 13 minutes at 285 degrees F.
10. Remove from air fryer and place the pie pan onto a wire rack to cool for about 10-15 minutes before serving.
11. Serve warm.

## Nutrition Values (Per Serving)

- Calories: 575
- Carbohydrate: 49.9g
- Protein: 6.9g
- Fat: 40.5g
- Sugar: 33.5g
- Sodium: 286mg

# Apple Tart

(**Yields:** 3 servings / **Prep Time:** 10 minutes / **Cooking Time:** 25 minutes)

## Ingredients

- 2½ ounces butter, chopped and divided
- 3½ ounces flour
- 1 egg yolk
- 1 ounce sugar
- 1 large granny smith apple, peeled, cored and cut into 12 wedges

## Instructions

1. In a bowl, add half of the butter, flour, and egg yolk and mix until a soft dough forms.
2. Now, put the dough onto a floured surface and roll into a 6-inch round circle.
3. Set the temperature of air fryer to 390 degrees F.
4. In a baking pan, add the remaining butter and sprinkle with sugar.
5. Top with the apple wedges in a circular pattern.
6. Place the rolled dough over apple wedges and gently press along the edges of the pan.
7. Arrange the pan into an air fryer basket.
8. Air fry for about 25 minutes.
9. Remove from the air fryer and serve warm.

### Nutrition Values (Per Serving)

- Calories: 382
- Carbohydrate: 45.2g
- Protein: 4.7g
- Fat: 21.1g
- Sugar: 17.3g
- Sodium: 140mg

---

# Fudge Brownies

**(Yields:** 8 servings / **Prep Time:** 15 minutes / **Cooking Time:** 20 minutes)

## Ingredients

- 1 cup sugar
- ½ cup butter, melted
- ½ cup flour
- 1/3 cup cocoa powder
- 1 teaspoon baking powder
- 2 eggs
- 1 teaspoon vanilla extract

## Instructions

1. Set the temperature of Air fryer to 350 degrees F. Grease a baking pan.
2. In a large bowl, add the sugar, and butter and whisk until light and fluffy.
3. Add the remaining ingredients and mix until well combined.
4. Place mixture evenly into the prepared pan and with the back of spatula, smooth the top surface.
5. Arrange the baking pan into an air fryer basket.
6. Air fry pan for about 20 minutes.
7. Remove the baking pan from air fryer and set aside to cool completely.
8. Cut into 8 equal-sized squares and serve.

## Nutrition Values (Per Serving)

- Calories: 250
- Carbohydrate: 33.4g
- Protein: 13g
- Fat: 13.2g
- Sugar: 25.2g
- Sodium: 99mg

# Walnut Brownies

**(Yields:** 4 servings / **Prep Time:** 15 minutes / **Cooking Time:** 22 minutes)

## Ingredients

- ½ cup chocolate, roughly chopped
- 1/3 cup butter
- 5 tablespoons sugar
- 1 egg, beaten
- 1 teaspoon vanilla extract
- A pinch of salt
- 5 tablespoons self-rising flour
- ¼ cup walnuts, chopped

## Instructions

1. In a microwave-safe bowl, add the chocolate and butter. Microwave on high heat for about 2 minutes, stirring after every 30 seconds.
2. Remove from microwave and set aside to cool.
3. Now, in a bowl, add the sugar, egg, vanilla extract, and salt and whisk until creamy and light.
4. Add the chocolate mixture and whisk until well combined.
5. Add the flour, and walnuts and mix until well combined.
6. Set the temperature of air fryer to 355 degrees F. Line a baking pan with a greased parchment paper.
7. Place mixture evenly into the prepared pan and with the back of spatula, smooth the top surface.
8. Arrange the baking pan into an air fryer basket.
9. Air fry for about 20 minutes.
10. Remove the baking pan from air fryer and set aside to cool completely.
11. Cut into 4 equal-sized squares and serve.

## Nutrition Values (Per Serving)

- Calories: 205
- Carbohydrate: 1g
- Protein: 3.1g
- Fat: 13.8g
- Sugar: 13.1g
- Sodium: 91mg

# Shortbread Fingers

**(Yields:** 10 servings / **Prep Time:** 15 minutes / **Cooking Time:** 12 minutes)

## Ingredients

- 1/3 cup caster sugar
- 1 2/3 cups plain flour
- ¾ cup butter

## Instructions

1. In a large bowl, mix together the sugar and flour.
2. Add the butter and mix until a smooth dough forms.
3. Cut the dough into 10 equal-sized fingers.
4. With a fork, lightly prick the fingers.
5. Set the temperature of air fryer to 355 degrees F. Lightly, grease a baking sheet.
6. Arrange fingers into the prepared baking sheet in a single layer.
7. Arrange the baking sheet into an air fryer basket.
8. Air fry for about 12 minutes.
9. Remove the baking sheet from air fryer and place onto a wire rack to cool for about 5-10 minutes.
10. Now, invert the short bread fingers onto wire rack to completely cool before serving.
11. Serve.

## Nutrition Values (Per Serving)

- Calories: 223
- Carbohydrate: 22.6g
- Protein: 2.3g
- Fat: 14g
- Sugar: 6.7g
- Sodium: 99mg

# Cream Doughnuts

(**Yields:** 8 servings / **Prep Time:** 15 minutes / **Cooking Time:** 16 minutes)

## Ingredients

**For Doughnuts:**

- ½ cup sugar
- 2 tablespoons butter, softened
- 2 egg yolks
- 2¼ cups plain flour
- 1½ teaspoons baking powder
- 1 teaspoon salt
- ½ cup sour cream
- 2 tablespoons butter, melted

**For Topping:**

- 1/3 cup caster sugar
- 1 teaspoon cinnamon

## Instructions

1. In a large bowl, add the sugar and 2 tablespoons of softened butter and whisk until crumbly mixture forms.
2. Add the egg yolks and whisk until well combined.
3. In another bowl, sift together the flour, baking powder, and salt.
4. Divide the flour mixture in 3 portions.

5. Add first portion of flour mixture and ½ of sour cream in the bowl of sugar mixture and mix well.
6. Add the second portion of flour mixture, and remaining sour cream and mix well.
7. Now, add the remaining portion and mix until a dough forms.
8. Refrigerate the dough before rolling.
9. Now, put the dough onto a lightly floured surface and roll into 2-inch thickness.
10. With a floured doughnut cutter, cut the dough.
11. Set the temperature of air fryer to 355 degrees F. Grease an air fryer basket.
12. Coat both sides of the doughnut with melted butter.
13. Arrange doughnuts into the prepared air fryer basket in 2 batches.
14. Air fry for about 8 minutes or until golden brown.
15. Meanwhile, in a bowl, mix together the sugar and cinnamon.
16. Remove from air fryer and transfer the doughnuts onto a platter to cool completely.
17. Sprinkle the doughnuts with cinnamon sugar and serve.

## Nutrition Values (Per Serving)

- Calories: 272
- Carbohydrate: 40.8g
- Protein: 4.8g
- Fat: 10.2g
- Sugar: 12.6g
- Sodium: 343mg

# Milky Doughnuts

(**Yields:** 12 servings / **Prep Time:** 15 minutes / **Cooking Time:** 24 minutes)

## Ingredients

**For Doughnuts:**

- 1 cup all-purpose flour
- 1 cup whole wheat flour
- 2 teaspoons baking powder
- Salt, to taste
- ¾ cup sugar
- 1 egg
- 1 tablespoon butter, softened
- ½ cup milk
- 2 teaspoons vanilla extract

**For Glaze:**

- 2 tablespoons icing sugar
- 2 tablespoons condensed milk
- 1 tablespoon cocoa powder

## Instructions

1. In a large bowl, mix well flours, baking powder, and salt.
2. In another bowl, add the sugar and egg. Whisk until fluffy and light.
3. Add the flour mixture and stir until well combined.
4. Add the butter, milk, and vanilla extract and mix until a soft dough forms.

5. Refrigerate the dough for at least 1 hour.
6. Now, put the dough onto a lightly floured surface and roll into ½-inch thickness.
7. With a small doughnut cutter, cut 24 small doughnuts from the rolled dough.
8. Set the temperature of air fryer to 390 degrees F. Grease an air fryer basket.
9. Place doughnuts into the prepared air fryer basket in 3 batches.
10. Air fry for about 6-8 minutes.
11. Remove from air fryer and transfer the doughnuts onto a platter to cool completely.
12. In a small bowl, mix together the condensed milk and cocoa powder.
13. Spread the glaze over doughnuts and sprinkle with icing sugar.
14. Serve.

## Nutrition Values (Per Serving)

- Calories: 166
- Carbohydrate: 33.4g
- Protein: 3.9g
- Fat: 2.3g
- Sugar: 16.2g
- Sodium: 34mg

---

# Apple Doughnuts

(**Yields:** 6 servings / **Prep Time:** 20 minutes / **Cooking Time:** 5 minutes)

## Ingredients

**For Doughnuts:**
- 1 cup apple cider
- 2½ cups plus 2 tablespoons all-purpose flour
- 1 teaspoon baking powder
- ½ teaspoon baking soda
- ½ teaspoon ground cinnamon
- ½ teaspoon salt
- ½ cup brown sugar
- 2 tablespoons unsalted butter, softened
- 1 egg
- ½ pink lady apple, peeled, cored and grated

**For Topping:**
- ½ cup sugar
- ½ tablespoon ground cinnamon
- 3 tablespoons butter, melted

## Instructions

1. In a medium pan, add the apple cider over medium-high heat and bring it to a boil.
2. Lower the heat and simmer for about 15 minutes or until the cider reduces to ¼ cup.
3. Remove the pan from heat and transfer the apple cider into a bowl. Refrigerate to cool.

4. In a large bowl, mix well flour, baking powder, baking soda, cinnamon, and salt.
5. In another bowl, add the brown sugar, and butter and with an electric hand mixer, whisk until light and fluffy.
6. Add the egg and whisk well.
7. Add the cooled apple cider and mix well.
8. Put the flour mixture and mix until well combined.
9. Add the grated apple and mix until a dough forms.
10. Now, put the dough onto a lightly floured surface and with your hands, knead until a soft dough comes together.
11. With a plastic wrap, wrap the dough and refrigerate for about 30 minutes.
12. Now, place the dough onto a lightly floured surface and roll into 1-inch thickness.
13. With a 3-inches doughnut cutter, cut the doughnuts.
14. Set the temperature of air fryer to 360 degrees F for about 2 minutes. Grease an air fryer basket.
15. Now, turn off the air fryer.
16. Arrange doughnuts into the prepared air fryer basket and let the dough rest in the turned off air fryer for about 5 minutes.
17. Again, set the temperature of air fryer to 360 degrees F.
18. Air fry for about 5 minutes, flipping once halfway through.
19. Meanwhile, in a shallow bowl, mix together the sugar, and cinnamon.
20. Remove from air fryer and transfer the doughnuts onto a platter.
21. Brush both sides of doughnuts with melted butter and then, coat with the cinnamon sugar.
22. Serve.

## **Nutrition Values (Per Serving)**

- Calories: 433
- Carbohydrate: 78.3g
- Protein: 6.8g
- Fat: 11g
- Sugar: 35g
- Sodium: 383mg

# **Chocolate Banana Pastries**

(**Yields:** 4 servings / **Prep Time:** 15 minutes / **Cooking Time:** 12 minutes)

## **Ingredients**

- 1 puff pastry sheet
- ½ cup Nutella
- 2 bananas, peeled and sliced

### Instructions

1. Cut the pastry sheet into 4 equal-sized squares.
2. Spread Nutella evenly on each square of pastry.
3. Divide the banana slices over Nutella.
4. Fold each square into a triangle and with wet fingers, slightly press the edges.
5. Then with a fork, press the edges firmly.
6. Set the temperature of air fryer to 375 degrees F. Lightly, grease an air fryer basket.
7. Arrange pastries into the prepared air fryer basket in a single layer.
8. Air fry for about 10-12 minutes.
9. Remove from air fryer and transfer the pastries onto a platter.
10. Serve warm.

### Nutrition Values (Per Serving)

- Calories: 205
- Carbohydrate: 30.3g
- Protein: 3.2g
- Fat: 8.9g
- Sugar: 14.4g
- Sodium: 96mg

---

## Pear Pastry Pouch

**(Yields:** 4 servings / **Prep Time:** 15 minutes / **Cooking Time:** 15 minutes)

### Ingredients

- 2 small pears, peeled, cored and halved
- 2 cups vanilla custard
- 4 puff pastry sheets
- 2 tablespoons sugar
- Pinch of ground cinnamon
- 1 egg, lightly beaten
- 2 tablespoons whipped cream

### Instructions

1. Carefully, make small cuts in each pear half.
2. In the center of each pastry sheet, place a spoonful of vanilla custard and top with a pear half.
3. In a bowl, mix together the sugar and cinnamon.
4. Sprinkle the sugar mixture evenly over pear halves.
5. Pinch the corners to shape into a pouch.
6. Now, coat each pear with egg.
7. Set the temperature of air fryer to 330 degrees F. Lightly, grease an air fryer basket.
8. Arrange pear pouches into the prepared air fryer basket in a single layer.

9. Air fry for about 15 minutes.
10. Remove from air fryer and transfer the pear pouches onto a platter.
11. Top with whipped cream and serve with the remaining custard.

## Nutrition Values (Per Serving)
- Calories: 467
- Carbohydrate: 56.1g
- Protein: 8g
- Fat: 24.4g
- Sugar: 36.5g
- Sodium: 140mg

---

# Apple Pastry Pouch

(**Yields:** 2 servings / **Prep Time:** 15 minutes / **Cooking Time:** 25 minutes)

## Ingredients
- 1 tablespoon brown sugar
- 2 tablespoons raisins
- 2 small apples, peeled and cored
- 2 puff pastry sheets
- 2 tablespoons butter, melted

## Instructions
1. In a bowl, mix together the sugar and raisins.
2. Fill the core of each apple with raisins mixture.
3. Place one apple in the center of each pastry sheet and fold dough to cover the apple completely.
4. Then, pinch the edges to seal.
5. Coat each apple evenly with butter.
6. Set the temperature of air fryer to 355 degrees F. Lightly, grease an air fryer basket.
7. Arrange apple pouches into the prepared air fryer basket in a single layer.
8. Air fry for about 25 minutes.
9. Remove from air fryer and transfer the apple pouches onto a platter.
10. Serve warm.

## Nutrition Values (Per Serving)
- Calories: 418
- Carbohydrate: 55.2g
- Protein: 3.1g
- Fat: 22.8g
- Sugar: 33.2g
- Sodium: 157mg

# Raspberry Wontons

**(Yields:** 12 servings / **Prep Time:** 20 minutes / **Cooking Time:** 16 minutes)

## Ingredients

**For Wonton Wrappers:**

- ½ cup powdered sugar
- 18 ounces cream cheese, softened
- 1 teaspoon vanilla extract
- 1 package of wonton wrappers

**For Raspberry Syrup:**

- ¼ cup water
- ¼ cup sugar
- 1 (12-ounces) package frozen raspberries
- 1 teaspoon vanilla extract

## Instructions

1. For wrappers: in a bowl, add the sugar, cream cheese, and vanilla extract and whisk until smooth.
2. Place a wonton wrapper onto a smooth surface.
3. Place one tablespoon of cream cheese mixture in the center of each wrapper.
4. With wet fingers, fold wrappers around the filling and then, pinch the edges to seal.
5. Set the temperature of air fryer to 350 degrees F. Lightly, grease an air fryer basket.
6. Arrange wonton wrappers into the prepared air fryer basket in 2 batches.
7. Air fry for about 8 minutes.
8. Meanwhile, for the syrup: in a medium skillet, add water, sugar, raspberries, and vanilla extract over medium heat and cook for about 5 minutes, stirring continuously.
9. Remove from the heat and set aside to cool slightly.
10. Transfer the mixture into food processor and blend until smooth.
11. Remove the wontons from air fryer and transfer onto a platter.
12. Serve the wontons with topping of raspberry syrup.

## Nutrition Values (Per Serving)

- Calories: 325
- Carbohydrate: 39.6g
- Protein: 7.1g
- Fat: 15.5g
- Sugar: 15.4g
- Sodium: 343mg

# Fruity Tacos

**(Yields:** 2 servings / **Prep Time:** 10 minutes / **Cooking Time:** 5 minutes)

## Ingredients

- 2 soft shell tortillas
- 4 tablespoons strawberry jelly
- ¼ cup blueberries
- ¼ cup raspberries
- 2 tablespoons powdered sugar

## Instructions

1. Set the temperature of air fryer to 300 degrees F. Lightly, grease an air fryer basket.
2. Arrange the tortillas onto a smooth surface.
3. Spread two tablespoons of strawberry jelly over each tortilla and top each with berries.
4. Sprinkle each with the powdered sugar.
5. Arrange tortillas into the prepared air fryer basket.
6. Air fry for about 5 minutes or until crispy.
7. Remove from the air fryer and transfer the tortillas onto a platter.
8. Serve warm.

## Nutrition Values (Per Serving)

- Calories: 272
- Carbohydrate: 63.4g
- Protein: 3.5g
- Fat: 1.8g
- Sugar: 34.8g
- Sodium: 26mg

---

# Raisin Bread Pudding

**(Yields:** 3 servings / **Prep Time:** 15 minutes / **Cooking Time:** 12 minutes)

## Ingredients

- 1 cup milk
- 1 egg
- 1 tablespoon brown sugar
- ½ teaspoon ground cinnamon
- ¼ teaspoon vanilla extract
- 2 tablespoons raisins, soaked in hot water for about 15 minutes
- 2 bread slices, cut into small cubes
- 1 tablespoon chocolate chips
- 1 tablespoon sugar

## Instructions

1. In a bowl, mix well milk, egg, brown sugar, cinnamon, and vanilla extract.
2. Stir in the raisins.

3. In a baking dish, spread the bread cubes and top evenly with the milk mixture.
4. Refrigerate for about 15-20 minutes.
5. Set the temperature of air fryer to 375 degrees F.
6. Remove from refrigerator and sprinkle with chocolate chips and sugar on top.
7. Arrange the baking dish into an air fryer basket.
8. Air fry for about 12 minutes.
9. Remove from the air fryer and serve warm.

## Nutrition Values (Per Serving)

- Calories: 143
- Carbohydrate: 21.3g
- Protein: 5.5g
- Fat: 4.4g
- Sugar: 16.4g
- Sodium: 104mg

---

# Apple Bread Pudding

(**Yields:** 8 servings / **Prep Time:** 15 minutes / **Cooking Time:** 44 minutes)

## Ingredients

**For Bread Pudding:**

- 10½ ounces bread, cubed
- ½ cup apple, peeled, cored and chopped
- ½ cup raisins
- ¼ cup walnuts, chopped
- 1½ cups milk
- ¾ cup water
- 5 tablespoons honey
- 2 teaspoons ground cinnamon
- 2 teaspoons cornstarch
- 1 teaspoon vanilla extract

**For Topping:**

- 1 1/3 cups plain flour
- 3/5 cup brown sugar
- 7 tablespoons butter

## Instructions

1. In a large bowl, mix well bread, apple, raisins, and walnuts.
2. In another bowl, add the remaining pudding ingredients and mix until well combined.
3. Add the milk mixture into bread mixture and mix until well combined.
4. Refrigerate for about 15 minutes, tossing occasionally.
5. For topping: in a bowl, mix together the flour and sugar.
6. With a pastry cutter, cut in the butter until a crumbly mixture forms.
7. Set the temperature of air fryer to 355 degrees F.
8. Place the mixture evenly into 2 baking pans and spread the topping mixture on top of each.
9. Place 1 pan into an air fryer basket.
10. Air fry for about 22 minutes.
11. Repeat with the remaining pan.

12. Remove from the air fryer and serve warm.

## Nutrition Values (Per Serving)
- Calories: 432
- Carbohydrate: 69.1g
- Protein: 7.9g
- Fat: 14.8g
- Sugar: 32g
- Sodium: 353mg

---

# Doughnuts Pudding

**(Yields:** 4 servings / **Prep Time:** 15 minutes / **Cooking Time:** 60 minutes)

## Ingredients
- 6 glazed doughnuts, cut into small pieces
- ¾ cup frozen sweet cherries
- ½ cup raisins
- ½ cup semi-sweet chocolate baking chips
- ¼ cup sugar
- 1 teaspoon ground cinnamon
- 4 egg yolks
- 1½ cups whipping cream

## Instructions
1. In a large bowl, mix together doughnut pieces, cherries, raisins, chocolate chips, sugar, and cinnamon.
2. In another bowl, add the egg yolks, and whipping cream and whisk until well combined.
3. Add the egg yolk mixture into doughnut mixture and mix well.
4. Set the temperature of air fryer to 310 degrees F. Line a baking dish with a piece of foil.
5. Place doughnuts mixture evenly into the prepared baking dish.
6. Arrange the baking dish into an air fryer basket.
7. Air fry for about 60 minutes.
8. Remove from the air fryer and serve warm.

## Nutrition Values (Per Serving)
- Calories: 786
- Carbohydrate: 9.3g
- Protein: 11g
- Fat: 43.2g
- Sugar: 60.7g
- Sodium: 419mg

# Chocolate Pudding

**(Yields:** 4 servings / **Prep Time:** 20 minutes / **Cooking Time:** 14 minutes)

## Ingredients

- ½ cup butter
- 2/3 cup dark chocolate, chopped
- ¼ cup caster sugar
- 2 medium eggs
- 2 teaspoons fresh orange rind, finely grated
- ¼ cup fresh orange juice
- 2 tablespoons self-rising flour

## Instructions

1. In a microwave-safe bowl, add the butter, and chocolate. Microwave on high heat for about 2 minutes or until melted completely, stirring after every 30 seconds.
2. Remove from microwave and stir the mixture until smooth.
3. Add the sugar, and eggs and whisk until frothy.
4. Add the orange rind and juice, followed by flour and mix until well combined.
5. Set the temperature of air fryer to 355 degrees F. Grease 4 ramekins.
6. Divide mixture into the prepared ramekins about ¾ full.
7. Air fry for about 12 minutes.
8. Remove from the air fryer and set aside to completely cool before serving.
9. Serve warm.

## Nutrition Values (Per Serving)

- Calories: 454
- Carbohydrate: 34.2g
- Protein: 5.7g
- Fat: 33.6g
- Sugar: 28.4g
- Sodium: 217mg

# Vanilla Soufflé

**(Yields:** 6 servings / **Prep Time:** 15 minutes / **Cooking Time:** 39 minutes)

## Ingredients

- ¼ cup butter, softened
- ¼ cup all-purpose flour
- ½ cup plus 2 tablespoons sugar, divided
- 1 cup milk
- 3 teaspoons vanilla extract, divided
- 4 egg yolks
- 5 egg whites
- 1 teaspoon cream of tartar
- 2 tablespoons powdered sugar plus extra for dusting

## Instructions

1. In a bowl, add the butter, and flour and mix until a smooth paste forms.
2. In a medium pan, mix together ½ cup of sugar and milk over medium-low heat and cook for about 3 minutes or until the sugar is dissolved, stirring continuously.
3. Add the flour mixture, whisking continuously and simmer for about 3-4 minutes or until mixture becomes thick.
4. Remove from the heat and stir in 1 teaspoon of vanilla extract.
5. Set aside for about 10 minutes to cool.
6. In a bowl, mix together the egg yolks and 1 teaspoon of vanilla extract.
7. Add the egg yolk mixture into milk mixture and mix until well combined.
8. In another bowl, add the egg whites, cream of tartar, remaining sugar, and vanilla extract and whisk until stiff peaks form.
9. Fold the egg whites mixture into milk mixture.
10. Set the temperature of air fryer to 330 degrees F. Grease 6 ramekins and sprinkle each with a pinch of sugar.
11. Place mixture evenly into the prepared ramekins and with the back of a spoon, smooth the top surface.
12. Arrange the ramekins into an air fryer basket in 2 batches.
13. Air fry for about 14-16 minutes.
14. Remove from air fryer and set aside to cool slightly.
15. Sprinkle with the powdered sugar and serve warm.

## Nutrition Values (Per Serving)

- Calories: 250
- Carbohydrate: 29.8g
- Protein: 6.8g
- Fat: 11.6g
- Sugar: 25g
- Sodium: 107mg

# Chocolate Soufflé

**(Yields:** 2 servings / **Prep Time:** 15 minutes / **Cooking Time:** 16 minutes)

## Ingredients

- 3 ounces semi-sweet chocolate, chopped
- ¼ cup butter
- 2 eggs, egg yolks and whites separated
- 3 tablespoons sugar
- ½ teaspoon pure vanilla extract
- 2 tablespoons all-purpose flour
- 1 teaspoon powdered sugar plus extra for dusting

## Instructions

1. In a microwave-safe bowl, put the butter, and chocolate. Microwave on high heat for about 2 minutes or until melted completely, stirring after every 30 seconds.
2. Remove from microwave and stir the mixture until smooth.
3. In another bowl, add the egg yolks and whisk well.
4. Add the sugar, and vanilla extract and whisk well.
5. Add the chocolate mixture and mix until well combined.
6. Add the flour and mix well.
7. In a clean glass bowl, add the egg whites and whisk until soft peaks form.
8. Fold the whipped egg whites in 3 portions into the chocolate mixture.
9. Set the temperature of air fryer to 330 degrees F. Grease 2 ramekins and sprinkle each with a pinch of sugar.
10. Place mixture evenly into the prepared ramekins and with the back of a spoon, smooth the top surface.
11. Arrange the ramekins into an air fryer basket.
12. Air fry for about 14 minutes.
13. Remove from air fryer and set aside to cool slightly.
14. Sprinkle with the powdered sugar and serve warm.

## Nutrition Values (Per Serving)

- Calories: 569
- Carbohydrate: 54.1g
- Protein: 6.9g
- Fat: 38.8g
- Sugar: 42.2g
- Sodium: 225mg

# Stuffed Apples

**(Yields:** 4 servings / **Prep Time:** 15 minutes / **Cooking Time:** 13 minutes)

## Ingredients

### For Stuffed Apples:
- 4 small firm apples, cored
- ½ cup golden raisins
- ½ cup blanched almonds
- 2 tablespoons sugar

### For Vanilla Sauce:
- ½ cup whipped cream
- 2 tablespoons sugar
- ½ teaspoon vanilla extract

## Instructions

1. In a food processor, add raisins, almonds, and sugar and pulse until chopped.
2. Carefully, stuff each apple with raisin mixture.
3. Set the temperature of air fryer to 355 degrees F. Line a baking dish with a parchment paper.
4. Now, place apples into the prepared baking dish.
5. Arrange the baking dish into an air fryer basket.
6. Air fry for about 10 minutes.
7. Meanwhile, for vanilla sauce: in a pan, add the cream, sugar, and vanilla extract over medium heat and cook for about 2-3 minutes or until sugar is dissolved, stirring continuously.
8. Remove the baking dish from air fryer and transfer the apples onto plates to cool slightly
9. Top with the vanilla sauce and serve.

## Nutrition Values (Per Serving)

- Calories: 329
- Carbohydrate: 60.2g
- Protein: 4g
- Fat: 11.1g
- Sugar: 46.5g
- Sodium: 9mg

# Crispy Banana Split

**(Yields:** 8 servings / **Prep Time:** 15 minutes / **Cooking Time:** 14 minutes)

## Ingredients

- 3 tablespoons coconut oil
- 1 cup panko breadcrumbs
- ½ cup corn flour
- 2 eggs
- 4 bananas, peeled and halved lengthwise
- 3 tablespoons sugar
- ¼ teaspoon ground cinnamon
- 2 tablespoons walnuts, chopped

## Instructions

1. In a medium skillet, heat the oil over medium heat and cook breadcrumbs for about 3-4 minutes or until golden browned and crumbled, stirring continuously.
2. Transfer the breadcrumbs into a shallow bowl and set aside to cool.
3. In a second bowl, place the corn flour.
4. In a third bowl, whisk the eggs.
5. Coat the banana slices with flour and then, dip into eggs and finally, coat evenly with the breadcrumbs.
6. In a small bowl, mix together the sugar and cinnamon
7. Set the temperature of air fryer to 280 degrees F. Grease an air fryer basket.
8. Arrange banana slices into the prepared air fryer basket in a single layer and sprinkle with cinnamon sugar
9. Air fry for about 10 minutes.
10. Remove from air fryer and transfer the banana slices onto plates to cool slightly
11. Sprinkle with chopped walnuts and serve.

## Nutrition Values (Per Serving)

- Calories: 216
- Carbohydrate: 26g
- Protein: 3.4g
- Fat: 8.8g
- Sugar: 11.9g
- Sodium: 16mg

# Fried Banana Slices

**(Yields:** 8 servings / **Prep Time:** 15 minutes / **Cooking Time:** 15 minutes)

## Ingredients

- 4 medium ripe bananas, peeled
- 1/3 cup rice flour, divided
- 2 tablespoons all-purpose flour
- 2 tablespoons corn flour
- 2 tablespoons desiccated coconut
- ½ teaspoon baking powder
- ½ teaspoon ground cardamom
- A pinch of salt
- Water, as required
- ¼ cup sesame seeds

## Instructions

1. In a shallow bowl, mix well 2 tablespoons of rice flour, all-purpose flour, corn flour, coconut, baking powder, cardamom, and salt.
2. Gradually, add the water and mix until a thick and smooth mixture forms.
3. In a second bowl, place the remaining rice flour.
4. In a third bowl, add the sesame seeds.
5. Cut each banana into half and then, cut each half in 2 pieces lengthwise.
6. Dip the banana slices into coconut mixture and then, coat with the remaining rice flour, followed by the sesame seeds.
7. Set the temperature of air fryer to 392 degrees F. Line an air fryer basket with a greased and floured piece of foil.
8. Arrange banana slices into the prepared air fryer basket in a single layer.
9. Air fry for about 10-15 minutes, flipping once halfway through.
10. Remove from air fryer and transfer the banana slices onto plates to cool slightly
11. Serve warm.

## Nutrition Values (Per Serving)

- Calories: 260
- Carbohydrate: 51.2g
- Protein: 4.6g
- Fat: 6g
- Sugar: 17.6g
- Sodium: 49mg

# Air Fryer Cooking Charts

## Air Fryer Cooking Chart

NOTE: All times and temperatures assume that the food is flipped over half way through the cooking time OR the basket is shaken to redistribute the ingredients once or twice.

| | | Temp (°F) | Time (Min) | | Temp (°F) | Time (Min) |
|---|---|---|---|---|---|---|
| **FISH AND SEAFOODS** | Calamari (8 oz.) | 400°F | 4 | Fish Fillet (1-inch, 8 oz.) | 400°F | 10 |
| | Shrimp | 400°F | 5 | Swordfish steak | 400°F | 10 |
| | Scallops | 400°F | 5 to 7 | Salmon, fillet (6 oz.) | 380°F | 12 |
| | Tuna steak | 400°F | 7 to 10 | | | |
| **BEEF** | Meatballs (1-inch) | 380°F | 7 | Burger (4 oz.) | 370°F | 16 to 20 |
| | Meatballs (3-inch) | 380°F | 10 | Filet Mignon (8 oz.) | 400°F | 18 |
| | Sirloin steaks (1-inch, 12 oz.) | 400°F | 9 to 14 | London Broil (2 lbs.) | 400°F | 20 to 28 |
| | Ribeye, bone in (1-inch, 8 oz.) | 400°F | 10 to 15 | Beef Eye Round Roast (4 lbs.) | 390°F | 45 to 55 |
| | Flank Steak (1.5 lbs.) | 400°F | 12 | | | |
| **FROZEN FOODS** | Onion Rings (12 oz.) | 400°F | 8 | Fish Sticks (10 oz.) | 400°F | 10 |
| | Mozzarella Sticks (11 oz.) | 400°F | 8 | Thin French Fries (20 oz.) | 400°F | 14 |
| | Pot Sticker (10 oz.) | 400°F | 8 | Fish Fillets (½-inch, 10 oz.) | 400°F | 14 |
| | Breaded Shrimp | 400°F | 9 | Thick French Fries (17 oz.) | 400°F | 18 |
| | Chicken Nuggets (12 oz.) | 400°F | 10 | | | |
| **PORK AND LAMB** | Bacon (regular) | 400°F | 5 to 7 | Tenderloin (1 lb.) | 370°F | 15 |
| | Bacon (thick cut) | 400°F | 6 to 10 | Sausages | 380°F | 15 |
| | Lamb Loin Chops (1-inch thick) | 400°F | 8 to 12 | Rack of lamb (1.5 – 2 lbs.) | 380°F | 22 |
| | Pork Chops, bone in (1-inch, 6.5 oz.) | 400°F | 12 | Loin (2 lbs.) | 360°F | 55 |

|  | | Temp (°F) | Time (Min) | | Temp (°F) | Time (Min) |
|---|---|---|---|---|---|---|
| **VEGETABLES** | Tomatoes (cherry) | 400°F | 4 | Brussels Sprouts (halved) | 380°F | 15 |
| | Asparagus (Sliced 1-inch) | 400°F | 5 | Carrots (sliced ½-inch) | 380°F | 15 |
| | Mushrooms (sliced ¼) | 400°F | 5 | Eggplant (1½-inch cubes) | 400°F | 15 |
| | Green Beans | 400°F | 5 | Fennel (quartered) | 370°F | 15 |
| | Broccoli (florets) | 400°F | 6 | Kale leaves | 250°F | 12 |
| | Corn on the cob | 390°F | 6 | Parsnips (½-inch chunks) | 380°F | 15 |
| | Tomatoes (halves) | 350°F | 10 | Peppers (1-inch chunks) | 400°F | 15 |
| | Onions (pearl) | 400°F | 10 | Potatoes (small baby, 1.5lbs) | 400°F | 15 |
| | Squash (½-inch chunks) | 400°F | 12 | Sweet Potato (baked) | 380°F | 30 to 35 |
| | Potatoes (1-inch chunks) | 400°F | 12 | Potatoes (baked whole) | 400°F | 40 |
| | Cauliflower (florets) | 400°F | 12 | Beets (whole) | 400°F | 40 |
| | Zucchini (½-inch sticks) | 400°F | 12 | | | |

|  | | Temp (°F) | Time (Min) | | Temp (°F) | Time (Min) |
|---|---|---|---|---|---|---|
| **CHICKEN** | Tenders | 360°F | 8 to 10 | Game Hen (halved – 2 lbs.) | 390°F | 20 |
| | Breasts, boneless (4 oz.) | 380°F | 12 | Thighs, bone in (2 lbs.) | 380°F | 22 |
| | Wings (2 lbs.) | 400°F | 12 | Breasts, bone in (1.25 lbs.) | 370°F | 25 |
| | Drumsticks (2.5 lbs.) | 370°F | 20 | Legs, bone in (1.75 lbs.) | 380°F | 30 |
| | Thighs, boneless (1.5 lbs.) | 380°F | 18 to 20 | Whole Chicken (6.5 lbs.) | 360°F | 75 |

# Measurement Conversion Charts

The charts you are seeing below will help you to convert the difference between units of volume in US customary units.

Please note that US volume is not the same as in the UK and other countries, and many of the measurements are different depending on your country.

It's very easy to get confused when dealing with US and UK units. The good thing is that the metric units never change.

All the measurement charts below are for US customary units only.

We have gone to great length in order to make sure that the measurements are on the following Measurement Charts are accurate.

| American and British Variances | | | | | |
|---|---|---|---|---|---|
| Term | Abbreviation | Nationality | Dry or liquid | Metric equivalent | Equivalent in context |
| **cup** | c., C. | | usually liquid | 237 milliliters | 16 tablespoons or 8 ounces |
| **ounce** | fl oz, fl. oz. | American | liquid only | 29.57 milliliters | |
| | | British | either | 28.41 milliliters | |
| **gallon** | gal. | American | liquid only | 3.785 liters | 4 quarts |
| | | British | either | 4.546 liters | 4 quarts |
| **inch** | in, in. | | | 2.54 centimeters | |
| **ounce** | oz, oz. | American | dry | 28.35 grams | 1/16 pound |
| | | | liquid | see OUNCE | see OUNCE |
| **pint** | p., pt. | American | liquid | 0.473 liter | 1/8 gallon or 16 ounces |
| | | | dry | 0.551 liter | 1/2 quart |
| | | British | either | 0.568 liter | |
| **pound** | lb. | | dry | 453.592 grams | 16 ounces |
| **Quart** | q., qt, qt. | American | liquid | 0.946 liter | 1/4 gallon or 32 ounces |
| | | | dry | 1.101 liters | 2 pints |
| | | British | either | 1.136 liters | |
| **Teaspoon** | t., tsp., tsp | | either | about 5 milliliters | 1/3 tablespoon |
| **Tablespoon** | T., tbs., tbsp. | | either | about 15 milliliters | 3 teaspoons or 1/2 ounce |

## Volume (Liquid)

| American Standard (Cups & Quarts) | American Standard (Ounces) | Metric (Milliliters & Liters) |
|---|---|---|
| 2 tbsp. | 1 fl. oz. | 30 ml |
| 1/4 cup | 2 fl. oz. | 60 ml |
| 1/2 cup | 4 fl. oz. | 125 ml |
| 1 cup | 8 fl. oz. | 250 ml |
| 1 1/2 cups | 12 fl. oz. | 375 ml |
| 2 cups or 1 pint | 16 fl. oz. | 500 ml |
| 4 cups or 1 quart | 32 fl. oz. | 1000 ml or 1 liter |
| 1 gallon | 128 fl. oz. | 4 liters |

## Volume (Dry)

| American Standard | Metric |
|---|---|
| 1/8 teaspoon | 5 ml |
| 1/4 teaspoon | 1 ml |
| 1/2 teaspoon | 2 ml |
| 3/4 teaspoon | 4 ml |
| 1 teaspoon | 5 ml |
| 1 tablespoon | 15 ml |
| 1/4 cup | 59 ml |
| 1/3 cup | 79 ml |
| 1/2 cup | 118 ml |
| 2/3 cup | 158 ml |
| 3/4 cup | 177 ml |
| 1 cup | 225 ml |
| 2 cups or 1 pint | 450 ml |
| 3 cups | 675 ml |
| 4 cups or 1 quart | 1 liter |
| 1/2 gallon | 2 liters |
| 1 gallon | 4 liters |

## Oven Temperatures

| American Standard | Metric |
|---|---|
| 250° F | 130° C |
| 300° F | 150° C |
| 350° F | 180° C |
| 400° F | 200° C |
| 450° F | 230° C |

## Weight (Mass)

| American Standard (Ounces) | Metric (Grams) |
|---|---|
| 1/2 ounce | 15 grams |
| 1 ounce | 30 grams |
| 3 ounces | 85 grams |
| 3.75 ounces | 100 grams |
| 4 ounces | 115 grams |
| 8 ounces | 225 grams |
| 12 ounces | 340 grams |
| 16 ounces or 1 pound | 450 grams |

## Dry Measure Equivalents

| | | | |
|---|---|---|---|
| 3 teaspoons | 1 tablespoon | 1/2 ounce | 14.3 grams |
| 2 tablespoons | 1/8 cup | 1 ounce | 28.3 grams |
| 4 tablespoons | 1/4 cup | 2 ounces | 56.7 grams |
| 5 1/3 tablespoons | 1/3 cup | 2.6 ounces | 75.6 grams |
| 8 tablespoons | 1/2 cup | 4 ounces | 113.4 grams |
| 12 tablespoons | 3/4 cup | 6 ounces | .375 pound |
| 32 tablespoons | 2 cups | 16 ounces | 1 pound |

# About the Author

As one of seven children, Rachel Collins grew up in Cleveland, Ohio before moving to the mountains of Colorado in her early teens. From a young age she dreamed of moving to LA and becoming a fashion stylist. But when Rachel was fifteen, her only sister was born. Ever determined to rein in the chaos of her big family...and have dinner on the table before midnight...Rachel began doing the cooking. She eventually discovered a new found freedom and a creativity she hadn't known existed. She began chronicling her fresh takes on old favorites and coupling them with her styling skills - only this time on tables and cutting boards - on her blog.

Since then, lots of people have fallen in love with her unique recipes, stunning photography, and charming life in her barn, which she has made into her home, high up in the snow-capped mountains.

Finally, before you go, I'd like to say "thank you" for purchasing my book and I hope that you had as much fun reading it as I had writing it.

I know you could have picked from dozens of books on air fryer recipes, but you took a chance with my guide. So, big thanks for purchasing this book and reading all the way to the end.

Now, I'd like to ask for a *small* favor. Could you please take a minute or two and leave a review for this book on Amazon by returning to your order history, the top right-hand side of your screen.

This feedback will help me continue to write the kind of books that will help you get results and help me to compete with other big publishers and authors.

**I bid you farewell and encourage you to move forward and find your true air fryer cooking spirit!**

Thank you and good luck!

—Rachel Collins

# RECIPE INDEX

## A

Apple
  Apple Bread Pudding, 308
  Apple Cake, 281
  Apple Chips, 60
  Apple Crumble, 292
  Apple Doughnuts, 302
  Apple Muffins, 35
  Apple Pastry Pouch, 305
  Apple Pie, 294
  Apple Tart, 297
  Chicken with Apple, 119
  Mini Apple Pies, 293
  Stuffed Apples, 313
  Zucchini & Apple Bread, 26

Asparagus
  Almond Asparagus, 258
  Parmesan Asparagus, 236
  Salmon with Asparagus, 181

Avocado Fries, 65

## B

Bacon
  Bacon & Egg Cups, 47
  Bacon & Hot Dogs Omelet, 45
  Bacon Croquettes, 74
  Bacon Wrapped Filet Mignon, 142
  Bacon Wrapped Pork tenderloin, 161
  Bacon Wrapped Scallops, 211
  Bacon Wrapped Shrimp, 87, 203
  Bread & Bacon Cups, 49
  Pork Tenderloin with Bacon & Veggies, 162

Banana
  Banana Bread, 21
  Banana Cake, 282
  Banana Chips, 60
  Banana Muffins, 34
  Chocolate Banana Bread, 24
  Chocolate Banana Pastries, 303
  Crispy Banana Split, 314
  Fried Banana Slices, 315
  Nutty Banana Bread, 21
  Peanut Butter Banana Bread, 23
  Yogurt Banana Bread, 22

Basil
  Basil Tomatoes, 250

BBQ
  BBQ Chicken Wings, 113
  BBQ Pork Ribs, 158

Beef
  Beef & Mushroom Meatloaf, 152
  Beef & Veggie Kebabs, 148
  Beef Cheeseburgers, 151
  Beef Jerky, 147
  Beef Roast, 144
  Beef Short Ribs, 143
  Beef Stuffed Bell Peppers, 149
  Beef Taco Wraps, 153
  Beef Tips with Onion, 145
  Cheesy Beef Meatballs, 151
  Herbed Beef Roast, 144
  Smoky Beef Burgers, 150

Beer Coated Duck Breast, 133

Beet
  Beet Chips, 62

Bell Pepper
  Oatmeal Stuffed Bell Peppers, 261
  Pork Tenderloin with Bell Peppers, 161
  Potato & Bell Pepper Hash, 54
  Rice & Beans Stuffed Bell Peppers, 238
  Steak with Bell Peppers, 141
  Veggie Stuffed Bell Peppers, 237

Biscuit
  Lemon Biscuits, 89

Blueberry
  Blueberry Muffins, 36

Bok
  Sesame Seeds Bok Choy, 250

Bread
  Apple Bread Pudding, 308
  Banana Bread, 21
  Bread & Bacon Cups, 49

Breadcrumbs Stuffed Mushrooms, 255
Breaded Chicken Tenderloins, 103
Breaded Flounder, 191
Breaded Hake, 195
Breaded Pork Chops, 154
Breaded Shrimp with Lemon, 202
Chocolate Banana Bread, 24
Chocolate Peanut Butter Bread, 29
Cream Bread, 18
Creamy Breaded Shrimp, 201
Date Bread, 20
Nutty Banana Bread, 21
Nutty Zucchini Bread, 25
Peanut Butter Banana Bread, 23
Pumpkin & Yogurt Bread, 27
Raisin Bread Pudding, 307
Sourdough Bread, 17
Spiced Pumpkin Bread, 28
Sunflower Seeds Bread, 19
Veggie Bread Rolls, 79
Yogurt Banana Bread, 22
Zucchini & Apple Bread, 26

Breast
Bacon Wrapped Chicken Breasts, 109
Beer Coated Duck Breast, 133
Buttered Duck Breasts, 132
Buttermilk Brined Turkey Breast, 128
Cheese Stuffed Chicken Breasts, 108
Cheesy Chicken Breasts, 106
Duck Breast with Figs, 134
Glazed Turkey Breast, 127
Herbed Turkey Breast, 126
Oats Crusted Chicken Breasts, 104
Sausage Stuffed Chicken Breasts, 106
Simple Turkey Breast, 125
Spiced Chicken Breasts, 105
Spinach Stuffed Chicken Breasts, 107

Broccoli
Broccoli with Cauliflower, 262
Broccoli with Olives, 228
Buttered Broccoli, 226
Cheesy Broccoli Bites, 69
Chicken & Broccoli Quiche, 53
Chicken with Broccoli & Rice, 123
Garlic Broccoli, 227
Parmesan Broccoli, 227
Salmon with Broccoli, 181
Spicy Broccoli Poppers, 68

Brownies
Brownies Muffins, 273
Fudge Brownies, 298
Walnut Brownies, 299

Brussel Sprout
Brussel Sprout Salad, 215
Cheesy Brussel Sprouts, 223
Leg of Lamb with Brussels Sprout, 175
Sweet & Sour Brussel Sprouts, 224

Buffalo
Buffalo Chicken Tenders, 110
Buffalo Chicken Wings, 114

Burgers
Beans & Veggie Burgers, 272
Crispy Chicken Burgers, 124
Prawn Burgers, 207

Butter
Butter Cake, 280
Buttered Corn, 63
Buttered Crab Shells, 212
Buttered Dinner Rolls, 243
Buttered Filet Mignon, 142
Buttered Rib Eye Steak, 146
Buttered Scallops, 207
Buttered Striploin Steak, 137
Buttermilk Biscuits, 88
Chocolate Peanut Butter Bread, 29
Peanut Butter Banana Bread, 23
Spiced Butternut Squash, 253

## C

Cajun
Cajun Coated Catfish, 192
Cajun Spiced Salmon, 177

Cake
Apple Cake, 281
Banana Cake, 282
Butter Cake, 280
Chocolate Cake, 283
Chocolate Cream Cake, 284
Chocolate Mug Cake, 285
Creamy Tuna Cakes, 198
Lava Cake, 285
Layered Cake, 286
Lemon Cheesecake, 290
Raspberry Cupcakes, 277
Red Velvet Cupcakes, 278

Semolina Cake, 279
Simple Cheesecake, 288
Strawberry Cheesecake, 289
Strawberry Cupcakes, 276
Tuna & Potato Cakes, 197
White Chocolate Cheesecake, 291

Calamari
Glazed Calamari, 211

Capers
Scallops with Capers Sauce, 208
Tofu with Capers Sauce, 241

Carrot
Caramelized Carrots, 222
Carrot Sticks, 67
Herbed Carrots, 246
Honey Glazed Carrots, 222
Savory Carrot Muffins, 38

Cashew
Roasted Cashews, 56

Catfish
3-Ingredients Catfish, 192
Southern Style Catfish, 193

Cauliflower
Broccoli with Cauliflower, 262
Cauliflower Poppers, 70
Cauliflower Salad, 218
Crispy Cauliflower Poppers, 70
Sweet & Spicy Cauliflower, 252
Tofu with Cauliflower, 268

Cheese
Beef Cheeseburgers, 151
Cheese Cookies, 91
Cheese Omelet, 43
Cheese Pastries, 84
Cheese Sandwich, 82
Cheese Stuffed Mushrooms, 233
Cheese Stuffed Tomatoes, 230
Cheesy Beef Meatballs, 151
Cheesy Broccoli Bites, 69
Cheesy Brussel Sprouts, 223
Cheesy Dinner Rolls, 244
Cheesy Mushroom Pizza, 234
Cheesy Mustard Toasts, 42
Cheesy Shrimp, 200
Cheesy Spinach, 235

Chicken
Bacon Wrapped Chicken Breasts, 109
BBQ Chicken Wings, 113
Breaded Chicken Tenderloins, 103
Buffalo Chicken Tenders, 110
Buffalo Chicken Wings, 114
Cheese Stuffed Chicken Breasts, 108
Cheesy Chicken Breasts, 106
Cheesy Chicken Cutlets, 103
Chicken & Broccoli Quiche, 53
Chicken & Scallion Kabobs, 115
Chicken & Veggie Kabobs, 116
Chicken Chilaquiles, 122
Chicken Nuggets, 75
Chicken Omelet, 44
Chicken with Apple, 119
Chicken with Broccoli & Rice, 123
Chicken with Carrots, 120
Chicken with Veggies, 121
Chicken with Veggies & Rice, 123
Chinese Chicken Drumsticks, 99
Crispy Chicken Burgers, 124
Crispy Chicken Drumsticks, 100
Crispy Chicken Tenders, 111
Crispy Chicken Thighs, 102
Crispy Chicken Wings, 112
Curried Chicken, 118
Gingered Chicken Drumsticks, 97
Herbed Roasted Chicken, 93
Honey Glazed Chicken Drumsticks, 98
Jerk Chicken, Pineapple & Veggie Kabobs, 117
Oats Crusted Chicken Breasts, 104
Roasted Chicken with Potatoes, 93
Sausage Stuffed Chicken Breasts, 106
Simple Chicken Wings, 112
Spiced Chicken Breasts, 105
Spiced Roasted Chicken, 94
Spicy Chicken Legs, 95
Spinach Stuffed Chicken Breasts, 107
Sweet & Sour Chicken Thighs, 101
Sweet & Spicy Chicken Drumsticks, 98
Sweet Chicken Kabobs, 115
Tandoori Chicken Legs, 96

Chickpea
Spicy Chickpeas, 58

Chips
Apple Chips, 60
Banana Chips, 60
Beet Chips, 62

Kale Chips, 61
Nacho Chips Crusted Prawns, 206
Potato Chips, 61
Tortilla Chips, 58

Chocolate
Chocolate Banana Bread, 24
Chocolate Banana Pastries, 303
Chocolate Cake, 283
Chocolate Cookie Dough Balls, 88
Chocolate Cream Cake, 284
Chocolate Mug Cake, 285
Chocolate Peanut Butter Bread, 29
Chocolate Pudding, 310
Chocolate Soufflé, 312
Chocolate Yogurt Muffins, 273
Double Chocolate Muffins, 274

Chops
Breaded Pork Chops, 154
Herbed Lamb Chops, 168
Herbed Pork Chops, 155
Lamb Chops with Veggies, 170
Lamb Loin Chops with Garlic, 169
Lamb Loin Chops with Lemon, 168
Pork Chops with Peanut Sauce, 156
Simple Lamb Chops, 167
Sweet & Sour Pork Chops, 154

Cinnamon Toasts, 41

Clafoutis, 287

Coconut
Coconut Cookies, 90
Coconut Crusted Shrimp, 202

Cod
Chinese Style Cod, 185
Cod & Veggie Parcel, 186
Cod Cakes, 188
Cod Nuggets, 76
Crispy Cod Sticks, 187

Corn
Buttered Corn, 63
Cornish Game Hens, 92
Pineapple Cornbread, 31
Simple Cornbread, 30
Sweet Jalapeño Cornbread, 32
Sweet Rosemary Cornbread, 31

Crab
Buttered Crab Shells, 212
Crab Cakes, 213
Wasabi Crab Cakes, 214

Cream
Cream Bread, 18
Cream Doughnuts, 300
Creamy Breaded Shrimp, 201

Croissant Rolls, 244

Croquettes
Bacon Croquettes, 74
Potato Croquettes, 73
Salmon Croquettes, 74

Crumble
Apple Crumble, 292
Fruity Crumble, 292

Curried Eggplant, 246

# D

Date Bread, 20

Dill Pickle Fries, 66

Dough
Apple Doughnuts, 302
Chocolate Cookie Dough Balls, 88
Cream Doughnuts, 300
Doughnuts Pudding, 309
Milky Doughnuts, 301

Drumstick
Chinese Chicken Drumsticks, 99
Crispy Chicken Drumsticks, 100
Gingered Chicken Drumsticks, 97
Honey Glazed Chicken Drumsticks, 98
Sweet & Spicy Chicken Drumsticks, 98

Duck
Beer Coated Duck Breast, 133
Buttered Duck Breasts, 132
Duck Breast with Figs, 134
Herbed Duck Legs, 135

# E

Egg
Bacon & Egg Cups, 47
Egg & Mushroom Scramble, 47
Egg Yolks with Squid, 55
Eggs & Tomatoes Scramble, 46
Spinach & Egg Cups, 48

Eggplant
- Crispy Eggplant Slices, 71
- Curried Eggplant, 246
- Eggplant Salad, 216
- Herbed Eggplant, 247
- Salsa Stuffed Eggplants, 249
- Spiced Eggplant, 224
- Spices Stuffed Eggplants, 248
- Veggies Stuffed Eggplants, 225

**F**

Figs
- Duck Breast with Figs, 134

Filet
- Bacon Wrapped Filet Mignon, 142
- Buttered Filet Mignon, 142

Finger
- Shortbread Fingers, 299

Flounder
- Breaded Flounder, 191

Flour
- Rice Flour Coated Shrimp, 205
- Rice Flour Crusted Tofu, 265

French
- French Toasts, 40
- Savory French Toasts, 41

Fries
- Avocado Fries, 65
- Dill Pickle Fries, 66
- French Fries, 63
- Fried Banana Slices, 315
- Fried Flatbreads, 33
- Squash Fries, 65
- Zucchini Fries, 64

Frittata
- Mushroom & Tomato Frittata, 50
- Sausage Frittata, 50
- Trout Frittata, 51

Fritters
- Zucchini Fritters, 39

Fruit
- Fruit Pastries, 86
- Fruity Crumble, 292
- Fruity Oreo Muffins, 275
- Fruity Tacos, 307

Fudge Brownies, 298

**G**

Garlic
- Garlic Broccoli, 227
- Garlic Lamb Roast, 176
- Lamb Loin Chops with Garlic, 169
- Lemon Garlic Shrimp, 200

Gingered Chicken Drumsticks, 97

Green Beans
- Green Beans & Mushroom Casserole, 259
- Lemony Green Beans, 237
- Okra with Green Beans, 260
- Salmon with Green Beans, 182
- Sautéed Green Beans, 258

**H**

Haddock
- Pesto Haddock, 190
- Sesame Seeds Coated Haddock, 194

Hake
- Breaded Hake, 195

Halibut
- Crispy Halibut Strips, 189
- Glazed Halibut, 188

Ham
- Glazed Ham, 166

Hash
- Potato & Bell Pepper Hash, 54

Hasselback Potatoes, 232

Hen
- Cornish Game Hens, 92

Herb
- Herbed Beef Roast, 144
- Herbed Carrots, 246
- Herbed Duck Legs, 135
- Herbed Eggplant, 247
- Herbed Lamb Chops, 168
- Herbed Leg of Lamb, 174
- Herbed Pork Chops, 155
- Herbed Potatoes, 253
- Herbed Roasted Chicken, 93
- Herbed Turkey Breast, 126
- Herbed Veggies Combo, 263

Herbs Crumbed Rack of Lamb, 171
Spiced & Herbed Skirt Steak, 139

Honey
Honey Glazed Carrots, 222
Honey Glazed Chicken Drumsticks, 98

Hot Dogs
Bacon & Hot Dogs Omelet, 45

Hummus Mushroom Pizza, 256

## J

Jacket Potatoes, 230

Jalapeño
Sweet Jalapeño Cornbread, 32

Jerk
Beef Jerky, 147
Jerk Chicken, Pineapple & Veggie Kabobs, 117

## K

Kabob
Chicken & Scallion Kabobs, 115
Chicken & Veggie Kabobs, 116
Jerk Chicken, Pineapple & Veggie Kabobs, 117
Sweet Chicken Kabobs, 115

Kale Chips, 61

Kebab
Beef & Veggie Kebabs, 148
Shrimp Kebabs, 205

## L

Lamb
Garlic Lamb Roast, 176
Herbed Lamb Chops, 168
Herbed Leg of Lamb, 174
Herbs Crumbed Rack of Lamb, 171
Lamb Chops with Veggies, 170
Lamb Loin Chops with Garlic, 169
Lamb Loin Chops with Lemon, 168
Leg of Lamb with Brussels Sprout, 175
Nut Crusted Rack of Lamb, 171
Pesto Coated Rack of Lamb, 172
Simple Lamb Chops, 167
Spiced Lamb Steaks, 173

Lava Cake, 285

Layered Cake, 286

Legs
Herbed Duck Legs, 135
Spicy Chicken Legs, 95
Tandoori Chicken Legs, 96
Turkey Legs, 127

Lemon
Lemon Biscuits, 89
Lemon Cheesecake, 290
Lemon Garlic Shrimp, 200
Lemony Green Beans, 237

Loin
Pork Loin with Potatoes, 163

## M

Maple Glazed Salmon, 179

Meatball
Cheesy Beef Meatballs, 151

Meatloaf
Turkey Meatloaf, 131

Mignon
Bacon Wrapped Filet Mignon, 142
Buttered Filet Mignon, 142

Milky Doughnuts, 301

Mozzarella Sticks, 77

Muffin
Apple Muffins, 35
Banana Muffins, 34
Blueberry Muffins, 36
Brownies Muffins, 273
Chocolate Yogurt Muffins, 273
Double Chocolate Muffins, 274
Fruity Oreo Muffins, 275
Raisin & Oat Muffins, 37
Savory Carrot Muffins, 38

Mug
Chocolate Mug Cake, 285

Mushroom
Beef & Mushroom Meatloaf, 152
Breadcrumbs Stuffed Mushrooms, 255
Cheese Stuffed Mushrooms, 233
Cheesy Mushroom Pizza, 234

Egg & Mushroom Scramble, 47
Green Beans & Mushroom Casserole, 259
Hummus Mushroom Pizza, 256
Mushroom & Tomato Frittata, 50
Mushrooms with Peas, 255
Tofu & Mushroom Omelet, 45
Wine Infused Mushrooms, 233

Mustard
Cheesy Mustard Toasts, 42

# N

Nacho Chips Crusted Prawns, 206

Neck Salad
Pork Neck Salad, 165

New York Strip Steak
Simple New York Strip Steak, 137

Nugget
Chicken Nuggets, 75
Cod Nuggets, 76

Nut
Nut Crusted Rack of Lamb, 171
Nutty Banana Bread, 21
Nutty Zucchini Bread, 25
Roasted Mixed Nuts, 57

# O

Oat
Oatmeal Stuffed Bell Peppers, 261
Oats Crusted Chicken Breasts, 104
Raisin & Oat Muffins, 37

Okra
Okra with Green Beans, 260
Stuffed Okra, 261

Olive
Broccoli with Olives, 228

Omelet
Bacon & Hot Dogs Omelet, 45
Cheese Omelet, 43
Chicken Omelet, 44
Tofu & Mushroom Omelet, 45
Zucchini Omelet, 43

Onion
Beef Tips with Onion, 145
Onion Rings, 68

Orange
Tofu with Orange Sauce, 242

Oreo
Fruity Oreo Muffins, 275

# P

Parmesan
Parmesan Asparagus, 236
Parmesan Broccoli, 227

Parsnip
Sweet & Spicy Parsnips, 245

Pasta
Salmon with Shrimp & Pasta, 183

Pastry
Apple Pastry Pouch, 305
Cheese Pastries, 84
Chocolate Banana Pastries, 303
Fruit Pastries, 86
Pear Pastry Pouch, 304
Veggie Pastries, 85

Patties
Salmon Patties, 184

Pea
Mushrooms with Peas, 255

Peanut
Chocolate Peanut Butter Bread, 29
Peanut Butter Banana Bread, 23
Roasted Peanuts, 56
Tofu with Peanut Butter Sauce, 267

Pesto
Pesto Coated Rack of Lamb, 172
Pesto Haddock, 190
Pesto Tomatoes, 229

Pie
Apple Pie, 294
Mini Apple Pies, 293
Pecan Pie, 296
Sweet Potato Pie, 295

Pineapple
Jerk Chicken, Pineapple & Veggie Kabobs, 117
Pineapple Bites, 59
Pineapple Cornbread, 31

Pizza
- Cheesy Mushroom Pizza, 234
- Hummus Mushroom Pizza, 256

Polenta Sticks, 78

Popper
- Cauliflower Poppers, 70
- Crispy Cauliflower Poppers, 70
- Spicy Broccoli Poppers, 68

Pork
- Bacon Wrapped Pork tenderloin, 161
- BBQ Pork Ribs, 158
- Breaded Pork Chops, 154
- Glazed Pork Shoulder, 158
- Herbed Pork Chops, 155
- Pork Chops with Peanut Sauce, 156
- Pork Loin with Potatoes, 163
- Pork Neck Salad, 165
- Pork Rolls, 164
- Pork Sausage Casserole, 164
- Pork Shoulder with Pineapple Sauce, 159
- Pork Spare Ribs, 157
- Pork Tenderloin with Bacon & Veggies, 162
- Pork Tenderloin with Bell Peppers, 161
- Sweet & Sour Pork Chops, 154

Potato
- Hasselback Potatoes, 232
- Herbed Potatoes, 253
- Jacket Potatoes, 230
- Potato & Bell Pepper Hash, 54
- Potato Chips, 61
- Potato Croquettes, 73
- Potato Rosti, 39
- Potato Salad, 217
- Roasted Chicken with Potatoes, 93
- Spicy Potatoes, 254
- Stuffed Potatoes, 231
- Sweet Potato Pie, 295
- Tuna & Potato Cakes, 197

Prawn
- Crispy Prawns, 86
- Nacho Chips Crusted Prawns, 206
- Prawn Burgers, 207

Pudding
- Apple Bread Pudding, 308
- Chocolate Pudding, 310
- Doughnuts Pudding, 309
- Raisin Bread Pudding, 307

Pumpkin
- Pumpkin & Yogurt Bread, 27
- Spiced Pumpkin Bread, 28
- Stuffed Pumpkin, 239

# Q

Quiche
- Chicken & Broccoli Quiche, 53
- Mini Tomato Quiche, 52

# R

Rack
- Herbs Crumbed Rack of Lamb, 171
- Nut Crusted Rack of Lamb, 171
- Pesto Coated Rack of Lamb, 172

Radish Salad, 219

Raisin Bread Pudding, 307

Ranch Tilapia, 196

Raspberry
- Raspberry Cupcakes, 277
- Raspberry Wontons, 306

Ratatouille, 264

Red Velvet Cupcakes, 278

Rib
- BBQ Pork Ribs, 158
- Beef Short Ribs, 143
- Buttered Rib Eye Steak, 146
- Easy Rib Eye Steak, 136
- Pork Spare Ribs, 157

Rice
- Chicken with Broccoli & Rice, 123
- Chicken with Veggies & Rice, 123
- Rice & Beans Stuffed Bell Peppers, 238
- Rice Bites, 78
- Rice Flour Coated Shrimp, 205
- Rice Flour Crusted Tofu, 265
- Veggie Rice, 271

Rings
- Onion Rings, 68

Roast
- Beef Roast, 144
- Garlic Lamb Roast, 176
- Herbed Beef Roast, 144

Herbed Roasted Chicken, 93
Roasted Cashews, 56
Roasted Chicken with Potatoes, 93
Roasted Mixed Nuts, 57
Roasted Peanuts, 56
Spiced Roasted Chicken, 94

Rolls
Buttered Dinner Rolls, 243
Cheesy Dinner Rolls, 244
Croissant Rolls, 244
Pork Rolls, 164
Spinach Rolls, 80
Spring Rolls, 81
Turkey Rolls, 130
Veggie Bread Rolls, 79

Rosemary Cornbread
Sweet Rosemary Cornbread, 31

Rosti
Potato Rosti, 39

# S

Salad
Brussel Sprout Salad, 215
Cauliflower Salad, 218
Eggplant Salad, 216
Mixed Veggie Salad, 221
Pork Neck Salad, 165
Potato Salad, 217
Radish Salad, 219
Zucchini Salad, 220

Salmon
Cajun Spiced Salmon, 177
Maple Glazed Salmon, 179
Salmon Croquettes, 74
Salmon Patties, 184
Salmon with Asparagus, 181
Salmon with Broccoli, 181
Salmon with Green Beans, 182
Salmon with Shrimp & Pasta, 183
Simple Salmon, 177
Spicy Salmon, 178
Sweet & Sour Glazed Salmon, 180
Zesty Salmon, 179

Salsa Stuffed Eggplants, 249

Sandwich
Cheese Sandwich, 82
Veggie Sandwich, 83

Sauce
Pork Chops with Peanut Sauce, 156
Pork Shoulder with Pineapple Sauce, 159
Tofu in Sweet & Spicy Sauce, 266
Tofu with Capers Sauce, 241
Tofu with Orange Sauce, 242
Tofu with Peanut Butter Sauce, 267

Sausage
Pork Sausage Casserole, 164
Sausage Frittata, 50
Sausage Stuffed Chicken Breasts, 106

Scallion
Chicken & Scallion Kabobs, 115

Scallop
Bacon Wrapped Scallops, 211
Buttered Scallops, 207
Crispy Scallops, 209
Scallops with Capers Sauce, 208
Scallops with Spinach, 210

Scramble
Egg & Mushroom Scramble, 47
Eggs & Tomatoes Scramble, 46

Semolina Cake, 279

Sesame
Sesame Seeds Bok Choy, 250
Sesame Seeds Coated Haddock, 194
Sesame Seeds Coated Tuna, 197

Shell
Buttered Crab Shells, 212

Shortbread Fingers, 299

Shoulder
Glazed Pork Shoulder, 158

Shrimp
Bacon Wrapped Shrimp, 87, 203
Breaded Shrimp with Lemon, 202
Cheesy Shrimp, 200
Coconut Crusted Shrimp, 202
Creamy Breaded Shrimp, 201
Lemon Garlic Shrimp, 200
Rice Flour Coated Shrimp, 205
Shrimp Kebabs, 205
Shrimp Scampi, 204
Spicy Shrimp, 199

Smoky Beef Burgers, 150

Soufflé
- Chocolate Soufflé, 312
- Vanilla Soufflé, 311

Sourdough Bread, 17

Southern Style Catfish, 193

Spice
- Spiced Butternut Squash, 253
- Spiced Chicken Breasts, 105
- Spiced Eggplant, 224
- Spiced Lamb Steaks, 173
- Spiced Pumpkin Bread, 28
- Spiced Roasted Chicken, 94
- Spiced Soy Curls, 270
- Spices Stuffed Eggplants, 248
- Spicy Broccoli Poppers, 68
- Spicy Chicken Legs, 95
- Spicy Chickpeas, 58
- Spicy Potatoes, 254
- Spicy Shrimp, 199
- Spicy Tofu, 264

Spinach
- Cheesy Spinach, 235
- Sautéed Spinach, 257
- Spinach & Egg Cups, 48
- Spinach Rolls, 80
- Spinach Stuffed Chicken Breasts, 107

Spring Rolls, 81

Squash Fries, 65

Squid
- Egg Yolks with Squid, 55

Steak
- Buttered Rib Eye Steak, 146
- Buttered Striploin Steak, 137
- Crispy Sirloin Steak, 138
- Easy Rib Eye Steak, 136
- Simple New York Strip Steak, 137
- Skirt Steak with Veggies, 140
- Spiced & Herbed Skirt Steak, 139
- Steak with Bell Peppers, 141

Stick
- Mozzarella Sticks, 77
- Polenta Sticks, 78

Strawberry
- Strawberry Cheesecake, 289
- Strawberry Cupcakes, 276

Strip
- Crispy Halibut Strips, 189

Sunflower Seeds Bread, 19

Sweet
- Sweet & Sour Brussel Sprouts, 224
- Sweet & Sour Chicken Thighs, 101
- Sweet & Sour Pork Chops, 154
- Sweet & Spicy Cauliflower, 252
- Sweet & Spicy Chicken Drumsticks, 98
- Sweet & Spicy Parsnips, 245
- Sweet Chicken Kabobs, 115
- Sweet Jalapeño Cornbread, 32
- Sweet Potato Pie, 295
- Sweet Rosemary Cornbread, 31

# T

Taco
- Beef Taco Wraps, 153
- Fruity Tacos, 307

Tandoori Chicken Legs, 96

Tart
- Apple Tart, 297

Tender
- Buffalo Chicken Tenders, 110
- Crispy Chicken Tenders, 111

Tenderloin
- Breaded Chicken Tenderloins, 103
- Pork Tenderloin with Bacon & Veggies, 162
- Pork Tenderloin with Bell Peppers, 161

Thigh
- Crispy Chicken Thighs, 102
- Sweet & Sour Chicken Thighs, 101

Tilapia
- Ranch Tilapia, 196

Toast
- Cheesy Mustard Toasts, 42
- Cinnamon Toasts, 41
- French Toasts, 40
- Savory French Toasts, 41

Tofu
- Crispy Marinated Tofu, 266
- Rice Flour Crusted Tofu, 265
- Spicy Tofu, 264
- Tofu & Mushroom Omelet, 45

Tofu in Sweet & Spicy Sauce, 266
Tofu with Capers Sauce, 241
Tofu with Cauliflower, 268
Tofu with Orange Sauce, 242
Tofu with Peanut Butter Sauce, 267
Tofu with Veggies, 269

Tomato
Basil Tomatoes, 250
Cheese Stuffed Tomatoes, 230
Eggs & Tomatoes Scramble, 46
Mini Tomato Quiche, 52
Mushroom & Tomato Frittata, 50
Pesto Tomatoes, 229
Stuffed Tomatoes, 251

Tortilla Chips, 58

Trout Frittata, 51

Tuna
Creamy Tuna Cakes, 198
Sesame Seeds Coated Tuna, 197
Tuna & Potato Cakes, 197

Turkey
Buttermilk Brined Turkey Breast, 128
Glazed Turkey Breast, 127
Herbed Turkey Breast, 126
Simple Turkey Breast, 125
Turkey Legs, 127
Turkey Meatloaf, 131
Turkey Rolls, 130
Turkey Wings, 129

# V

Vanilla Soufflé, 311

Veggie
Beans & Veggie Burgers, 272
Beef & Veggie Kebabs, 148
Chicken & Veggie Kabobs, 116
Chicken with Veggies, 121
Chicken with Veggies & Rice, 123
Cod & Veggie Parcel, 186
Glazed Veggies, 240
Herbed Veggies Combo, 263
Jerk Chicken, Pineapple & Veggie Kabobs, 117
Lamb Chops with Veggies, 170
Mixed Veggie Bites, 72
Mixed Veggie Salad, 221
Pork Tenderloin with Bacon & Veggies, 162
Skirt Steak with Veggies, 140
Tofu with Veggies, 269
Veggie Bread Rolls, 79
Veggie Pastries, 85
Veggie Rice, 271
Veggie Sandwich, 83
Veggie Stuffed Bell Peppers, 237
Veggies Stuffed Eggplants, 225

Velvet
Red Velvet Cupcakes, 278

# W

Walnut Brownies, 299

Wasabi Crab Cakes, 214

White Chocolate Cheesecake, 291

Wine Infused Mushrooms, 233

Wings
BBQ Chicken Wings, 113
Buffalo Chicken Wings, 114
Crispy Chicken Wings, 112
Simple Chicken Wings, 112
Turkey Wings, 129

Wontons
Raspberry Wontons, 306

# Y

Yogurt
Pumpkin & Yogurt Bread, 27
Yogurt Banana Bread, 22

# Z

Zesty Salmon, 179

Zucchini
Nutty Zucchini Bread, 25
Zucchini & Apple Bread, 26
Zucchini Fries, 64
Zucchini Fritters, 39
Zucchini Omelet, 43
Zucchini Salad, 220